Ilona Horwath, Swetlana Schweizer (eds.)
Climate Protection, Resource Efficiency, and Sustainable Engineering



**Science Studies**

**Ilona Horwath** (Prof. Dr. rer. soc. oec.), born in 1977, is a sociologist employed as a junior professor for technology and diversity in engineering at the Faculty of Mechanical Engineering, Universität Paderborn.
**Swetlana Schweizer** (Dr.-Ing.), born in 1986, is a researcher at Universität Paderborn working on the use of renewable materials in vehicle bodies. In her research work and as coordinator of the NRW Forschungskolleg "Leicht-Effizient-Mobil", she is committed to the sustainable use of resources and materials.

Ilona Horwath, Swetlana Schweizer (eds.)

# Climate Protection, Resource Efficiency, and Sustainable Engineering

## Transdisciplinary Approaches to Design and Manufacturing Technology

[transcript]

Funded by the Ministry of Culture and Science of the State North Rhine-Westphalia.

**Bibliographic information published by the Deutsche Nationalbibliothek**
The Deutsche Nationalbibliothek lists this publication in the Deutsche Nationalbibliografie; detailed bibliographic data are available in the Internet at http://dnb.d-nb.de



Cover layout: Kordula Röckenhaus, Bielefeld
Proofread: Johanna Ellsworth
Typeset: Jan Gerbach, Bielefeld
Printed by: Majuskel Medienproduktion GmbH, Wetzlar
https://doi.org/10.14361/9783839463772
Print-ISBN: 978-3-8376-6377-8
PDF-ISBN: 978-3-8394-6377-2
ISSN of series: 2703-1543
eISSN of series: 2703-1551

Printed on permanent acid-free text paper.

# Contents

# Introduction

*Ilona Horwath, Swetlana Schweizer, Thomas Tröster*

> "Carried out at the interface of society and science, transdisciplinary research explores and finds solutions for societal problems by making these problems, and the societal actors involved, a central reference point of research and by further developing the scientific research tools it has employed."
> *(Bergmann et al., 2012, p. 14)*

Increasingly, interdisciplinary and transdisciplinary research and teachings are considered to be crucial approaches for solving complex problems (Gibbs et al., 2018), such as big societal challenges (Wissenschaftsrat, 2015; Riegraf & Berscheid, 2018b). Transdisciplinary research draws on the assumption that effective solutions to complex problems require exchanging knowledge and experience among a diversity of disciplines with stakeholders in both public and private spheres (Gibbs et al., 2018, p. 3). Thus, it aims to produce more socially robust knowledge and to bridge knowledge and practise gaps between science and society (Gibbons & Nowotny, 2001).

Scholars of transdisciplinarity distinguish between two modes of transdisciplinary research. Mode 1: research is practised within the traditional boundaries of scientific disciplines, institutions and epistemologies; it integrates epistemics from different branches of a discipline (Scholz & Steiner, 2015, p. 527). Mode 2 goes further in that it integrates or relates different epistemics from science and practise (Scholz & Steiner, 2015, p. 527). In addition to disciplinary perspectives, standards, validity, and quality, Mode 2 research also assesses the potential social impact of results and solutions (Scholz & Steiner, 2015, p. 530). In order to do so, the inclusion of societal stakeholders and practitioners into the problem definition, the research process and the formulation of results and solutions as well as mutual learning among scientists and practitioners is key for transdisciplinary Mode 2 processes (Scholz & Steiner, 2015). In short, Mode 2 *"makes it harder to say where science ends and society begins"* (Gibbons & Nowotny, 2001, p. 77). Hence, while traditional communication between science and the public assumes that there is a one-sided knowledge gap that has to be filled with information ("science to public"), transdisciplinary Mode 2 research is transgressive: "*If knowledge is transgressive, then we need to open up the process to the whole range of reverse communication*" (Gibbons & Nowotny, 2001, p. 80), that is: public to science. Scholz & Steiner (2015, p. 531) define Mode 2 transdisciplinarity as "(...) a facilitated process of *mutual learning* between science and society that relates a *targeted multidisciplinary or interdisciplinary research process* and *a multi-stakeholder discourse* for developing *socially robust orientations* about a specific real-world issue (either a problem or a case)."

The quality of transdisciplinary research and results then goes beyond scientific excellence (which, of course, remains one criterion of quality control) in that it should also integrate societal value into the definition of "good science" (Gibbons & Nowotny, 2001, p. 71; Pohl, 2011). It aims to produce not only reliable but also socially more robust knowledge and thus better technological solutions as well. In lightweight design, this touches the question of social acceptance of such technologies and potential future controversies of whether, how and where such methods and materials may be applicable and accepted by the public, and where other approaches may be more sustainable and less harmful to the environment. However, it is important to note that our research group did not use transdisciplinarity as a means to gain acceptance for lightweight methods and materials, though this might be one effect of our work (and a frequent expectation in traditional engineering work environments). Rather, it served to explore the contexts, implications, and limitations for a sustainable use of lightweight design regarding products and processes, and to develop better technical solutions (Gibbons & Nowotny, 2001, p. 79) which meet the needs of society. The results of these endeavours are presented in this book. The first main part introduces the development of our research context, aims, methods and transdisciplinary research strategy. The second part presents our case studies and results. Finally, we assess the scientific and societal outcomes and provide our conclusions in the last chapter.

## Research context: Transdisciplinary lightweight design, complexity, and big societal challenges

The approaches, methodological strategies and results presented in the following chapters were elaborated within the research network of the Forschungskolleg "Light-Efficient-Mobile" (FK-LEM). Founded in 2014 (under its previous name "Fortschrittskolleg"), the FK-LEM is a PhD programme for the development of lightweight construction technology, but with a special emphasis on how lightweight design connects to different areas of society, to various societal actors and technology users, and to the needs of a diversity of social groups. During its second research period 2019-2022, thirteen PhD candidates from the natural sciences, engineering and social science worked on that topic. Thereby, we could draw on lessons learned from a first generation of FK-LEM researchers (2014-2018, see Riegraf & Berscheid [2018a], Berscheid [2019]).

Lightweight design refers to an optimisation of technological solutions, either in a way that reduces the weight of a product while maintaining its full functionality, or in a way that maintains the weight of the product but extends its particular functionality and/or improves its properties (see Lightweight Design in this book). Thus, lightweight design can be considered a strategy to increase the resource efficiency in production processes, and to reduce the energy required for the use of a product. Lightweight design can be used in many areas of application, entailing a vital and creative development of materials, structures, and processes. Currently, a main focus of application is automotive construction. However, proponents and researchers in lightweight design are also looking for new fields of application, and it is an open discussion as well as an empirical question to which degree and in which areas lightweight design can also be considered a (more) sustainable solution compared to conventional approaches – for instance, to supply assisted-living technologies in order to improve the everyday life of humans with specific needs. This raises profound scientific and societal questions regarding the reu-se and recycling potential of materials, the efficiency of processes and the consequences for the environment in addition to the economic and social sustainability of particular areas of lightweight application. Against this background, the FK-LEM sought to explore the potential and limitations of sustainable lightweight design as a solution to societal challenges. In order to achieve this, the FK-LEM research and development approach was grounded in transdisciplinarity.

The aim to combine lightweight design with transdisciplinary research is as innovative as it is challenging. Particular challenges regarding transdisciplinary research on lightweight design refer to the complex and multi-layered topics which are difficult to convey to lay people, and to the culture in engineering, trained to focus on technological and economic aspects rather than societal effects. The FK-LEM provided the space and the resources to overcome such traditional limitations and to bring together science and society (Horwath et al., 2018). Traditionally, engineering education is very compact and specialised. Critics claim that it does not encourage students to acknowledge ethical and social responsibilities or public welfare concerns – nor does it provide students with the skills to reflect upon how their work and engineering more generally may influence society and diverse social groups both positively and negatively (Cech, 2014; Cech, 2013). Although lightweight design requires interdisciplinary cooperation between natural sciences and engineering, the contributing disciplines are highly specialised, and disciplinary or topical specialisation entails a fragmentation of thought and action (Neuhauser, 2018).

However, the problem with specialisation and fragmentation of thought and action are also true for sociology, philosophy and cultural studies. In addition, members of these disciplines face the challenge of gaining a basic understanding of lightweight design and engineering, materials and properties, and the complexity of bringing technological and societal issues together. This requires time, continuous involvement, and a preparedness to learn about unfamiliar topics as well as to participate in and contribute to the mutual learning and research process. Social scientific education tends to focus on theoretical expertise; graduates have limited experience regarding empirical research. Their motivation to expand empirical research competence, to participate in the time-consuming interdisciplinary collaboration, and to embark on untraditional pathways with open outcome is further limited by the highly individualistic and competitive academic culture. In addition to the structural underrepresentation of social sciences in the FK-LEM setting (see below, Structural and Cultural Challenges), this meant that the elaboration of social-scientific research dimensions and methods (which are essential for conceptualising and conducting the transdisciplinary research agenda) entailed a significant extra effort from the rest of the team to compensate this lack.

Thus an expectation often posed by funding agencies that transdisciplinarity can simply be "added" as a research dimension within the processes and practises of traditional research approaches is bound to be disappointed. Transdisciplinarity requires professional skills, resources, methods and a willingness and commitment to collaborate and to learn from each other in a culture of openness and mutual respect. A solid research strategy in order to advance the methods, results, and to achieve meaningful transdisciplinarity in lightweight engineering is necessary (see also Berscheid (2018, p. 241)). We could draw on the experience and results of a first generation of transdisciplinary research in lightweight design (Riegraf & Berscheid, 2018a; Berscheid, 2019) in the development of our particular transdisciplinary research strategies and methods.

## Lessons learned from the first generation

We started our transdisciplinary work in the second funding period by evaluating the results of the first funding period, or generation of FK-LEM, respectively. Over the course of four years, the research group had established a common understanding of a transdisciplinary research process among the participating disciplines (Riegraf & Berscheid, 2018a; Berscheid, 2019). However, there were some challenges in the process of putting the concept into research practise (for a detailed analysis see Berscheid (2018)).

As Berscheid (2018) describes: The main challenges and obstacles included a high workload for participants who, in addition to their daily workload, should also perform transdisciplinary research in an attempt to extend and advance their PhD topics by questions of how their work can contribute to solve the so-called "Big Societal Challenges". Moreover, regular meetings were dominated by organisational tasks and topics rather than scientific exchange and advancement of transdisciplinary research. This was also due to the lack of a methodological framework as a prerequisite to enable advances in transdisciplinary research, and methodological strategies as well as theoretical approaches to integrate the manifold forms of knowledge arising in the process of transdisciplinary work. Finally, to find and gain societal partners in order to build up transdisciplinary research cooperation turned out to be difficult, not in the least due to a certain des-orientation regarding the who, why and how of such collaborations (ibid).

In order to address these obstacles faced by the first generation and to enable a more prosperous interdisciplinary and transdisciplinary research collaboration for the second generation we took the following measures:

- **Introduction of a Research Seminar on interdisciplinary and transdisciplinary collaboration:** The seminar was held fortnightly during each term of the funding period of FK-LEM. It served to introduce participants to the societal, political and scientific background of transdisciplinary research (Riegraf & Berscheid, 2018b; Wissenschaftsrat, 2015; Grunwald, 2015; Schneidewind, 2015; Schneidewind & Singer-Brodowski, 2014; Strohschneider, 2014), to provide insights regarding the philosophy of science (Fleck, 2012; Schiebinger & Schraudner, 2011; Barad, 2007; Haraway, 1988; Harding, 1986) and to elaborate theoretical and epistemic concepts which enable transdisciplinary cooperation (Pohl et al., 2017; Pohl, 2011; Pohl & Hirsch Hadorn, 2008; Pohl et al., 2008; Bergmann et al., 2012; Harding, 2015), and to provide participants with a range of transdisciplinary and social-scientific research methods (and the related methodologies; Rosenthal, 2018; Atteslander, 2010; Kirchhoff et al., 2010; Di Guilo & Defila, 2018) in order to enable the participants' transdisciplinary ambitions to strive towards successful collaboration with societal partners connected to their PhD topics. The Research Seminar also served to develop three research clusters, where participants worked together on the transdisciplinary elaboration of the topics of climate protection, resource efficiency, and mobility. The assignment to each cluster was based on the particular relationship to the participants' individual PhD topics. This way, the synergetic development of individual and collective research was enhanced. The seminar proved to provide the appropriate space for discussion, for the elaboration of the transdisciplinary case studies of our research clusters, and for developing common scientific practises, mutual understanding and learning opportunities as well as, to a certain degree, a common identity and orientation as transdisciplinary researchers.

- **Introduction workshop into interdisciplinary writing:** To provide an introduction into interdisciplinary writing techniques and start the wrap-up and writing of the results of the research clusters.
- **Advancement of the concept of the "Thought School"** ("Denkschule"): The Thought School was introduced by the first generation of FK-LEM to provide a dialogue forum for scientists, societal stakeholders, and industry. Drawing on the Documentary Method (Bohnsack, 2008), we advanced the "Thought School" from a "science to public" event to a format which allows reverse communication – "public to science" - as well, and which could be used as a transdisciplinary research method (Horwath et al., 2018; Horwath & Terhechte, 2018). During the course of FK-LEM, the "Thought School" enhanced our joint problem formulation, the production of new knowledge, and it helped to continuously render our research activities socially relevant and to build up networks and common activities with societal stakeholders such as Fridays4Future and Lippe Zirkulär (a regional consortium to foster and advance circular economy)[1].
- **Networking activities and active membership:** In order to establish meaningful cooperation with relevant societal organisations during the second funding period, we not only cooperated with societal partners, but several participants of the FK-LEM also became active members of relevant networks themselves. For instance, FK-LEM participants founded Engineers Without Borders Paderborn, acted as firefighters and members of firefighting networks or joined the Lippe Zirkulär consortium. This not only allowed a continuous transdisciplinary collaboration and exchange with societal partners, but also the build-up of new infrastructures for knowledge transfer and engagement.
- **Evaluation of the research results and processes of the first generation:** Drawing on Pohl's (2011) concept of progress in transdisciplinary research, we evaluated the results and the research progress of – and together with – the first generation of FK-LEM. Pohl defines four areas of progress in the development of transdisciplinary research: to analyse and process issues in a way that (1) grasps the complexity of the issue, (2) takes the diverse perspectives on the issue into account, (3) links abstract and case-specific knowledge and (4) develops descriptive, normative, and practical knowledge that promotes what is perceived to be the common good (Pohl, 2011, p. 620). We found that 12 PhD candidates of the first generation had achieved a common understanding of the complexity of the issues in their PhD theses, the transdisciplinary research topics respectively (1); that they were able to take diverse perspectives on the issues into account (2) and, at least to some degree, managed to link abstract

1 https://www.lippe-zirkulaer.de/

and case-specific knowledge. However, there was room to improve results on (3) and (4) through the work of the second generation. This was a task, which required advanced methods and skills of transdisciplinary research as well as more time for elaboration. As the aim was to develop the research of the second generation towards advances in (3) and (4), we implemented three research clusters to enable participants to focus on the task. It should be stated that progress on (3) and (4) is only possible through extensive collaboration and time resources. Therefore it is not surprising that the first generation could not achieve comprehensive results in these dimensions as, compared to the second generation, they had to start their research on how lightweight design can contribute solutions to the big societal challenges from scratch. In addition, literature on transdisciplinary methods, learning, research practises and dimensions as well as quality criteria advanced tremendously since the first generation had started its work. Thus, the first generation provided us with a solid base of knowledge and experience (Riegraf & Berscheid, 2018a) to start our work, and the joint evaluation of the results of the first period facilitated the transfer of the most important "lessons learned" to the second generation.

- **Lecture series:** Another helpful kick-off for our work was the lecture series "Crossing Borders. Inter- and Transdisciplinarity in the Context of Sustainability and Transformation" (Grenzüberschreitungen - Inter- und Transdisziplinarität im Kontext von Nachhaltigkeit und Transformation), which marked the transition from the first to the second generation of FK-LEM researchers in the academic year of 2017/18.

## Structural and cultural challenges for interdisciplinary and transdisciplinary collaboration

The structural conception of the FK-LEM posed further challenges to interdisciplinary and transdisciplinary collaboration. There was a major imbalance in the construction of the professional positions of the participating disciplines: the eight participants from engineering got full positions (100%), whereas the three participants from the natural sciences got 75% positions, and the two from sociology, philosophy and cultural studies got 65% positions. In addition, a certain degree of fluctuation amongst participants was to be expected as some only participated at FK-LEM for a couple of months, others longer, in addition to colleagues from science and engineering who participated as associated members but without being employed at the FK-LEM. Hence, we developed a research design based on research clusters responsible for the common topics to strengthen the continuity of the elaboration of our research.

The structural imbalance amongst the participating disciplines implied a quantitative and cultural "dominance" of the engineering disciplines (Berscheid,

2018), while the research questions of the FK-LEM suggested that a major contribution from social scientists was necessary to ensure a successful performance. This might be one reason why it turned out to be extremely difficult to fill the 65% positions (for a critical discussion see also Bahr et al. (2022), pp. 80-81). In an attempt to mitigate the imbalance and to provide the FK-LEM with expertise in interdisciplinary and transdisciplinary methodologies, a junior professorship for technology and diversity in engineering was implemented in 2017 to facilitate the work of FK-LEM.

With regard to the first generation, the structural imbalance also entailed a cultural and epistemic imbalance in that the research logic and strong orientation towards industries and markets prevailed (Berscheid, 2018). For sociologists, such environments can come with expectations or even demands to deliver "socially relevant" results to accompany the work of engineers and contribute to the social acceptance of their products, respectively. In contrast, participants from social and cultural studies tended to focus on their individual PhD topics and were hard to motivate to contribute to the common topics. Thus, the structural imbalance and the narrow disciplinary cultures as well as the dogmatic conventions typical for the organisation of science and research at neoliberal universities had to be overcome in order to enhance substantial interdisciplinary and transdisciplinary collaboration and to create research spaces where innovative thinking could thrive.

A last challenge refers to a meaningful commitment to interdisciplinary and transdisciplinary cooperation aiming to tackle the big societal challenges with lightweight design – a willingness to cooperate is essential, especially from the side of the participating professors (Berscheid, 2018, p. 242). As stated above, the transdisciplinary research dimension requires additional work to the daily tasks and to the work related to the PhD thesis of the participating PhD candidates and supervising professors which not everyone associated with FK-LEM was ready to perform (Berscheid, 2018, p. 243). However, most professors participated actively in the workshops, the Thought School and thus the elaboration of our transdisciplinary research; in addition, the work within our research clusters, particularly during the Research Seminar, fostered a culture of collaboration and identification with the transdisciplinary goals of FK-LEM among most of our PhD candidates. It provided the space to develop our own research community and culture of transdisciplinary cooperation, similar to what Klein (2018, p. 18) describes as a "*Transdisciplinary Orientation in Team Science*", a "*(...) synergistic combination of values, attitudes, beliefs, skills, knowledge, and behaviours that predisposes individuals to collaboration. They promote team participation marked by willingness to learn about unfamiliar theories and methods and to adjust individual disciplinary schema to fit the demands of teamwork*" (Klein 2018, p. 13).

## A Model and a strategy for transdisciplinary research in lightweight design

The ISOE Model of Transdisciplinary Research (Bergmann et al., 2012, Jahn et al. 2012, see Figure 1) served to illustrate the general idea of a transdisciplinary research strategy, and our work draws strongly on the integrative approach of transdisciplinary research. It defines transdisciplinary research as

> "(...) a reflexive research approach that addresses societal problems by means of interdisciplinary collaboration as well as the collaboration between researchers and extra-scientific actors: its aim is to enable mutual learning processes between science and society: integration is the main cognitive challenge of the research process" (Jahn et al., 2012, p. 4).

*Figure 1: ISOE Model of Transdisciplinary Research (Bergmann et al., 2012, p. 35)*

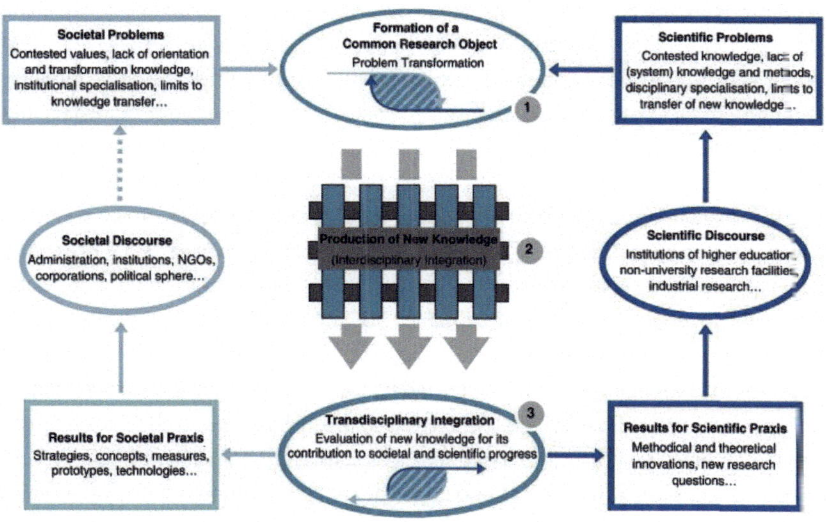


An integrative approach to transdisciplinary research means to pursue two epistemic paths simultaneously: first, the real-world approach defining real-world problems, often with practitioners and experts in the fields; the research goal here is to produce knowledge that can be used to solve a practical problem (Bergmann et al., 2012, p. 32f). Second, the science-focused approach addresses complex internal scientific issues (which can be part of an overarching real-world problem), not the least of which problems are those which arise during the research process; here the goal is to improve scientific research and results, and/or to define new research needs (Bergmann et al., 2012, p. 33). As the integrative approach to transdisciplinary research implies

> "(...) striving for research results serving two totally different purposes, it is particularly important to come up with a careful design of the concept at the very beginning of a research project" (Bergmann et al., 2012, p. 35f).

The design of our concept was realised continuously within a series of formats. The Thought School as a public dialogue forum served to examine the complexity of the issues, to capture diverse perspectives and descriptions of real-world problems, and to analyse values and practical knowledge that promote what is perceived to be the common good in our areas of concern (for a detailed description of the methodology and results of this approach see Horwath et al. (2018), Horwath & Terhechte (2018)). The second and internal part of the Thought School served the FK-LEM research group to integrate these results, identify gaps in knowledge and methods, and revise the research concept iteratively. The theories and methods required were then provided and applied in the Research Seminar. Finally, the Thought School also served as a continuous forum of dialogue between FK-LEM scientists and the public and to fill specific knowledge gaps on sustainable mobility through public expert workshops (Thought School 2018), particular materials and sustainable and responsible engineering (Thought School 2019). Importantly, the Thought School also entailed opportunities to respond to societal needs in a more immediate fashion than research processes would allow; for instance, we provided a workshop on the reflection of social privilege for members of Fridays4Future and developed and promoted a catalogue of requirements together in order to move Paderborn University towards a sustainable, $CO_2$ -neutral University. In addition to the Thought School, science cafés for pupils were also provided. This was a format to promote exchange with young potential future scientists and to provide insights into the work of FK-LEM, which required us to present our research topics in an accessible manner and through "hands-on" exercises. A further format, the PhD colloquium, focused on the discussion and advancement of the individual PhD topics in FK-LEM in terms of disciplinary perspectives and quality criteria.

The first phase of a transdisciplinary research process consists of the formation of a common research object derived from societal and scientific problems. In transdisciplinary research, problems are formulated from the very beginning within a dialogue among a large number of different actors and their perspectives (Gibbons & Nowotny, 2001, p. 69). Against this backdrop, transdisciplinary research coined the term "problem transformation", which means that both aspects, the contribution to practical problem solutions for actors and to scientific progress, are understood as essential parts of the research dynamic (Becker & Jahn, 2006, p. 290, in: Bergmann et al. 2012, p. 42). In other words, a societal and a scientific problem are linked to form a common research object (Jahn et al., 2012), the so-called boundary object. Boundary objects are then *"transformed into epistemic objects by means of developing or applying theories or concepts"*, and epistemic objects are the basis from which research questions are derived (Jahn et al. 2012, p. 5). The process of problem transformation proved to be one of intense collaboration both with societal partners and within the research communities and supported the process of team formation for our three research clusters.

Once a problem description and the formulation of the research questions have been accomplished, the second phase is to plan the research concept, including the design of the integration, which requires a consideration of which actors must work together, when and how (Bergmann et al., 2012, p. 40). In this phase, the production of new knowledge is crucial, which we understood and realised as

> "an interplay of specialized work in subteams (e.g. including both researchers and extra-scientific actors) and dedicated stages of integration of the epistemologically pluralistic [...] outcomes of the work" (Jahn et al., 2012, p. 5).

Transdisciplinarity focusing on societal problems mainly aims at producing three types of knowledge: system knowledge (the knowledge involved in the understanding of an issue); orientation knowledge (required for determining the possibilities and boundaries of decision-making); and transformation knowledge (knowledge of the ways and means of practically realising such decisions). However, a diversity of knowledge including practical experience has to be integrated in order to gain transdisciplinary results (Jahn et al., 2012, p. 8).

The requirement for integration work is shown in the middle column of Figure 1. According to Bergmann et al. (2012, p. 43), the integration work needs to combine both the practical path aimed at action to solve societal problems and the scientific path aimed at producing new theoretical and empirical knowledge. With regard to the broad yet highly specialised nature of interdisciplinarity related to FK-LEM research, the integration of social and natural science was additionally challenging, not because of "cultural differences" but because of the heterogeneity of the knowledge bases. Hence, we had to take into account that a technologically reasonable solution can usually be found – but that the question remains as to whether the solution is also reasonable according to criteria such as practicability, social acceptability or sustainability. Technologies that do not comply with the structures, practises and values in the particular societal field of application may not be accepted and used whereas a societally desirable solution might come with restrictions and constraints related to technology or natural sciences (Bergmann et al., 2012, p. 46).

To address these issues, we designed a "circular" or – a term more familiar for engineers – an "iterative" approach to knowledge production and integration, which facilitated a reflective monitoring of the research process and helped to maintain close ties between scientific and societal problem descriptions throughout the whole research process (Jahn et al., 2012). A reflexive approach

> "proactively considers the dynamics, interests and concerns, roles and responsibilities, the collaboration culture within a project, and the connectivity to the context of action addressed" (Lux et al., 2019, p. 183).

This process is very time-consuming and could only be realised through continuous and engaged collaboration of FK-LEM researchers within the various formats developed for the second generation of FK-LEM, in particular the Research Seminar, where the production of new knowledge (in collaboration with the societal partners) could unfold under constant (peer) reflection and revision of the societal and scientific dimensions of our epistemic objects and the related research activities.

The third and last phase of the transdisciplinary research process is the transdisciplinary integration of results. Transdisciplinary integration can be understood as a form of assessment of the integrated results, asking for their possible contribution to both societal (validity and relevance for the original global issue) and scientific progress (new insights within and beyond disciplines). Assessment procedures can involve mutual critique among all process participants, to examine what is the "added value", an assembly of products for science and society, or to measure the impact of the project on the societal and scientific discourses. It also includes a targeted or non-targeted knowledge transfer by both scientists and societal actors (Jahn et al., 2012, p. 7).

It should be mentioned that due to the diverse nature of the epistemic objects derived and elaborated within our research clusters, and due to the consequential variety of knowledge gaps to be closed and methods to be applied in order to do so, as well as the following differences in time scales and schedules of the cluster projects, we did not (yet) conduct a comprehensive evaluation of the second generation of FK-LEM. At the time of writing this book, one cluster concerned with Re-Use and Recycling (Re-Use and Recycling Cluster) had gone through the whole cycle of (an ideal) transdisciplinary research process, including the evaluation of the collaboration process and the critical assessment of results. The research cluster on Emergency and Recue Equipment for First Responders (Rescue Cluster), in contrast, had already generated a myriad of new empirical knowledge but was still occupied with the integration of this knowledge and the transformation into new prototypes of rescue tools, i.e., the construction of demonstrators. The cluster on additive manufacturing of medical devices (Medicin Cluster), with its great possibilities to respond to the demands of societal members in a very immediate way – at least as far as the mere production of 3D printed assistive technologies is concerned – focused on doing exactly that, thereby examining the legal requirements and technological challenges related to their collaborative activities systematically.

Compared to the ideal-typical model of a transdisciplinary research process, in a research practise which draws on an iterative research design, the ideal phases and the production and integration of both disciplinary and transdisciplinary knowledge are much more interwoven. In addition, the intensity and the role of the involvement of societal partners in transdisciplinary projects can differ, as the type of involvement depends on the particular problem, the specific lack of knowledge and the agreement on knowledge and values (Jahn et al., 2012, p. 8).

The societal impact is hard to measure as it can contain short term and long term effects, depends on framework conditions, the historicity (of the problem), the heterogeneity of actors, the general environment, the funding conditions (Lux et al., 2019, p. 185). The framework conditions in which transdisciplinary research processes are embedded are of high relevance in fostering or hindering the societal effectiveness of transdisciplinary research (Lux et al., 2019, see also Lam et al. 2021).

## Formation of a common research object

### a) Big societal challenges

"Big Societal Challenges" refers to a complex of problems which are reflected in politics, science policy and governance (e.g. Wissenschaftsrat, 2015; European Union, n.d.). The solutions we, as scientists and members of society, develop in order to tackle the "Big Societal Challenges" will crucially determine not only the quality of life of future generations but also the habitability of the planet in general. Science policy calls for a transformation of these pressing societal challenges into research topics and questions and thereby promotes a transformation of the role of science in society. The goal is that by the joint forces of scientists and practitioners in order to address the challenges, innovative scientific, technological as well as social solutions can be found and implemented. This way, science is expected to contribute to "the common good" (Wissenschaftsrat, 2015). However, what that "common good" actually is or should be, in particular from the perspective of a multitude of participants in transdisciplinary research and development processes, is an empirical question involving ecological, economic, technological and social dimensions (see below for the empirical results from our workshops).

In North Rhine-Westphalia (NRW), where our research took place, the „Forschungsstrategie Fortschritt NRW" (MIWF, 2013) focused on the following challenges:

- Climate protection
- Resource efficiency and raw materials
- Secure, clean and efficient energy

- Food security, sustainable agriculture
- Smart, green and integrated transport
- Health, demographic change and wellbeing
- Participation, inclusive, innovative and reflective societies in a changing world

A series of projects, regional networks and funding opportunities were implemented to set up an infrastructure and processes to tackle the challenges (MIWF, 2013). The FK-LEM is one of these projects. In addition to taking up research questions and providing technological and scientific approaches to solutions, we also aimed to contribute by educating a new generation of engineers equipped with professional competence and experience in interdisciplinary and transdisciplinary sustainability research.

Against this backdrop, the areas of climate protection, resource efficiency, and mobility were predefined as the main fields of activity in the FK-LEM research design (see Figure 2). Thought School and Research Seminar served to refine the research programme iteratively based on systematic exchange with the public and practitioners specialised in the relevant areas, occupations, and professions.

Of immense value, the research design for the second generation was designed in the transition period from the first to the second generation FK-LEM. Even though some challenges for teamwork arose through the fluctuation, the

*Figure 2: Spheres of activity (Handlungsfelder) and research cluster: general research framework*

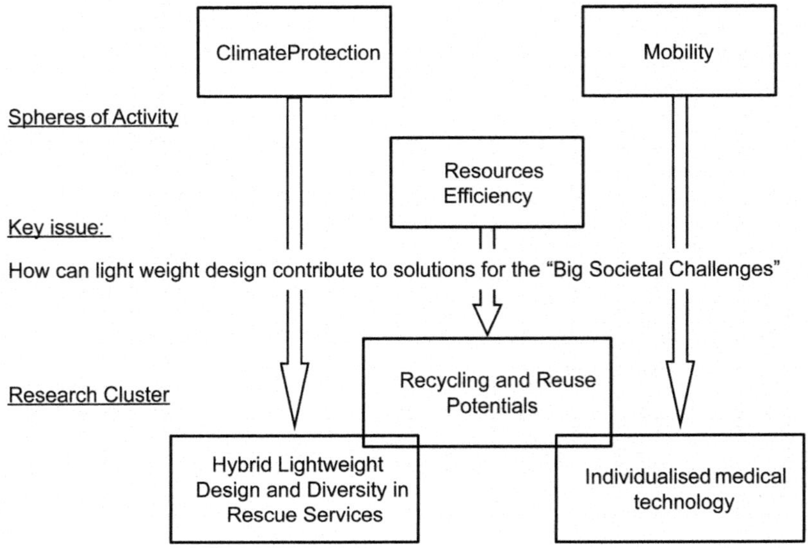

transition period still permitted us to involve the insights, findings, experience, and advice of the former FK-LEM participants.

From the general question of how to apply lightweight design "for the common good" in the predefined areas of action, we derived specific, empirically grounded research topics.

As a first step, we invited the interested public to discuss perceived urgencies and related problems in the three areas from the perspective of practitioners at the Thought School. In 2017, the public forum of the Thought School focused on climate protection and the workshops, where problem formation took place, addressed the societal areas of rescue and security services, medical care, mobility and assisted living, and sustainable resources and climate protection (for a detailed description of the methodology and results of the workshops see Horwath et al. (2018), Horwath & Terhechte (2018)[2]).

To dismantle barriers of lay people regarding their participation in transdisciplinary exchange with engineers and scientists, we applied the principles of openness and communication (Bohnsack, 2008; Rosenthal, 2018) deduced from the requirements and quality criteria established in qualitative research methodology, which we transferred to our particular workshop settings as follows: we addressed participants as experts in their area of practise and experience, pointed out that their experience and expertise are crucial for scientists to fully comprehend the problem and that science or technology skills are not necessary to make meaningful contributions to the workshops discussion. In addition, through the appreciative moderation of the discussions we ensured an open, respectful and non-hierarchical discussion climate. To encourage and structure the discussions, we asked three basic questions in each workshop:

1. What are the biggest challenges you currently perceive in your professional field?
2. What would good solutions to these problems look like?
3. What could science and engineering contribute to solve these problems?

## b) Rescue and security services

At the Rescue and Security Workshop, ten participants from rescue and security organisations, i.e. fire service, medical emergency service, and from research institutions attended. The main challenges they discussed were related to the rescue of people, i.e. the location and exploration of areas, rescue and transport of vic-

2 The following section sums up empirical findings and results presented in Horwath et al. 2018. In favour of the readability of sections a) to e) we refrain from pointing out identical wording as direct quotes. Instead, we aim to state here that the main content of section a) to e) can also be found in more detail in Horwath et al. 2018.

tims from collapsed buildings, natural disasters, and – most frequently – transport of adipose people or victims of car accidents.

Participants described the **main challenge** of such scenarios in keeping the required rescue time short: victims have to be located and provided with first aid, have to be stabilised and kept alive, and they have to get prepared for the transport from a site of accident or disaster. Ironically, the issue of the rescue time is also caused by advances in vehicle engineering and the construction of cars such as improved material strength or a myriad of electronic features, which increase the time required to reach victims of car accidents (see Case Study III). As a consequence, complex rescue strategies have to be performed, tailored to the particular on-site conditions and the technologies that are available and can be applied in the particular environment. Thereby, first responders have to proceed with great caution and care in order to avoid putting victims, members of the rescue teams or the public at any further risk. Another challenge participants discussed was the weight of the rescue equipment itself. Paradoxically, despite significant technical progress and new options available through lightweight technologies, rescue tools and vehicles tend to become even heavier. For instance, in many cases a fully equipped fire truck actually exceeds its legally permitted weight limits.

Discussing **solutions**, participants perceived that lightweight technologies could contribute to develop lighter rescue equipment and optimise tools and vehicles for rescue and emergency operations. However, reflecting on the above-mentioned paradoxical situation and the fact that technological advancement always entails new challenges or downsides, they also pointed out that lighter and optimised technologies may not necessarily lead to better solutions for rescue services. Importantly, responding to emergencies or disasters and the rescue of those affected requires rescue teams to perform an integration of organisational, technological, medical, and other procedures necessary to achieve their tasks. Hence, the development of rescue and security technologies has to take the complexity of such processes into account in order to develop applicable solutions. Specifically, in the case of firefighters (and technological rescue services), any approaches to optimise tools have to take the significance of a frequent "misuse" of tools into account: As each rescue scenario poses different challenges, firefighters need to be creative and often use the available tools in ways that quite diverge from their originally intended functions (Hanses & Horwath, 2021; Hanses & Horwath, 2022, Hanses et al., 2020); for a general discussion of how tools and their use relate to gender and diversity in firefighting organisations see also Horwath (2013), Horwath et al. (2021a), Horwath et al. (2021b), Kastein et al. (2022); for insights into the intimate but also gendered relationship between firefighters and their tools see Harrison & Olofsson (2016).

To address these issues, two (then) associated FK-LEM members explored the potential of lightweight design for firefighting and rescue technology under consideration of important practises of "misuse" (Neuser, 2019), and the potential to optimise tools and practises for the case of rescue scenarios in car accidents (Hanses, 2019). Therefore, both candidates were trained and supported to apply expert interviews and participant observation. Thus, empirical findings on user practises enriched their technological and material analysis. As a result, we were able to identify a range of tools with a high potential to be optimised in line with the practical experience, needs and requirements of practitioners in the field. In a later research phase, the transfer of expert knowledge for the optimisation of firefighting rescue tools was also supported by the master thesis of the associated FK-LEM member Kathiri (2022).

However, participants also researched creative solutions in our workshop. Regarding the question of how to reduce rescue time, one antagonist in the struggle against time that first responders face is the prevalence of ever more complex materials and structures in the design of modern cars, which ironically often serve the purpose of making the vehicle safer (see Case Study III). In order to tackle this problem, the participants discussed the implementation of predetermined and standardised "breaking points" in the construction of new cars: *"Optimised for a quick rescue"*, a "breaking point" would allow first responders to open cars more easily, e.g. by lifting the roof. A standardisation of predetermined "breaking points" independent of particular car models, companies or branches was seen as a potential path to ensure that first responders can start their operation quickly. Another suggestion was to extend standard crash tests by developing and including indicators for rescue features and test results on rescue time for frequent rescue scenarios. Finally, participants stressed that new evaluation systems should be designed to promote such rescue features in cars, i.e. data which help to assess additional costs of such features but also to explain their potentially lifesaving value.

Reflecting on challenges related to international disaster control, participants encouraged the development of a further innovation: lightweight rescue tools for lay people. In the face of catastrophic events, increasingly due to the effects of climate change, the involvement of lay people and untrained volunteers can be crucial to saving lives. Therefore, rescue tools that are lightweight enough to facilitate easy transport and simple enough to enable lay people to handle them safely would be of immense value. The availability of such tools would allow people who are affected and volunteers to rescue themselves and others.

Participants made several suggestions on how **research and development** should contribute to solving the discussed challenges: vehicle engineers, some claimed, should actively promote rescue features, extend crash test scenarios and elaborate on new rescue-related safety standards. They should actively promote the use of lighter and safer materials for the construction of cars, and get actively involved so as to change standardised priorities of the vehicle industry and marketing, i.e. push for the establishment of new standards, norms and marketing concepts regarding material and structure-related rescue and safety features. Concerning rescue and safety equipment more generally, participants concluded that for any new solution to be practicable and potentially established within rescue and security organisations, it has to match the complexity of emergency realities and facilitate emergency rescue strategies. Consequently, the optimisation of rescue tools by means of lightweight design in the FK-LEM research cluster started with an empirical analysis of organisational contexts, practical demands and experience with particular rescue scenarios and tools. Based on the results, crucial criteria to link practical, functional and technological improvements for a safe performance could be identified and addressed.

### c) Nursing care, mobility, and assisted living

At the workshop dedicated to **nursing care**, mobility & assisted living, fourteen participants from public and private care homes, various health institutions, hospitals, medical technology companies, civil society and people with care needs attended.

Against the background of the demographic development towards an agingsociety, the major **challenge** perceived by practitioners was how to provide increasing numbers of people with sufficient care facilities and services. Ideally, *"people should be provided with as much technology as necessary – but not necessarily more technology than actually required"* (participant, public health institution) in order to enable them to live as independently as possible within their chosen social and/or family environment. Practitioners criticised the current trend to compromise elderly or disabled people's autonomy by sending them to care homes instead of prioritising options for a more autonomous assisted living. Assisting technologies could change such practises and support the normative establishment of a care-at-home-priority. However, assisting technologies come with further challenges.

Smart assisting technologies, for instance, hold a huge potential to enhance the freedom and autonomy of individuals in need of care and assistance – but also for surveillance, control, and violation of privacy.[3] Hence, people who could benefit tremendously from such technologies often refuse to use them for a perceived

3 For a detailed analysis of the fundamental change of the priorities guiding privacy policies of assisted care settings see also Zuboff (2019). She describes the shift from the initial principle that the rights to access and use the data created in such environments belong exclusively to the people who live in the house, and should serve exclusively to improve their own lives. This principle has been reflected in early assisted living concepts, such as the famous Georgia Tech "Aware Home" from the year 2000. However, two decades later the now exploding market for smart homes, devices and data extraction in the U.S. has fundamentally limited data scarcity and privacy protecting approaches to assisting technologies (Zuboff, 2019, 5-7; Zuboff, 2019, 233-234; Zuboff, 2019, 246).

lack of trustworthiness of technologies and their providers. Another problem causing barriers to the acceptance of new technologies is limited technological affinity and understanding on the side of potential users, resulting in a lack of confidence or motivation with respect to becoming skilled enough to learn how to use assisting technologies efficiently. Workshop participants cautioned that social acceptance and practical applicability of highly effective technologies in care contexts cannot be taken for granted, even if these technologies would bring about a great degree of improvement to people's daily lives.

Some participants suggested that certain gaps between existing technologies and their social acceptance, desirability and applicability are also related to prevailing funding terms and to typical procedures of research and development in engineering: funding policies tend to foster research practises which focus on highly specialised topics and deal with abstract problem definitions. As a consequence, the process of technology development unfolds rather isolated from the social contexts, needs and practical expectations of future users. Instead of analysing the particular social preconditions and how they can be used to improve both technology and its social embedding in the user context, engineers are expected to focus on the production of new technology in terms of models or prototypes. Usually, funding for technological research does not allow for an exhaustive analysis of social environments, user's needs, for comprehensive usability tests, or the development of socio-technological strategies for the transfer of assisting technologies into living environments.

In stark contrast, practitioners stressed the importance of acknowledging individuals and their particular needs as the appropriate starting point for a definition of the requirements for socially sustainable assisting and care technologies. Even though the effort to analyse such needs may be challenging for all people involved – researchers, engineers, elderly and/or disabled persons as well as their caregivers – the process was considered crucial to determine *"which support is really needed, and (how) could it be realised by technological means"* (participant, caregiver). Eventually, the results of a thorough analysis would justify the investment as they allow for the construction of socially relevant and suitable technologies. The example of an individualised cutlery set (Hemme, 2018) and substantial previous work from Schramm et al. (2017, 2018) served to highlight the potential of lightweight solutions and additive manufacturing designed from individual needs.

However, in the experience of our workshop participants, effective norms, laws and standards often undermine their aims to exhaust the enormous potential of additive manufacturing to provide individualised assisted living solutions swiftly. Although the current state of 3D printing technologies allows engineers to produce various artefacts or products at relatively low cost and effort, the inherent risk is their legal liability for such devices. Producers of such 3D items can be held accountable for any damage potentially related to their technology, i.e. accidents or defective materials. While norms and standards are recognised as important means to make technologies safe, participants find it increasingly challenging to deal with areas where (legal) standards lag behind technological advancement. As a consequence, many existing technologies for assisted living, care and mobility cannot be provided to those who would benefit immediately; instead they remain what participants called *"drawer solutions"* or *"technologies for the drawer"*, respectively.

Public health institutions and private insurance companies play a crucial role in the development and transfer of assisting technologies. Individuals in need of assistance have to apply for support in official procedures, and public health institutions have the power to allow or refuse these applications for assistance regarding both technological assistance and human assistance by a caregiver. For each case, they grant permission and financial support or deny them. Practitioners heavily criticised the quality and length of the administrative procedures to assess care needs and to authorise entitlement to receive the assisting technology. Public health institutions as cost objectives also decide on the materials and standard components used for the production of assisting technologies, such as wheelchairs, for instance. Hence, institutional decisions determine the potential as well as the limits and the quality of assisting and care technologies to a large degree – sometimes with severe consequences for the people affected.

Conflicting values and competing norms have also been pointed out as a further challenge. Various disadvantaged social groups, their needs as well as their legitimate values and social norms are perceived to be played off against each other, for instance the needs related to individual mobility of disabled people vs. the requirements of fire protection norms, privacy vs. mobility needs related to the use of smart wheelchairs, cheap materials to provide more people with assisting technologies vs. exploitation of humans and resources in globalised production chains culminated in the metaphor of *"wheelchairs made by children's hands"* (participant).

Regarding **solutions**, participants stressed the need to improve transparency, exchange of information, technology transfer, administrative procedures, education, and awareness of professionals. Solutions to improve technology transfer should include changes of funding policies in a way that would enable researchers to take future application contexts, individual needs, and issues of technology transfer into account. Participants emphasised that such requirements should be promoted as important dimensions of care and assisting technology development if transfer and applicability are to be successful. In addition, case studies to focus on the topic of technology transfer into care contexts would be helpful in order to design effective strategies. Another approach to enhance transferability of technological innovations was to form syndicates for technology development involving researchers, cost objectives, stakeholders, civil society, and engineers. This way *"drawer solutions"* could be avoided by a collaborative development and decision-making based on the consolidation of relevant proficiencies and responsibilities.

Generally, participants described a lack of transparency regarding the range of currently available technologies and trends in technological development. Although a myriad of information on care and assisting technologies can be found online, user-friendly, understandable explanations that include assessment of risks and benefit or details on availability are hard to find. Hence, participants suggested the creation of specific information platforms for the people affected. This way, their particular questions, interests and needs could be better addressed. Participants also suggested that more *"objective"* information on assisting technologies should be provided. By objective, they referred to information independent of the specific interests and corporate perspectives of technology providers, companies, and health institutions.

Practitioners urgently called for measures to improve the administrative procedures and current practises of health institutions that serve to assess the care needs of individuals. Significantly, they point out that changes also need to be made within the educational systems of health care professionals and engineers of assisting technologies. In the opinion of our participants, health care professionals and engineers should be trained in a way that would enable them to critically reflect on the impact of the decisions they make concerning assisting technology, be it the decision on applications to receive assistance, or a decision on which materials to use, or a decision on the data policy of smart assisting items.

Participants see the path to advance the (social) acceptability of assisting technologies in an open dialogue among stakeholders. Such a dialogue should also address the ambiguities inherent to technologies and take the concerns of users and caregivers seriously. Ambiguities of smart technologies, i.e. autonomy vs. coercion and surveillance, are important issues as elderly and disabled people are particularly vulnerable to privacy violations and patronising treatment. Hence, ambiguities as well as the above competing needs and values should be actively reflected upon, balanced, and dealt with. Such aspects – ambiguity and values – should also form part of standard information on technology for lay people as a basic understanding of how a technology works and transparency provided on related risks contribute to create trust and acceptance.

Participants **expected researchers and developers** to get involved in the establishment of a continuous open dialogue, to pay attention to concerns related to the ambiguities of technologies, and to provide understandable and transparent information on care and assisting technologies.

Importantly, researchers and developers should be accountable to members of civil society, receptive to their criticism and concerns, and reflective on the social dimensions and impact of technologies. To achieve this, participants considered interdisciplinary and transdisciplinary research essential to grasp the complexity of care and assisting technologies within their particular social and institutional contexts of application.

### d) Sustainable resources & climate protection

Twenty participants from a variety of public and private institutions, politics, civil society, and industry attended the workshop **Sustainable Resources & Climate Protection.** Climate protection and progress toward sustainable resources require changes in individual behaviour that often appear inconvenient. Accordingly, participants started by discussing the **challenge** of how to gain broader acceptance for sustainable behaviours and technologies. However, they also pointed out that sustainability is not only a question of (dis)comfort but also of social class – not everyone is able to afford new technologies or behavioural changes.

The second challenge was described as a *"competition of materials"*, where more often costs and economic interests rather than the best or most sustainable material available to solve a given problem determine whether materials are used and standardised. Once established, norms and standards in turn determine which materials prevail in engineering and construction. As effective standards and norms tend to favour conventional materials and practises, new approaches are difficult to establish, and innovative engineers have to make greater efforts to ensure their competitiveness.

In the private sector, insecure market developments resulting in high development pressure were perceived as another major challenge. For example, the future of mobility could take several directions as various trends concerning materials, energy and construction can be observed in different markets. Companies respond with high investments in order to be prepared for changes in unknown directions. Such practises result in a huge waste of resources for research and development with potentially no outcome or progress toward environment protection. Hence, participants raised questions about responsibility.

Related to the challenge of how to bring about change, the question of responsibility was perceived as a major challenge. "Market rules", "customers", "providers/engineers" and "politics" appeared to be entangled in a way that each group assigned "responsibility" for changes to the other group, thus inhibiting progress and improvements.

Yet, even where commitment to sustainability and climate protection existed, participants still found it challenging to decide what sustainability actually is. For instance, the lightweight construction industry uses and creates a variety of materials to reduce the weight of conventional products in order to save energy. But little is known about decomposition and recycling possibilities of such combined materials. Generally, participants criticised a lack of transparent evaluations and specifically evaluations that cover the whole life cycle and all components of a particular technology or product.

Finally, participants discussed a perceived change that technologies that are prevalent in everyday life, such as washing machines, were designed to last for as long as possible in former decades, whereas today opportunities for updates or replacement through advanced models are guiding principles.

Participants suggested a number of approaches for **solutions.** The trend to short life cycles should be addressed by new combinations of re-use and recycling models.

To bring about meaningful changes for climate protection and resource efficiency, **solutions** and areas *"where small changes have huge effects"* (participant, public service) must be identified and promoted. Such areas are not only found in everyday practises, but also in agricultural and industrial processes. The increasing availability of suitable technologies, such as e-bikes, may help to boost sustainable behaviour. In addition, new business models need to be developed and promoted in order to demonstrate that sustainability and economic success are not mutually exclusive. Consequently, new sales and marketing strategies should be implemented to generate awareness for actual product costs as opposed to the market price, i.e. the costs of a product drawing on the whole life cycle from resource mining to decomposition. Awareness and comparability of market prices and the actual costs which individuals and society have to pay for a product or technology may make sustainable products more attractive for costumers.

Finally, participants called for politics to take responsibility for future generations. Strategies need to be implemented top down (by laws and incentives) as well as bottom up (by engineer's attitudes and decisions). Importantly, politics should also draw on current trends to foster sustainable practises instead of forcing solutions which may not be practicable, i.e. reinforce current trends to use public transport instead of individual mobility with cars.

To achieve the outlined solutions, participants made the following suggestions about what **research and development** could contribute: researchers should be encouraged to keep the "the bigger picture" in mind. In a profession characterised by highly specialised expert profiles and research topics, it is easier to lose the social and ecological embedding and consequences of technologies; they become out of sight. Participants called for research and development to actively create that "bigger picture" by reflecting on the social impact of engineering topics, strategies, and practises. According to the participants, a systematic reflection should take place routinely at the beginning of every research project. Also, researchers were prompted not to hide behind catch phrases like *"the costumers' expectation and needs"* to legitimate decisions in engineering processes. Rather, they were expected to critically reflect and question such assumptions and arguments, as *"expectations and needs"* are socially constructed, and they are heterogeneous among diverse social groups.

A topic intensely discussed was education for sustainability. Here, more basic research is needed to develop technologies in line with social values instead of insisting on a dubious "market orientation" as the guiding norm. Sustainability issues and social values need to be included in education as well as in the training of engineers in order to create a generation of engineers that is professionally capable of reflecting on social and ecological values and developing technologies from there.

Researchers should acknowledge the need for transparency and information and develop new concepts to illustrate the complexity of production and life cycles. There was a strong need for scientific models to demonstrate that and how sustainability and economic success are not mutually exclusive. The promotion of such models should not only motivate individuals but also create incentives for companies to apply them. Finally, participants argued for the development of new combined recycling and re-use strategies: the life cycle of some products could be extended by designs that allow broken components to be fixed; products designed to be updated or to have a short life cycle should be re-usable, at least their particular components if recycling of the whole product is not possible. Therefore, norms and standards for elements and for groups of components to be re-used in further products (by customers or companies) need to be implemented.

### e) General Conclusions

In addition to the empirical findings and the problem descriptions from the societal areas of interest, the methodology developed for the Thought School 2017 also enabled us to derive some general conclusions for our transdisciplinary work, in particular from the discussion about societies' expectations and needs with respect to sustainable and responsible science and engineering:

- The need for transparency and exchange of information between science and society
- The need for new models and strategies
- The need to respond to challenges resulting from complex and competing norms and values, and to reflect upon the impact for the social groups affected
- The need to recognise the ambiguity inherent to technologies and to find strategies to deal with it
- The need to take responsibility and act on that base – also in science and engineering

Thus, we could take a variety of interests, needs and value orientations from different societal and scientific actors into account and formulate our research questions and strategies accordingly. Didactically, we found that the intense discussion with a variety of actors and exchange of various forms of knowledge, of experience, ideas and practises, the process of documenting and analysing the discussions, and reflection upon results and implications for engineering during the internal workshop of the Thought School enabled our PhD candidates and the participating FK-LEM professors to gain deep insights with respect to the complex entanglement of apparently abstract engineering topics with social welfare and justice (Horwath et al., 2018).

The results in terms of research and development approaches as well as research partners and networks served as a base to advance the establishment of sustainable mobility initiatives at the Faculty of Engineering. The Thought School proved to be of immense importance for the development of a common problem definition and supported us in finding research partners and strengthening the transdisciplinary network. With the progress of our research, the Thought School not only served to exchange ideas with the public but increasingly created a framework for the production of new knowledge and the establishment and institutionalisation of new topics. For instance, the Thought School 2018 was dedicated to "New Approaches for Sustainable Mobility", providing a keynote and three workshops on "Transdisciplinary Mobility Projects", "Mobility Support through Additive Manufacturing" and "Sustainable Mobility and the Reduction of $CO_2$- Emissions". The discussion of a variety of innovative approaches to sustainable mobility, in particular with various external partners like the Wissenschaftszentrum Berlin für Sozialforschung (WZB), inspired the development of further research and development initiatives, such as "NeMo Paderborn – Neue Mobilität, die verbindet" (https://nemo-paderborn.de/). In addition, newly designed projects at the Faculty of Mechanical Engineering, such as HyOpt – Optimierungsbasierte Entwicklung von Hybridwerkstoffen (NW-2-2-008a), started to include comprehensive interdisciplinary research not only on acceptance of hybrid materials among various stakeholder groups but also on the influence of societal and economic conditions on the establishment of specific norms of construction and materials in automotive design (see also Triebus et al., 2022). Another example is the new Re2Pli project, which is about establishing a sustainable production process for lightweight components using only renewable energies. Our work at the FK-LEM also sparked a successful constitution of further initiatives, i.e. Engineers without Borders Paderborn, the elaboration of a data base on re-use and recycling materials as a teaching resource for lecturers of our faculty, or the newly established emphasis on responsible and sustainable engineering, including lectures and the focus of development of the faculty itself. However, it should be mentioned that the rise of the climate protection movement was an unexpected external force which helped to legitimate and boost the faculties' engagement with more sustainable approaches to engineering, materials and design.

In 2019, the Thought School focused on "Sustainable and Responsible Engineering". In close cooperation with members of the Fridays4Future movement, we developed a list of demands for a sustainable Paderborn University. The list of demands was presented at the Thought School where we also discussed how climate protection could be put into practise within our everyday work environments. After the public discussion, we handed the list over to the Executive Board of Paderborn University. In addition, we also provided a workshop for members (pupils, parents, teachers) of the Fridays4Future movement to reflect on privilege and how it enables or hampers active commitment, participation, and societal change.

## Production of new knowledge

As a next step, within the FK-LEM research team, the internal part of the Thought School served to integrate results from the workshops with scientists and the public and to derive new knowledge with respect to the constituting research topics (Table 1). Therefore, we translated the insights gained in the public part of the Thought School into research questions and revised the concepts for our research clusters iteratively. In doing so, we also connected the cluster research to the individual PhD topics. Thus, we were able to link the topics to their societal relevance (see Pohl et al., 2017) and to identify multiple societal and industrial stakeholders for transdisciplinary cooperation. FK-LEM PhD candidates, associate members and professors worked together to examine the following questions for the individual PhD topics and each of the three research clusters:

General question: How can lightweight design contribute to solutions for the "Big Societal Challenges"?

Detailed questions:

1. Which disciplinary knowledge and which methods could enable the development of the individual PhD thesis in a way that contributes to solve the general question?
2. What can the three research clusters contribute to solve the general question?
3. What knowledge and which methods are missing? Which societal (and industrial) actors do we need to involve into the research processes?

The results were adjusted (disciplinary) research plans for the individual PhD projects and for their coordination within each of the three research clusters (Table 1).

The examination and subsequent discussion of the research strategies was guided by the 10-Step Approach to render research socially relevant (Pohl et al., 2017). A further result was a clear picture of the methodologies, epistemologies and theories necessary to enable FK-LEM participants to realise their envisioned research plans, in other words: the programme to be provided in our Research Seminar.

## Transdisciplinary research partners and the formation of boundary objects

In the next step we established stakeholder networks and invited selected members of society/practitioners to participate in each cluster. In line with the strategy of the MIWF (2013), one criterion for the selection was the potential to contribute to the formation of new networks and infrastructure to promote lightweight design as an approach to solve the "Big Societal Challenges".

*Table 1: Key Issues, research cluster and individual PhD topics*

| **Key Issue** | | **How can lightweight design contribute to solutions for the "Big Societal Challenges"?** |
|---|---|---|
| **Climate Protection** | Hybrid Lightweight Design and Diversity in Rescue Services | Diversity and technology in emergency and rescue services |
| | | Hybrid lightweight design in the field |
| | | Differential phase contrast in the scanning transmission electron microscope on interface-dominated materials |
| **Resources Efficiency** | Re-Use & Recycling Potential | Analysis of the effectiveness of governance processes using the example of lightweight design |
| | | Integration of technology, sustainability and economic efficiency criteria for the development of products and value networks |
| | | Production, characterisation and recycling of wood-plastic composites |
| | | Functionalisation of carbon fibres |
| | | Stochastic finite element method for wood-plastic composites |
| | | Friction-induced approach to further processing of recyclable metallic materials |
| **Mobility** | Personalised medical technology | Laser sintered mobility aids |
| | | Reducing the stiffness of the implant plates |
| | | Influence of the combination of surface chemistry and hierarchical structure of oxide-coated biomaterials on bio adhesion |

The Re-Use and Recycling Cluster started to cooperate with "Lippe zirkulär", a regional network of stakeholders from political, societal and industrial/economic sectors working together to develop, promote and implement new models of circular economy in the district Lippe.[4] Through this involvement, the contact with the company Hebie GmbH & Co.KG arose and the common research object could be designed. The Rescue Cluster cooperated with the German Network of Female Firefighters[5] and the Weber-Hydraulik GmbH.[6] The Medicine Cluster found its cooperation partners

4 https://www.lippe-zirkulaer.de/

5 https://www.feuerwehrfrauen.de/english/

6 https://www.weber-hydraulik.com/en/company/locations/

mainly through being accountable for enquiries from society and health professionals and responded to more immediate needs of the public, for instance by producing shields to protect health professionals at the beginning of the pandemic.

Bringing people from various areas of society into the research process and knowledge productions entails a contextualisation as researchers move into the context of application and think about the implications of what they are doing, of formulating problems in particular ways and of legitimate ways to conceptualise the position of the people in transdisciplinary research (Gibbons & Nowotny, 2001, p. 75). There are many ways to conceptualise that position, for instance people as a statistical aggregate (e.g. the survey study of the Rescue Cluster), as active agents (e.g. addressed through participating observation, the Thought School or the research cooperation of the Re-Use and Recycling Cluster), or as participating observers in research activities (e.g. Case Study I). However, we reflected upon and modified the "place of the people" in our research continuously rather than reducing the participatory potential by prescribing it through our research design.

Together with our societal partners, we envisioned which artefacts and services, according to their practical experience, would be appropriate to be created or optimised in a way that also contributes to solving a real-world problem and to integrating the knowledge from science and practise (Bergmann et al., 2010, p. 64f), in other words: the "boundary objects" we aimed to co-design, co-construct or co-produce by joining forces from science and practise. The Re-Use and Recycling Cluster decided to design a bicycle stand, the Rescue Cluster[7] focused on the optimisation of two selected standard tools for rescue operations, and the Medicine Cluster started to examine the legal and (inter)disciplinary requirements for the production of 3D printed products.

As Bergmann et al. (2012, p. 108) point out, artefacts, "*(...) due to their nature as materialized focal points of research and some specific properties, are well suited as boundary objects within transdisciplinary problem-solving processes*". The concept of "boundary objects" stems from science and technology studies (Star & Grisemer 1989; Star, 2010), where it serves to highlight that objects such as tools, information, prototypes, demonstrators or research objects can have different meanings for different communities, i.e. scientists, engineers, practitioners, etc. Boundary objects are

7 Due to our confidentiality agreement with Weber-Hydraulik GmbH, we cannot give any details about the particular tools and the criteria applied for the optimisation. However, we aim to provide insights into research methods, processes and empirical findings from the field that form the transdisciplinary approach to derive technologically and socially relevant criteria for technology optimisation.

> "both plastic enough to adapt to local needs and the constraints of the several parties employing them, yet robust enough to maintain a common identity across sites. [...] (Star & Griesemer, 1989, p. 393).

This interpretive flexibility is a main characteristic of boundary objects. They have different meanings in different social worlds but their structure is common enough to more than one world to make them recognisable (Star & Griesemer, 1989, p. 393). Thus, boundary objects enable action and cooperation among various actors and across various social sites. The creation and management of boundary objects is considered a key process in developing and maintaining coherence across intersecting social worlds (Star & Griesemer, 1989, p. 393).

Two further "boundary objects" emerged during the research process: the "Big Societal Challenges" and "the transmission electron microscope (TEM)". "Big Societal Challenges"– as outlined above – is a complex of challenges that also come with interpretive flexibility, have different meanings in different social worlds and are intended to stimulate action and collaboration. Therefore, by examining the challenges, perceptions and interpretations empirically, differentiating between social worlds and actors, and by exploring and discussing related concepts, such as the 17 Sustainable Development Goals, defined and adopted by all United Nations Member States in 2015,[8] we transformed the "Big Societal Challenges" into an epistemic object.

The transmission electron microscope (TEM) as a scientific object attracted much interest within our research group. However, a conclusive strategy to include it into the work of the research clusters, or the question of how this object could be used for transdisciplinary research was hard to discover. Therefore, we turned the latter question into the research question (see Case Study I).

## Transdisciplinary Integration

During the research process, multiple actors bring an essential heterogeneity of skills and expertise to the problem-solving process (Gibbons & Nowotny, 2001, p. 69). This sort of interdisciplinary and transdisciplinary research, as a consequence, requires dealing with different knowledge bases (e.g. theoretical knowledge, tacit knowledge, practical experience, etc.), thought styles, and communities.

The integration of different forms of knowing and knowledge (Bergmann et al., 2012) took place in the Thought School and the Research Seminar primarily. A first step was the empirical examination described above and an explication of interpretations regarding the big societal challenges, transdisciplinary research and the expectations of the public towards science and engineering, as well as the

8 https://sdgs.un.org/goals

development of common definitions for the research process, first with the wider public (joint formulation of relevant research topics in lightweight design, see also Horwath et al. (2018)), then transferred and elaborated on within the FK-LEM and the contributing disciplines (integration through interdisciplinary conceptual work, see Bergmann et al. (2012)).

In this phase, the Research Seminar also served as a research forum for screening, introducing, discussing, advancing, applying and integrating appropriate interdisciplinary and transdisciplinary methods for each cluster; it allowed data collection, analysis, continuous reflection of the collaborative process and technology development towards our boundary objects. Importantly, it also served as a forum to develop a transdisciplinary research and collaboration culture which differed from the prevailing (highly competitive, disciplinary-focused and gendered) scientific cultures (Cech, 2013; Cech, 2014; see also Horwath et al., 2018). Importantly, this culture includes accountability

> "(...) to different stakeholders, to different users, that the way to understanding how scientific knowledge is produced opens up. Once there is awareness, which has to penetrate even to curricula and the way we educate future scientists and engineers – once you open this up – then accountability becomes a way to broaden the horizon of those for whom you are producing knowledge" (Gibbons & Nowotny, 2001, p. 71).

To foster transdisciplinary integration, we emphasised education and mutual learning processes both among the members of FK-LEM and between researchers and practitioners. Education is a key approach of transdisciplinarity. It is linked to the idea of changing the role of science in society through changing higher education and its relationship to society (Thompson Klein, 2008, p. 399). In order to provide a research environment which allows – at least to a certain degree – overcoming the constraints of the narrowly defined competition and practise in science collaboratively, we provided formats such as the Research Seminar and the PhD colloquium to ensure that both transdisciplinary and interdisciplinary research of the PhD candidates receives professional support. This proved to be essential for the commitment to contribute to both streams of research. As Jahn et al. (2012, p. 8) describe:

> "Transdisciplinarity requires an uncommon willingness of individual scientists to learn and to think outside the disciplinary box. This willingness, in return, crucially depends on the extent to which individual interests are recognised and supported."

Processes of quality assurance are vital for transdisciplinary research. As stated above, quality control in transdisciplinary research goes beyond scientific excellence (which, of course, remains one criterion). In that it should also integrate societal value in the definition of "good science" (Gibbons & Nowotny, 2001, p. 71), it aims to produce not only reliable but also socially more robust knowledge and thus better technological solutions as well. Although to this date, we are not able to provide a full evaluation of the quality of our work, we can point to the evaluation of the Re-Use and Recycling Cluster (see Case Study II), to a multitude of disciplinary (peer reviewed and thus quality-controlled) publications of our PhD candidates, and to the successful collaborations established within and between cluster groups. The FK-LEM allowed us to practise collaborative learning, which goes beyond cooperation:

> "Cooperative learning typically entails divisions of labor, with each participant being responsible for part of a shared goal. In contrast, collaboration is a coordinated synchronous activity resulting from continued attempts to construct and maintain a shared conception of a particular problem. Cooperation helps facilitate collaboration. However, collaboration assumes a high degree of joint attention, communication, interaction, mutual engagement, and co-elaboration of knowledge." (Klein, 2018, p. 15).

## References

Atteslander, P. (2010). *Methoden der empirischen Sozialforschung.* Erich Schmidt Publisher (ESV Verlag), 13. Edition. ISBN: 978-3-503-12618-7

Bahr, A., Eichhorn, K. & Kubon, S. (2022). *#IchBinHanna. Prekäre Wissenschaft in Deutschland.* Suhrkamp Publisher. ISBN: 978-3-518-02975-6

Barad, K. (2007). Agential Realism: How Material-Discursive Practices Matter. In K. Barad (2007). *Meeting the Universe Halfway.* Duke University Press. https://doi.org/10.1515/9780822388128-006

Becker, E., & Jahn, T. (Eds.) (2006). *Soziale Ökologie. Grundzüge einer Wissenschaft von den gesellschaftlichen Naturverhältnissen.* Campus Publisher. ISBN: 978-3-5933-7993-7

Bergmann, M., Jahn, T., Knobloch, T., Krohn, W., Pohl, C., & Schramm, E. (2012). *Methods for Transdisciplinary Research. A Primer for Practice.* Campus Publisher. ISBN: 978-3-5933-9647-7

Berscheid, A.-L. (2018). Die Bedeutung transformativer Forschung für die wissenschaftliche Praxis. Ein Fallbeispiel. In B. Riegraf, & A.-L. Berscheid (Eds.) (2018). *Wissenschaft im Angesicht „großer gesellschaftlicher Herausforderungen". Das Beispiel der Forschung an hybriden Leichtbaumaterialien (pp. 227 – 248).* transcript Publisher. ISBN: 978-3-8376-4099-1

Berscheid, A.-L. (2019). *Arbeit an der Grenzfläche: Inter- und Transdisziplinarität in der Forschungspraxis.* Springer VS Wiesbaden. https://doi.org/10.1007/978-3-658-28636-1

Bohnsack, R. (2008). *Rekonstruktive Sozialforschung. Einführung in qualitative Methoden.* 7. Ed., Publisher Barbara Budrich. ISBN: 978-3-8252-8242-4

Bowker, G. C., & Star, S. L. (1999): *Sorting Things Out. Classification and its Consequences.* The MIT Press Cambridge. ISBN: 9780262522953

Cech E. A. (2013). The (Mis)Framing of Social Justice: Why Meritocracy and Depoliticization Hinder Engineers' Ability to Think About Social Injustices. In J. Lucena (Eds.). *Engineering Education for Social Justice. Philosophy of Engineering and Technology,* Vol. 10, 67–84, Springer, Dordrecht Publisher. https://doi.org/10.1007/978-94-007-6350-0_4

Cech E. A. (2014). Culture of Disengagement in Engineering Education? *Science, Technology, & Human Values,* Vol. 39, Issue 1, 42-72. https://doi.org/10.1177/0162243913504305

Di Guilo, A., & Defila, R. (2018). *Transdisziplinär und transformativ forschen. Eine Methodensammlung.* Springer Publisher. https://doi.org/10.1007/978-3-658-21530-9

European Union (n.d.). *Societal Challenges.* European Commission, Research and Innovation. https://open-research-europe.ec.europa.eu/gateways/societal-challenges/about

Fleck, L. (2012). *Entstehung und Entwicklung einer wissenschaftlichen Tatsache. Einführung in die Lehre vom Denkstil und Denkkollektiv.* Suhrkamp Publisher, 9. Edition. ISBN: 978-3-518-27912-0

Gibbons, M., & Nowotny, H. (2001). The Potential of Transdisciplinarity. In J. Thompson Klein, R. Häberli, R. W. Scholz, W. Grossenbacher-Mansuy, A. Bill, & M. Welti (Eds.). *Transdisciplinarity: Joint Problem Solving among Science, Technology, and Society. An Effective Way for Managing Complexity (pp. 67-80).* Springer Publisher. ISBN: 978-3-0348-8419-8

Gibbs, P., Neuhauser, L., & Fam, D. (2018). Introduction – The art of Collaborative Research and Collective Learning: Transdisciplinary Theory, Practice and Education. In D. Fam, L. Neuhauser, & P. Gibbs (Eds.). *Transdisciplinary Theory, Practice and Education. The Art of Collaborative Research and Collective Learning (pp. 3-9),* Springer Cham. https://doi.org/10.1007/978-3-319-93743-4_1

Grunwald, A. (2015). Transformative Wissenschaft – eine neue Ordnung im Wissenschaftsbetrieb? *GAIA - Ecological Perspectives for Science and Society.* Vol. 24, Issue 1, 17-20. https://doi.org/10.14512/gaia.24.1.5

Hanses, H. (2019). *Verfahrensoptimierung bei der Personenrettung aus Fahrzeugen mit verstärkten Strukturen und alternativen Antriebstechnologien* (Optimisation of tools and practices for rescue scenarios in car accidents). [Unpublished master's thesis]. Paderborn University, Germany.

Hanses, H., Akbuluk Irmak, E. F., & Horwath, I. (2020). *Lightweight Rescue Scissor optimized for the demands of the Emergency Services to Rescue People After Traffic Accidents.* Accepted for presentation at the 37th Danubia-Adria Symposium on Advances in Experimental Mechanics and Postponed to 2021 due to COVID-19

Hanses, H., & Horwath, I. (2021, September 21-24). *Project for the development of operational and demandoriented firefighting equipment.* Extended Abstracts to 37th Danubia Adria Symposium on Advances in Experimental Mechanics, JKU Linz, Austria.

Hanses H., & Horwath I. (2022). Development of operational and demand-oriented firefighting equipment. *Materials Today: Proceedings, Vol. 62, Part 5, 2684-2688.* https://doi.org/10.1016/j.matpr.2022.06.031

Haraway, D. (1988). Situated Knowledges: The Science Question in Feminism and the Privilege of Partial Perspective. *Feminist Studies,* Inc., Vol. 14, No. 3, 575-599. https://doi.org/10.2307/3178066

Harding, S. (1986): *The science question in feminism.* Cornell University Press. ISBN: 978-0-8014-1880-8

Harding, S. (2015). *Objectivity and Diversity. Another Logic of Scientific Research.* The University of Chicago Press. ISBN: 9780226241364

Harrison, K., & Olofsson, J. (2016). Becoming-a-firefighter – on the intra-active relationship between firefighters and their tools. *NORMA - International Journal for Masculinity Studies,* Vol. 11, Issue 3, 158-173. https://doi.org/10.1080/1890 2138.2016.1217693

Hemme, L. (2018). [Drei, zwei, d]EINS für ALLE! Alle für einen Tablettwagen. Erfahrungen mit inter- und transdisziplinärer Zusammenarbeit. In B. Riegraf, & A.-L. Berscheid (Eds.) (2018). *Wissenschaft im Angesicht „großer gesellschaftlicher Herausforderungen". Das Beispiel der Forschung an hybriden Leichtbaumaterialien (pp. 219-226).* transcript Verlag. ISBN: 978-3-8376-4099-1

Horwath, I. (2013). *Gleichstellung im Feuerwehrwesen. „Gut Wehr!" und die HeldInnen von heute.* Springer VS Wiesbaden. https://doi.org/10.1007/978-3-658-00914-4

Horwath, I., Dohmeier-Fischer, S., Weiß-Borkowski, N., & Tröster, T. (2018). From Empowerment to Innovation: Inter- and Transdisciplinary Research Methods in Lightweight Engineering. *INTED2018 Proceedings,* 7060-7068. https://doi.org/10.21125/inted.2018.1651

Horwath, I., & Terhechte, J. (2018). Bedarfsorientierte Technikentwicklung und gesellschaftliche Akzeptanz. Das Modell der „Denkschule". In R. Weidner, & A. Karafillidis (Eds.) (2018). *Proceedings der 3. Transdisziplinäre Konferenz „Technische Unterstützungssysteme, die die Menschen wirklich wollen" (pp. 473-481).* ISBN: 978-3-86818-245-3

Horwath, I., Kastein, M., & Dağlar-Sezer, N. (2021a). Feuerwehren im Spiegel gesellschaftlicher Diversität. In N. Eschenbruch, S. Kaufmann, & P. Zoche (Eds.) (2021). *Vielfältige Sicherheiten. Gesellschaftliche Dimensionen der Sicherheitsforschung (pp. 107-131).* SiFo Fachdialog Sicherheitsforschung des BMBF Deutschland, Band 20. LIT-Publisher.

Horwath, I., Kastein, M., & Finke, J. (2021b). *Herausforderungen und Chancen von Diversität für Sicherheit, Effizienz und Zukunft des deutschen Feuerwehrsystems.* Final report of the project FORTESY – Organisation, Technik, Diversität: Neue Ansätze für Sicherheit, Effizienz und soziale Integration im Feuerwehrwesen (Organisation, Technology, Diversity: New Approaches to Safety, Efficiency and Social Integration in the Fire Service). Funded by Federal Ministry of Education and Research (Bundesministerium für Bildung und Forschung - BMBF) as part of the Innovation and Technology Analysis (16ITA208).

Jahn, T., Bergmann, M., & Keil, F. (2012). Transdisciplinarity: Between mainstreaming and marginalization. *Ecological Economics*, Vol. 79, 1-10. https://doi.org/10.1016/j.ecolecon.2012.04.017

Jahn, T., & Keil, F. (2015). An Actor-Specific guideline for quality assurance in transdisciplinary research. *Futures Publisher*, Vol. 65, 195-208. https://doi.org/10.1016/j.futures.2014.10.015

Kastein, M., Finke, J., & Horwath, I. (2022). Waschen, Warten, Wege ebnen. Ambivalente Fürsorge und der männliche Heldenmythos in der Feuerwehr. In M. Kastein, & L. Weber (Eds.) (2022). *Care-Arbeit und Gender in der digitalen Transformation (pp. 119-134)*. Juventa Beltz. ISBN: 978-3-7799-6739-2

Khatiri, F. (2022). *Transfer von ExpertInnenwissen zur Optimierung feuerwehrtechnischer Ausrüstung* (Transfer of expert knowledge for the optimisation of firefighting rescue tools). [Unpublished master's thesis]. Paderborn University, Germany.

Kirchhoff, S., Kuhnt, S., Lipp, P., & Schlawin, S. (2010). *Der Fragebogen. Datenbasis, Konstruktion und Auswertung*. Verlag für Sozialwissenschaften, Springer, 5. Edition. https://doi.org/10.1007/978-3-531-92050-4

Klein, J.T. (2018). Learning in Transdisciplinary Collaborations: A Conceptual Vocabulary. In Fam, D., Neuhauser, L. & Gibbs, P. (Eds.) *Transdisciplinary Theory, Practice and Education. The Art of Collaborative Research and Collective Learning* (11-23). Springer Publisher. https://doi.org/10.1007/978-3-319-93743-4_2

Lam, D. P.M., Freund M. E., Kny, J., Marg, O., Mbah, M., Theiler, L., Bergmann, M., Brohmann, B., Lang, D. J. & Schäfer, M. (2021). Transdisciplinary research: towards an integrative perspective. *GAIA - Ecological Perspectives for Science and Society*. Vol. 30, Issue 4, 243-249. https://doi.org/10.14512/gaia.30.4.7

Lux, A., Schäfer, M., Bergmann, M., Jahn, T., Marg, O., Nagy, E., Ransiek, A.-C., & Theiler, L. (2019). Societal effects of transdisciplinary sustainability research—How can they be strengthened during the research process? Environmental Science & Policy, Vol. 101, 183-191. https://doi.org/10.1016/j.envsci.2019.08.012

MIWF – Ministerium für Innovation, Wissenschaft und Forschung des Landes

Neuhauser, L. (2018). Practical and Scientific Foundations of Transdisciplinary Research and Action. In Fam, D., Neuhauser, L. & Gibbs, P. (Eds.) *Transdisciplinary Theory, Practice and Education. The Art of Collaborative Research and Collective Learning* (25-38). Springer Publisher. https://doi.org/10.1007/978-3-319-93743-4_3

Neuser, M. (2019). *Potenzialanalyse von Leichtbauanwendungen im Feuerwehr- und Rettungswesen* (Exploring the potential of light weight design for firefighting and rescue technology). [Unpublished master's thesis]. Paderborn University, Germany.

Nordrhein-Westfalen (2013). *Forschungsstrategie „Fortschritt NRW". Forschung und Innovation für nachhaltige Entwicklung 2013 – 2020.* http://www.onlines3.eu/wp-content/uploads/RIS3_strategy_repository/D_Broschuere_Fortschritt_NRW.pdf

Pohl, C., van Kerkhoff, L., Hadorn, G.H. & Bammer, G. (2008). Integration. In Hirsch Hadorn, G., Hoffmann-Riem, H., Biber-Klemm, S., Grossenbacher-Mansuy, W., Joye, D., Pohl, C., Wiesmann, U. & Zemp, E. (Eds.) *Handbook of Transdisciplinary Research* (411- 424). Springer, Dordrecht. https://doi.org/10.1007/978-1-4020-6699-3_27

Pohl, C., & Hirsch Hadorn, G. (2008). Methodological challenges of transdisciplinary research. *Natures Sciences Sociétés*, Vol. 16, 111-121. https://www.cairn.info/revue-natures-sciences-societes-2008-2-page-111.htm

Pohl, C. (2011). What is progress in transdisciplinary research? *Futures*, Vol. 43, Issue 6, 618–626. https://doi.org/10.1016/j.futures.2011.03.001

Pohl, C., Krütli P., & Stauffacher M. (2017). Ten Reflective Steps for Rendering Research Societally Relevant. *GAIA - Ecological Perspectives for Science and Society*, Vol. 26, No.1, 43–51. https://doi.org/10.14512/gaia.26.1.10

Riegraf, B., & Berscheid, A.-L. (Eds.) (2018a). *Wissenschaft im Angesicht „großer gesellschaftlicher Herausforderungen". Das Beispiel der Forschung an hybriden Leichtbaumaterialien.* transcript Verlag. ISBN: 978-3-8376-4099-1

Riegraf, B., & Berscheid, A.-L. (2018b). Wissenschaft im Angesicht „großer gesellschaftlicher Herausforderungen": Zur Einführung. In B. Riegraf, & A.-L. Berscheid (Eds.) (2018). *Wissenschaft im Angesicht „großer gesellschaftlicher Herausforderungen". Das Beispiel der Forschung an hybriden Leichtbaumaterialien (pp. 9-16).* transcript Verlag. ISBN: 978-3-8376-4099-1

Rosenthal, G. (2018). *Interpretive Social Research. An Introduction.* Göttingen University Press. https://doi.org/10.17875/gup2018-1103

Schiebinger, L., & Schraudner, M. (2011). Interdisciplinary Approaches to Achieving Gendered Innovations in Science, Medicine, and Engineering. *Interdisciplinary Science Reviews*, Vol. 36, No. 2, 154–167. https://doi.org/10.1179/030801811X13013181961518

Schneidewind, U., & Singer-Brodowski, M. (2014). *Transformative Wissenschaft. Klimawandel im deutschen wissenschafts- und Hochschulsystem.* Metropolis Publisher. ISBN 978-3-7316-1057-1

Schneidewind, U. (2015). Transformative Wissenschaft – Motor für gute Wissenschaft und lebendige Demokratie. *GAIA - Ecological Perspectives for Science and Society*, Vol. 24, Issue 2, 88-91. https://doi.org/10.14512/gaia.24.2.5

Scholz, R. W., & Steiner, G. (2015). The real type and ideal type of transdisciplinary processes: part I – theoretical foundations. *Sustainability Science*, Vol. 10, Issue 4, 527-544. DOI 10.1007/s11625-015-0326-4

Schramm, B.; Rupp, N.; Risse, L.; Brüggemann, J.-P-; Riemer, A.; Richard, H.A.; Kullmer, G. (2017): Medizintechnische Anwendungen der additiven Fertigung. In: Richard, H.A.; Schramm, B.; Zipsner, T. (Eds.): *Additive Fertigung von Bauteilen und Strukturen*. Springer Vieweg.

Schramm, B.; Risse, L.; Brüggemann, J.-P.; Richard, H.A.; Kullmer, G. (2018): Overview of structural mechanical investigations on additively manufactured medical products. *Journal of 3D Printing in Medicine* Vol. 2, Issue 2, DOI: doi.org/10.2217/3dp-2017-0020.

Star, S. L., & Griesemer, J. R. (1989). Institutional Ecology, `Translations' and Boundary Objects: Amateurs and Professionals in Berkeley's Museum of Vertebrate Zoology, 1907-39. *Social Studies of Science*, Vol. 19, Issue 3, 387–420. https://doi.org/10.1177/030631289019003001

Star, S. L. (2010). This is Not a Boundary Object: Reflections on the Origin of a Concept. *Science, Technology, & Human Values*. Vol. 35, Issue 5, 601-617. https://doi.org/10.1177/0162243910377624

Strohschneider, P. (2014). Zur Politik der Transformativen Wissenschaft. In Brodocz, A., Herrmann, D., Schmidt, R., Schulz, D., Schulze Wessel, J. (Eds.) *Die Verfassung des Politischen* (175-192). Springer Publisher. https://doi.org/10.1007/978-3-658-04784-9_10

Thompson Klein, J. (2008). Education. In Hirsch Hadorn, G., Hoffmann-Riem, H., Biber-Klemm, S., Grossenbacher-Mansuy, W., Joye, D., Pohl, C., Wiesmann, U. & Zemp, E. (Eds.), *Handbook of Transdisciplinary Research* (pp. 399-410). Springer Publisher. ISBN: 978-1-4020-6699-3

Triebus, M., Ostermann, M., Tröster, T. & Horwath, I. (2022, July 5-6): *Advanced Automotive Components by Fiber-Metal-laminates* [Conference Presentation]. *Materials in Car Body Engineering*, Automotive Circle, Bad Nauheim.

Wissenschaftsrat (2015). *Zum wissenschaftspolitischen Diskurs über Große gesellschaftliche Herausforderungen*. Positionspapier (Drs. 4594-15). https://www.wissenschaftsrat.de/download/archiv/4594-15.pdf

Zuboff, S. (2019). *The age of surveillance capitalism. The fight for a human future at the new frontier of power*. Public Affairs. ISBN: 978-1-78125-685-5

# Lightweight Design: Background and Challenges

*Swetlana Schweizer, Thomas Tröster*

The most significant driver of technological developments, innovations and technical progress are human needs, or rather the fulfilment of these needs. At the same time, different needs are not all of equal value. The most popular model that summarises the hierarchical relationship of human needs was established by Abraham Maslow in the 20th century. His social-psychological model divides human needs into five levels: physiological needs (air, water, food, sleep), security needs (work, family, health), social needs (social exchange), individual needs (esteem, freedom) and self-realisation (realising one's own potential). Unlike most other creatures, humans have learned to help fulfil their needs through technical creations: making a fire, building a house, producing and using electricity, exploring the universe. At the same time, the perception of what our basic needs include changes with time and technological progress.

Above all, time plays an important role. In an increasingly fast-paced society, people don't want to spend any of their precious lifetime on mostly boring, worthless travel time to visit family, see famous landmarks, relax and swim in the ocean and everything else there is to experience and marvel at. So it is only too logical that the need for free and comfortable mobility is increasing and will continue to do so in the future. Our understanding of how we want to experience mobility is closely linked to our current living conditions. The currently existing mobility models (i.e., the interaction of all means of transport) are causing increasingly dramatic consequences for our environment and as a result are being critically examined more and more.

What would today's ideal mobility model look like? No one can answer this question unequivocally because our mobility is multi-layered and can be greatly influenced by technological developments in a short time. In addition to the necessary technological progress, a multitude of other aspects are decisive with regard to how we discover our world. These are, for example

- the availability and linkage between the different modes of transport: Air transport, rail transport, water transport, public transport and individual transport,

- an optimised road infrastructure, which is what makes free and individual mobility possible in the first place,
- the level road surface, the quality of which significantly influences the adhesion of the vehicle tires,
- the road traffic regulations, which govern the behaviour of individual participants,
- the test centres and certification bodies that test and approve our vehicles and remove life-threatening technology from the road,
- supplying our vehicles with the necessary energy. For instance, in order to switch to electrically powered vehicles, a corresponding supply infrastructure must first be established.

This list certainly offers room for further aspects, but it already shows the complexity of the requirements for an idealised future mobility model. In addition, each individual aspect is built, operated and further developed by different institutions / organisations / economic sectors. For an optimal solution, close cooperation among all partners and society is necessary. Thus, it is obvious how vital collaboration between interdisciplinary (with the participation of different disciplines) and transdisciplinary (with the additional participation of society) is in order to solve this challenge.

According to the German Federal Statistical Office (Statistisches Bundesamt), the automobile is the most common means of transport in motorised passenger traffic in Germany, with a share of over 80 %. More than half of all Germans own a vehicle, producing over 60 % of the emissions in road traffic. This means that there is enormous potential for development and reduced emissions.

One of the possible fields of development is the vehicle itself. Three aspects must remain in focus when developing vehicles:

The **safety** of a vehicle's occupants is the top priority. The car manufacturers are faced with technical challenges in vehicle development. Not only load weight occurring during the journey but, above all, all passengers should survive any collision with other road users or objects without damage.

The **economic efficiency** of a product, i.e. a vehicle, often determines its chances of successfully surviving on the market and asserting itself against the competition. The modern vehicle is a product for the masses and, as such, must also be affordable for the masses in the population.

Only through **sustainable management** of existing resources and preservation of ecosystems can a sustainable supply of the materials a population needs be guaranteed. Above all, the shift from finite to renewable resources promotes sustainable management. The consequences of the currently only partially sustainable economy are becoming increasingly visible, which is why a rethinking process has been taking place within the population in this regard, especially in recent years. There is a growing demand for sustainably produced products; therefore, technological developments in this area also increase rapidly. Legislators are also reacting to this and are promoting them through new regulations and targeted subsidies.

Taken on their own, these requirements seem manageable and feasible. On closer inspection, the numerous interactions among safety, economy and sustainability become apparent. For example: ensuring the safety of vehicle occupants often leads to the increased use of higher-quality materials. This increases the development and production effort, which is ultimately reflected in the price. A higher price reduces the economic efficiency of the product. If sustainability is sacrificed in order to increase profitability, it can have fatal negative effects on our ecosystem. Here it is essential to find a balance among these requirements.

Other important influencing factors primarily concern the demographic development of the population. Not only the constant population growth on the entire planet, but also the increasing prosperity of the population have a negative impact on the environmental balance. The growing number of vehicles pollutes our environment in several ways: through the energy and materials used in their manufacture and through the exhaust gases emitted during their use phase. By means of statutory recycling quotas of over 95 %, much has already been done regarding recycling of materials. Increasingly advanced technology in vehicles is also reducing the amount of exhaust gases emitted. The German Association of the Automotive Industry (Verband der Automobilindustrie) states that between 2007 and 2017, a 25-%-reduction in $CO_2$ average values for newly registered vehicles was achieved. Car manufacturers are required to provide the safest and most environmentally friendly technology in each new vehicle model. The goal of $CO_2$ neutral mobility is thus getting closer but is still not within reach.

## Driving resistance as an energy consumer

To start the development process for car manufacturers, the physical basics of a moving vehicle must be clarified. The vehicle drive generates energy that is transferred to the road via the tyres; the type of energy generation is initially irrelevant. The amount of energy required depends on the vehicle's driving resistance. From a physical point, there are four types of driving resistance: rolling resistance, acceleration resistance, air resistance and gradient resistance. Air resistance increases quadratically with driving speed. Thus, the faster a vehicle travels, the more energy it must continuously expend in order to maintain the driving speed.

The vehicle mass is an important influencing factor for the other three types of driving resistance. If the vehicle mass changes, e.g., due to larger engines with more power or additional passengers with luggage, this additional mass is directly included in the required energy demands. This correlation is far greater for car manufacturers than just the extra energy consumption. If, for example, the safety of the passengers is increased by using more material, a larger and thus heavier chassis is also needed, which in turn requires a bigger and heavier engine, which results in a larger fuel tank. In this way, the weight of the vehicle continues to increase. This so-called weight spiral can also be seen in reverse order: lighter body – lighter chassis – smaller engine – smaller fuel tank. Therefore, car manufacturers deliberately pursue lightweight construction in the area of the car body in order to reverse this weight spiral. A lower vehicle weight not only has an effect on the energy input and thus on fuel consumption. Among other things, this also has a positive impact on the vehicle's agility, which in turn contributes to increased safety and driving pleasure.

## Minimisation of the energy demand

Lightweight construction is competing with consumer demands for more safety, space, comfort, functionality and torque of the engine and the demands of legislators for better compatibility of the vehicle's weight with respect to the energy needed to be reduced in a crash situation, low emissions/fuel consumption and more pedestrian protection. This increases the complexity of the task at hand enormously for car manufacturers and their suppliers.

With regard to the total energy requirements of a vehicle, a priority list of possible measures was drawn up: (Friedrich, 2017)

- Minimising the energy required to fulfil the driving task, for example by reducing the vehicle weight,
- Optimising the efficiency of energy conversion, e.g., by optimising the engine and the drive train,
- Energy management according to demand, e.g., through start-stop operation,
- Energy recuperation in electric-powered vehicles for partial energy recovery.

From these possible measures, technical measures are derived from developing and optimising vehicle areas, such as engine, transmission, chassis, air conditioning, on-board network and body in white. But operating strategies, aerodynamics and thermal management are also revised. In each of these areas, attention is paid to the weight of the installed components, among other things. After all, a 10 % reduction in the weight of a vehicle with an internal combustion engine leads to a decrease in energy requirements of about 6 % (Friedrich, 2017).

In an electrically driven vehicle, energy recuperation also recovers about 85 % of the braking energy. The braking energy is a part of the energy demands of a vehicle that remains in the system after deducting the energy required for the electrical consumption and for overcoming the driving resistance. Thus, the energy demands of these vehicles are reduced by the amount of recuperated energy. This partly offsets the greater energy requirement of vehicles with internal combustion engines, resulting from the higher vehicle mass. The reduction in vehicle weight also has a positive effect on driving resistance. This energy gain can be used to increase the range or, if the range remains the same, to reduce the battery capacity.

Another positive effect is the influence of weight reduction on driving dynamics. Better acceleration values and cornering behaviour, but also shorter braking distances, allow for more stable driving behaviour and contribute to increased safety in road traffic.

Automobile manufacturers, as well as their suppliers and research institutions, are working on the development of lightweight design principles and lightweight design strategies in all areas. In this context, it is essential to note that lightweight construction should only be pursued where it is necessary and makes sense. Changes to one part of such a complex system as a vehicle always have an impact on the entire system and also on the value chain associated with the vehicle. (Friedrich, 2017)

## Lightweight construction as a solution: But how should it be implemented?

Lightweight construction is not a new phenomenon. As early as the Bronze Age, people had an understanding of energy and material efficiency that was adapted to the general state of knowledge at the time. An example of this is the wheel. The first wheels were made of a solid material: a round wooden element surrounded by a metallic ring. Further development of this was the spoke model. Materials were used that were available, whose properties were known and whose processing was possible, i.e., wood as light basic construction and metal as a stronger component in particularly stressed areas. In addition, there was construction. The materials should only be used where they are needed. The connexion between the belt and the hub was realised from a full wheel with thin spokes. Materials, production technology and design are still the drivers of lightweight innovations today.

With the development of the combustion engine, the race in vehicle construction and also in lightweight construction has picked up speed. This is because developers quickly realised that vehicle weight has a significant influence on speed, acceleration and handling. Ferdinand Porsche, who developed the "Sascha" car in the 1920s, is considered a lightweight pioneer. All developers made use of technological trends from aircraft construction. Porsche built his car with a small-volume engine with increased compression and applied lightweight principles in body construction, e.g., the body was made of aluminium and not steel. At this time, innovations were driven primarily by the developers' desire for recognition and prestige.

After the automobile became more and more a product for the masses, fuel became scarcer. The harmful consequences for the environment became more and more apparent; consistent mass reductions were among the most critical areas of leverage for automotive engineers from around the 1970s onwards. The aim is to make vehicles more economical, more fuel-efficient and thus also more favourable in terms of emissions. From the predecessor model to the successor model, carmakers have to "double their efforts" in order to successfully counteract the weight spiral. From one vehicle model to the next, there is initially an increase in comfort options, which is reflected in an increase in weight. So if the weight of the successor model is to be reduced, the additional weight must first be compensated for by the additional contents. Only then can a weight reduction be generated by the further implementation of lightweight construction measures during the model change.

Reductions in weight are always accompanied by additional development and production costs, especially if novel manufacturing processes or materials have to be used. In industry, however, the economic efficiency of products or measures is decisive in determining whether the product exists on the market or planned measures are implemented. This is why the term "lightweight construction economics" was introduced in lightweight construction. In lightweight construction economics, reductions in weight are divided into four categories depending on the costs involved. The method used to reduce weight is not taken into account. Only the costs in relation to the weight reductions are taken into account. A distinction is made between economy, eco, purpose and ultra-lightweight construction. With low-cost, only the economy lightweight variant can be implemented. The greater the desired reduction in weight, the higher the costs. In ultra-lightweight construction, the lightest variant is chosen regardless of the costs. This process is usually exponential and is only limited upwards by the physical boundary conditions. (Friedrich, 2017)

When implementing lightweight construction in the area of vehicle bodies, lightweight construction strategies, lightweight construction methods and lightweight construction principles are used as development methods. The lightweight construction strategies include lightweight material construction, lightweight form construction, lightweight operating construction, lightweight concept construction and lightweight production construction. All five lightweight design strategies are to be understood as complementary to each other and are not considered individually. On the contrary, lightweight construction methods are different approaches to solving a specific problem. Only in this way can the potential of lightweight construction be fully exploited. Lightweight construction methods include modular, integral or hybrid construction. Only one construction method can be used to find a solution to a particular situation. There can be overlaps in the methods of lightweight construction strategies and lightweight construction methods. So, lightweight construction methods can be classified under lightweight construction strategies. The third method includes lightweight construction principles. Here, other objectives are also considered in addition to reduction in weight, such as dynamic behaviour. Here, parameters such as shape, topology, materials and construction method are used, however, not precisely defined. (Friedrich, 2017)

In addition to the technical and economic aspects, the ecological consequences of lightweight construction must also be precisely quantified and evaluated since not all lightweight construction measures are equally favourable for our environment. This is because the production, use and recycling of products are included in balancing the equation. In order to carry out efficient lightweight construction, all materials and production techniques are first taken into consideration. Depending on the materials used and the production technique employed, more or less environmentally harmful emissions are produced for the same product. To evaluate all emissions with one characteristic value, the $CO_2$ equivalent was introduced. The effect of all greenhouse gases is converted here to the impact of $CO_2$ and added up in the equivalent. In the automotive industry, due to the predominance of the internal combustion engine, most emissions are generated in the use phase. By reducing the weight of the vehicle, emissions in this phase can be reduced directly. Even the possibly higher emissions in the manufacturing phase of lighter components or vehicles can still lead to a positive overall balance through the savings in the use phase. However, this must already be taken into account in the development of the components. Only lightweight construction measures with a positive eco-balance over the entire life cycle should and will be implemented.

With e-mobility, the focus of lightweight construction is shifting from the use phase to the manufacturing phase. This is subject to the proviso that the energy supply in the entire utilisation phase is completely generated from renewable energies. The technology for generating and distributing this energy is also $CO_2$-neutral. In the long term, the aim is to conserve energy and materials resources. This future vision is closely linked to energy production and use and can only be realised when exclusively renewable energies are used across the board. Until then, the aim is to steadily increase the share of renewable energy in the use phase and the share of vehicles that can be operated with this energy as well.

It is now up to everyone to do their utmost to make this future vision a reality. The government must promote the corresponding infrastructure for energy distribution and remove the legal hurdles to the transformation of energy production and use. It is the duty of industry and science to provide technical innovations, i.e., to present an affordable alternative. But consumers should also reconsider their prejudices against these developments and get involved in this adventure for the sake of our environment.

## References

Friedrich, H. E. (Ed.) (2017). *Leichtbau in der Fahrzeugtechnik* (2nd Edition). ISBN 978-3-658-12295-9 (eBook)

# Case Study Profiles

*Ilona Horwath, Swetlana Schweizer*

> "Case studies are of special importance for transdisciplinary processes as they embody the complexity, multi-layeredness of trade-offs and conflicts, uncertainty, and incompleteness, which relate to any form of scientific knowledge for which real-world contexts and structures are the underlying basis."
> *(Scholz & Steiner, 2015, p. 528)*

This chapter presents the case studies conducted at the FK-LEM. The structure of description follows the model of an idealtypical transdisciplinary research (Bergmann et al., 2012, p. 35; see Figure 1 in the Introduction of this book) so that a brief illustration of the transdisciplinary profile serves to introduce the work of each research cluster. Subsequently, the case studies are presented. In addition to the three main research cluster in FK-LEM, Re-Use and Recycling Potentials (Re-Use and Recycling Cluster), Hybrid Lightweight Design and Diversity in Rescue Services (Rescue Cluster), Individualised medical technology (Medicine Cluster), where several empirical studies were realized, Bürger and Linder (Case Study I in this book) provide a conceptual contribution in which they explore the challenges and prospects of implementing transmission electron microscopy as a highly specialized technology in transdisciplinary research approaches to solve societal problems. Case Study II is dedicated to the work of the Re-Use and Recycling Cluster. As the Case Study of this cluster has gone through the whole cycle of (an ideal) transdisciplinary research process, we are able to close the section with the results of a critical evaluation of the collaboration process and the critical assessment of results from the perspective of both, FK-LEM researcher and their societal project partner.Case Study III provides selected insights to the work of the Rescue Cluster. As mentioned in the introduction, the research of this cluster, in particular its disciplinary and interdisciplinary advances, are subject to a confidentiality agreement between FK-LEM researcher and industrial partner Weber-Hydraulik GmbH. However, the transdisciplinary approach of the cluster is comprehensive.

The researcher in this cluster, all engineers, identified a major lack of knowledge concerning the particular scenarios and user practices where the two standard tools under investigation are used, the diversity of practitioners using rescue tools, and their experience as well as perspectives for the optimisation of the tools (weight, functionality, price). To address this lacuna, the engineers were trained to apply a range of methods from the social sciences in addition to their engineering research topics. Drawing on an explorative approach, a survey study and several participant observations were conducted. Although they can only present selected findings of their work in this book, their contribution shows that a transdisciplinary approach to the development of rescue tools is a promising path to include the diversity of practitioners experience as a central criterion for optimisation or the construction of new tools.Case study IV is concerned with the aim to enhance the mobility and quality of life of individuals with health related needs. While additive manufacturing provides the technological power to respond to such individual needs rather immediately, the technological potential currently faces strong limitations not at least due to the challenges to embed the technology in the dynamic landscapes of economic and legal (trans-)formation. In an area where advances in technology, in this case Additive Manufacturing (AM), unfold way more rapidly than the societal structures required to embed its procedures and use within established medical, legal, economic and further organizational frameworks, gaps between practices and responsibilities inevitably will arise. The authors are concerned with the question what it takes to close these gaps, or to achieve approximations on the way – solutions that allow to respond to the needs of individuals who would benefit greatly from individualized AM products. Finally, drawing on the revised and advanced model of an ideal transdisciplinary research process (Lam et al. 2021), we will sum up our reflections on the success and limitations of our transdisciplinary work at the FK-LEM in the conclusion of the book.

## Case Study I

The societal problem addressed by the authors was, generally, the question how to merge science (in this case: physics and engineering) with societal needs and knowledge in a way that supports solving social issues. Research related to the TEM focusses on highly specialized topics involving a range of complex apparatuses and procedures. Hence, the aim was to find ways to lower the barrier (for both lay people and scientists) to participate in transdisciplinary research with TEM.

The scientific challenge Bürger & Linder took up was that TEM, to our knowledge, had not yet been applied in transdisciplinary research or rendered as a transdisciplinary method. To bring TEM and transdisciplinary approaches together requires to reflect on different epistemic concepts. In particular, concepts of objectivity. Natural sciences work in a certain way to achieve objectivity, but within the social sciences there are quite different concepts of objectivity which also feed into transdisciplinary methods. In addition, the image formation and the interpretation of results related to TEM is highly complex.

In this particular project, stakeholders from society were not involved. However, the authors responded to societal discourses that promote to advance traditional approaches of science communication (i.e., that there is a one-sided knowledge gap that has to be filled with information, Kronberger (2016), see also Introduction in this book) as they aimed to conceptualize and facilitate mutual learning processes between science and society tackling the specific case of the TEM. And they included self-reflectivity, with a focus on the question of objectivity and the transformation of a highly abstract apparatus into a boundary object more accessible and relatable for lay people.

Regarding scientific discourses, the authors had to reflect on different approaches to objectivity. This required to bridge epistemic gaps between social scientific approaches, in particular feminist epistemology, Science and Technology Studies, and the epistemologies established in Physics and Natural Science – gaps, that are traditionally difficult to overcome as approximation requires a critical reflection of knowledge bases, position of the researcher, and partial perspectives. An integration of the different strands of epistemologies, theories and methodologies poses further challenges.

However, the results of Bürger and Lindner in terms of societal practice include suggestions on how to embed the TEM in transdisciplinary research, images that can be shown, examples where TEM helped to solve societal questions, an exploration of the tremendous prospects of TEM to contribute essentially to the solvation of societal problems, and the identification and analysis of the challenges in the process. With regard to results for scientific practise, the authors formulate new research questions and reflect on methodical and theoretical innovations. The examples given, where TEM helped to solve societal questions are also of scientific value. Finally, the kind of self-reflectivity applied in the elaboration of the contribution helped the researchers to understand that research should be based on a certain freedom and autonomy, but should also lead to valuable results for society.

The formation of a common research object was realized in the exploration of TEM and its transdisciplinary potentials as an "epistemic object" which allowed a problem transformation of the TEM from a "too complex and abstract" apparatus to one that can be made comprehensible in its workings and limitations to lay people. The production of new knowledge, primary through interdisciplinary integration, consisted in the combination and synthesis of epistemic and theoretical approaches that, from a theoretical stance, may initially appear immensurable Transdisciplinary integration, in terms of an evaluation of the new knowledge, was prepared through an interdisciplinary integration. Therefore, a TEM streaming session was provided for FK-LEM researcher and associates from chemistry and mechanical engineering. The authors presented images generated with TEM and discussed, what can actually be seen on an image without knowing/explaining the physics behind the image formation. While this discussion incited vivid interdisciplinary exchange, an event where this approach is demonstrated and tested with the public is still to perform. We hope that the case study is a step on this way.

## Case Study II

The research in this cluster had to deal with a range of societal problems. To start with, the impact of microplastics on the environment and human health has become a widely discussed topic in many areas of society, as well as the development and implementation of new rules on waste management. Driven by the rise of Fridays4Future and the climate protection movement, the relevance, value and urgency of research that contributes to a comprehensive, valid assessment of materials, products and processes, for instance, approaches such as Life Cycle Assessment or models for circular economy, has gained significantly in the public. On the other side, citizens remain sceptical regarding certain technologies (Nanotechnology, Synthetic biology) and trust in certain branches, actors and methods are low (Gaskell et al., 2010). Against this backdrop, the cluster addressed a strong societal demand for ecologically improved design, support (both financial and scientific) for the development and implementation of innovative procedures, quality standards, expansion and modernization of recycling capacity, and the creation of viable markets for recycled plastics.

Scientific problems identified in this context are the conceptualization of comprehensive approaches to the modelling and assessment of ecological footprints for products and processes, or how to design for recyclability including the questions of established norms and the development of quality standards for recycled plastics. The letter aspect is particularly important, not at least as the market demand for recycled materials is considered low. Hence, innovation and investment in circular economy solutions are required.

During the FK-LEM research period, societal discourses focussed on issues such as legislative initiatives to avoid single-use of plastics, the creation of policies and incentives to enhance re-use and recycling strategies and the creation of more durable products. More generally, a quick implementation of circular economy structures and processes emerged as a priority, also in the regional context of FK-LEM. In order to contribute to that goal, scientists are challenged to improve the economics and quality of plastic recycling and to be accountable for societal actors or initiatives.

The scientific discourses of the contributing disciplines were characterized by attempts to respond to the newly established urgency of the climate protection movement. For instance, the building up of collaborations with industry, NGOs and educational institutions or discussion on appropriate interventions, instruments, and quality assessment. Other strands of discourse focussed on economic questions, i.e. better pricing, taxes and subsidies, and the question of materials, i.e. bio-based and compostable products. The question of how to create awareness and behavioural change, finally, was salient in both societal and scientific discourses.

Through the intense transdisciplinary collaboration with Lippe Zirkulär and Hebie GmbH & Co.KG, the research cluster was able to achieve results for both social and scientific practice. The first cover educational materials, e.g. a data base on re-use and recycling materials as a teaching resource for the Faculty of Mechanical Engineering at Paderborn University, concepts for green alternatives, the contribution of expertise and research services to the establishment of circular plastic economy and, last but not least, the alternative TURRIX stand as a demonstrator. The latter refer to a better product design in terms of using recycled plastic and to a critical assessment of the ecological impact and limitations of the product, i.e. a circular life cycle assessment. Importantly, mutual learning effects between science and society have been achieved (for more details, please see Conclusion in this book).

## Case Study III

Firefighters and public services for technical support are at the forefront when it comes to tackling the disruptive realities of climate change. While fire services record increased emergencies also due to climate change, structural changes in society lead to decreases of active memberships in the respective volunteer organizations – which form a major pillar of the German fire service system (Horwath et al., 2021; Kastein et al., 2021). Another societal problem is the weight of much of contemporary rescue equipment, leading to an overload of emergency trucks as well as physical and health impact on force members. An additional issue for first responders is the use of new materials and structures in the construction of vehicles entailing further challenges for rescue operations regarding accidents.

Several scientific problems were rather clear, the cluster had to deal with a lack of knowledge concerning a range of topics: a lack of knowledge about the actual use of rescue equipment, on actual user practices, about the kinematic of particular tools, the load distribution on tools and on the performance capacity of particular tools.

With regard to societal discourses, the question of diversity in fire services turned out to be contested terrain. On the one hand, the promotion of diversity is part of strategies to modernize fire services in Germany and internationally, on the other hand, this strategy is of course not universally endorsed (Horwath et al., 2021; Kastein et al., 2021). A main reason is scepticism about the physical constitution, the effective power and thus the safety of, and provided by a more diverse workforce. The question is, then, how technology design – not only regarding the weight of tools but also aspects such as the ergonomic and functional design – can help to facilitate the inclusion of a more diverse workforce. And how considering "diversity" as a central criterion in the development of new, and the optimisation of established tools could contribute to reducing the physical power required for particular operations and hence the number of staff required to perform them. This approach was met with explicit interest by developers of firefighting technology who underscored its relevance for innovation and safety. Importantly, diversity in this context has to be considered as a dimension that far exceeds the common associations of diversity as a solely sociodemographic or identity related category. Rather, the consideration of the diversity of bodies, experience, occupational practices and routines with the use of certain tools, but also the diversity of challenges each new emergency situation poses has to be taken into account.

Scientific discourse or preliminary work on diversity as a criterion for the development of firefighting equipment was scarce. To a large degree, tools are developed by industrial companies and consequently, data access is limited. Though relatively little research information was available to the public in the field of technical rescue, the cluster could draw on the practical experience and work of Hanses (2019) and advance it (Hanses & Horwath, 2021; Hanses & Horwath, 2022). A general idea of how to design diversity sensitive aspects into mechatronic or engineering artefacts was available, as well as a best practice example to prove its benefits of the potential for innovation (Holl et al., 2018).

Although the projects in this cluster were not finished at the time of writing this book, results for society and science have already been achieved. As regards society and practice, criteria for an optimized light weight design of two rescue tools based on empirical insights into the actual practice of the use of the tools were elaborated. Still under construction is the production of the respective prototypes, a guide with general conclusions for the optimisation of firefighting equipment drawing on diversity and practical experience as a starting point. Furthermore, the ongoing integration of the development and optimisation of technical rescue equipment aims toward a more ergonomically designed equipment to protect practitioners physical health. Ecologically, a result could also be to conserve natural resources with a lightweight equipment design.

For scientific practise, the research of the cluster delivers an examination of the technical relationship between equipment performance and weight, equipment designed for highest performance with the help of kinematic analysis as well as an experimental and numerical analysis of the equipment mechanism.

Out of the empirical complexity of the research context, the formation of common research objects focussed on the development of tools oriented towards innovative approaches to the design of rescue spreaders, and a second widely established standard tool. The formation required to adhere to norms and equipment classification data sheet, and to close the knowledge gaps through an inter- and transdisciplinary mixed method approach.

## Case Study IV

The societal problems from which the cluster departed are embedded in wider changes in societies, and markets respectively. The transformation of societies through Individualization, Globalization and Digitalization is entangled with a transformation of markets and economy, from markets for industrialized mass production to markets for heterogeneous products which fit individual needs. In this process, additive manufacturing plays a key role as it allows to respond to increasing demands for individualized (medical) products at relatively low prices – a development captured in the slightly paradoxical category of "individualized mass customization" (for a detailed discussion see Josupeit & Schmid (2018)).

In settings of additive manufacturing, customers frequently become "co-designers", as the technology allows for the implementation of individually desired properties and, in many cases, provides access to interactive services to (co-) design an item or a product. Hence, the technology invites transdisciplinary collaboration and to interact and respond with the social (and medical) needs of individuals. In addition, a decentral production is possible: given data is available, additive manufacturing allows the production of artefacts independent of the particular location or time scheme of the customers and producers.

However, the ambivalence with the technology of additive manufacturing in this context is that successful collaboration with societal members in need has the potential for realizing immense improvements of the quality of everyday life in terms of gained mobility, autonomy, and so on. Thus, rehabilitation processes can also be facilitated. But it also entails questions of privacy and data protection regarding highly sensitive data (e.g. biomedical, biometric, physical, or data on private environments and behavioural patterns), and data availability. Furthermore, there are significant gaps between the technological and the societal possibilities to realize solutions for individuals in need as many medical artefacts require a legal classification and legitimation, are subject to medical device regulations, and application procedures for the coverage of costs through insurance companies.

Scientific problems in this context are manifold. One aspect is the necessity of interdisciplinary cooperation between science, medicine, and engineering. Further challenges include the development of new procedures and products for patients to apply medical technologies for individual bodies, the distinctive requirements concerning materials where a variety of properties, mechanical, chemical and biological, have to be taken into account, as well as biocompatibility. On a more general level, the standardization of additive manufacturing procedure entails questions of quality criteria. Also, printed products often need to be manually refined and reworked.

Societal discourses primarily address issues of public health, insurance policies, and the quality of medical products. However, as pointed out by workshop participants and research partners, the procedures underlying the processes of the development of products, quality standards and distribution need to be improved. This backdrop is reflected in scientific discourses, too, as they are concerned with conflicting norms and competing values (see also Introduction in this book) and the legal terms and conditions for individualized technologies.

Results for scientific practise gained through the work of the cluster refer to technology transfer and the educational and learning effects produces, in particular to raise awareness among the professionals involved in the projects. The formation of the common research object focussed on two aspects: to provide understandable and transparent information on care and assisting technology, and to pay attention to concerns related to ambiguities of technologies. In sum, the research and development process of this cluster was driven by the premise to be accountable for members of civil society, receptive for their critics and concerns, and reflective on the social dimensions and impact of technologies. The aim was to balance social expectations with scientific possibilities, not at least regarding the materials and processes used for the additive manufacturing of individualized assistive tools and artefacts.

## References


Bergmann, M., Jahn, T., Knobloch, T., Krohn, W., Pohl, C., & Schramm, E. (2012). Methods for Transdisciplinary Research. A Primer for Practice. Campus Publisher. ISBN: 978-3-5933-9647-7

Gaskell, G., Stares, S., Allansdottir, A., Allum, N., Castro, P., Esmer, Y., Fischler, C., Jackson, J., Kronberger, N., Hampel, J., Mejlgaard, N., Quintanilha, A., Rammer, A., Revuelta, G., Stoneman, P., Torgersen, H., & Wagner, W. (2010). *Europeans and biotechnology in 2010. Winds of change?* A report to the European Commission's Directorate-General for Research. https://data.europa.eu/doi/10.2777/23393.

Hanses, H. (2019). Verfahrensoptimierung bei der Personenrettung aus Fahrzeugen mit verstärkten Strukturen und alternativen Antriebstechnologien (Optimisation of tools and practices for rescue scenarios in car accidents). [Unpublished master's thesis]. Paderborn University, Germany.

Hanses, H., & Horwath, I. (2021, September 21-24). Project for the development of operational and demandoriented firefighting equipment. Extended Abstracts to 37th Danubia Adria Symposium on Advances in Experimental Mechanics, JKU Linz, Austria.

Hanses H., & Horwath I. (2022). Development of operational and demand-oriented firefighting equipment. *Materials Today: Proceedings*, Vol. 62, Issue 5, 2684-2688. https://doi.org/10.1016/j.matpr.2022.06.031

Holl, H., Horwath, I., Cojocaru, G., Hehenberger, P., & Ernst, W. (2018): Integration of gender in the design process of mechatronic products: An interdisciplinary approach. *Materials Today: Proceedings*, Vol. 5, Issue 13, 26673–26679. https://doi.org/10.1016/j.matpr.2018.08.134

Horwath, I., Kastein, M., & Dağlar-Sezer, N. (2021). Feuerwehren im Spiegel gesellschaftlicher Diversität. In N. Eschenbruch, S. Kaufmann, & P. Zoche (Eds.): *Vielfältige Sicherheiten. Gesellschaftliche Dimensionen der Sicherheitsforschung (107-131)*, Schriftenreihe SiFo Fachdialog Sicherheitsforschung des BMBF Deutschland, Band 20. LIT-Verlag.

Josupeit, S., & Schmid, H.-J. (2018). Individualisierung mit und durch additive(r) Fertigung. In B. Riegraf, & A.-L. Berscheid (Eds.). *Wissenschaft im Angesicht „großer gesellschaftlicher Herausforderungen". Das Beispiel der Forschung an hybriden Leichtbaumaterialien (19-34).* transcript Publisher. ISBN: 978-3-8376-4099-1

Kastein, M., Finke, J., & Horwath, I. (2021). Florian braucht Mehmet mehr als umgekehrt: Herausforderungen und Potenziale für Inklusion in der Freiwilligen Feuerwehr. *Voluntaris*, Vol. 9, Issue 1, 135-151. https://doi.org/10.5771/2196-3886-2021-1-135

Kronberger, N. (2016): Of worlds and objects: scientific knowledge and its publics. In G. Sammut, E. Andreouli, G. Gaskell, J. Valsiner (Eds.). *The Cambridge Handbook of Social Representations (358-368).* Cambridge University Press. https://doi.org/10.1017/CBO9781107323650.029

Lam, D. P.M., Freund M. E., Kny, J., Marg, O., Mbah, M., Theiler, L., Bergmann, M., Brohmann, B., Lang, D. J. & Schäfer, M. (2021). Transdisciplinary research towards an integrative perspective. GAIA - Ecological Perspectives for Science and Society. Vol. 30, Issue 4, 243-249. https://doi.org/10.14512/gaia.30.4.7

Scholz, R. W., & Steiner, G. (2015). Transdisciplinarity at the crossroads. Sustainability Science, Vol. 10, Issue 4, 521-526. https://doi.org/10.1007/s11625-015-0338-0

# Case Study I: Transmission Electron Microscopy and Transdisciplinary Research

*Julius Bürger, Jörg K.N. Lindner*

Each of us sees an unimaginably large number of atoms every day, as we can already see about $10^{27}$ of them when looking in the mirror. But we are not able to resolve them with the naked eye. However, as functional components of devices become smaller, the precise control of individual atoms, which are the building blocks of all matter, is not only important for state-of-the-art computers, but also for green energy harvesting and a variety of other applications that contribute to solving societal problems. To improve the devices and also to develop the materials of tomorrow, it is important to be able to look at and investigate all possible structures down to atomic resolution.

The fact that we cannot resolve individual atoms without further tools is due to the resolving power of the eye. To overcome this limitation, which depends on the individual quality of the eye lens and its maximum flexion as well as the maximum diameter of the iris (Hartridge, 1922), the visual light microscope (VLM), which was already invented in the 16th century, increases the maximum possible resolution by adding further magnifying glass lenses in front of the human eye (Bardell, 2004). Before entering the lens system, light as a probe is either reflected by or transmitted through the analysed structure. Thus, the eye sees a magnified image of the analysed object or, in particular, the interaction result of light with the specimen.

A modern VLM resolves features in the range of hundreds of nanometers, which are roughly 10 000 000 times smaller than a human being. This, for example, facilitates analysing biological samples such as the human hair, cells, and bacteria. Virions, which possess a diameter in the range of several tens of nanometers, cannot be visualised since their size is below the wavelength-limited resolution limit. Additionally, smaller substructures of the virions, which are also responsible for docking to human cells, and thus also single atoms cannot be resolved. This resolution limit arises from the wave characteristic of light and especially diffraction. In this context, Ernst Abbe developed his theory on the diffraction limit of resolution, describing a linear proportionality of obtainable resolution to the wavelength. As a consequence of the Abbe diffraction limit (Abbe, 1873), the maximum obtainable resolution when using visible light of 400 nm is approximately 200 nm despite using a highly optimised optical lens system. However, the typical atomic spacing is in the range of 0.5 nm. To overcome this limit, a different type of probe must be considered.

In 1923 De Broglie postulated that an accelerated electron has wave properties, such as a wavelength, similar to light (Kubli, 1970). As the accelerating voltage of the electrons increases, the wavelength decreases, which ultimately leads to an increase in resolution according to Abbe's theory. In addition to the finding that the resolution limit can be overcome by using electrons, rotational-symmetric magnetic fields exhibit focusing properties similar to those of an optical lens (Knoll & Ruska, 1932a; Knoll & Ruska, 1932b). By arranging such magnetic lenses in a similar fashion as the arrangement of lenses in a VLM, Ernst Ruska and Max Knoll built the first electron microscope (EM) (Knoll & Ruska, 1932b) at the Technische Hochschule in Berlin in 1932. Ernst Ruska was awarded the Nobel Prize in 1986, which was already a statement about the significance of TEM for society. By definition, Nobel Prizes are awarded only for outstanding contributions benefitting humankind (Nobel Media, 2022). Today's electron microscopes are able to visualise nanometer-sized features (Carenco et al., 2015) and even single atoms (Gamm, 2012; Mishra, 2017). They can be divided into two major types quite similar to the VLM by the way of detection, i.e. in transmission or reflection. Thus, EMs can be mainly divided into the scanning electron microscope (SEM) and the (scanning) transmission electron microscope ((S)TEM). However, this comparison of light and electron microscopes is an oversimplification. In the SEM, various interactions of the electron beam with the sample occur, and thus, for example, secondary or backscattered electrons can be detected. The resolution of the SEM is limited mainly by the interaction of the electrons with the sample in a large interaction volume. This problem is automatically circumvented in the TEM, since the samples must be exceptionally thin and thus typically have a thickness below 100 nm to be electron transparent.

A modern TEM readily enables us to resolve structures in the range of several tenth of picometer (Erni et al., 2009) and therefore even single atoms. The capability of resolving unimaginably tiny features, which are approximately 50 000 000 000 times smaller than a human being, in addition to further analytical methods to detect the chemical composition and other physical properties as the plasmonic structure inside the specimens (Williams & Carter, 2009), today makes TEM one of the commonly applied analytical techniques in the fields of physics, chemical engineering, material science, chemistry, and biology. This already makes TEM a multidisciplinary tool, which is mainly enabled by its instrumentation branching (Marcovic, 2017). For different applications, a variety of modes of operation are needed and readily accessible. Thus, each discipline works preferably with a certain set of modes, such as cryo-TEM in biology, in which the specimen is cooled down to temperatures of liquid nitrogen or helium. Cryo-TEM is mainly applied when investigating biological specimens to prevent disintegration in a vacuum. Therefore, virions and their behaviour in cells can be studied. This already shows how important TEM is and why the development of new TEM methods is inevitable. Otherwise, the visualisation of Corona virions without previous inventions and developments in the field of cryo-electron microscopy would not have been possible, as we will see later.

Not only transmission electron microscopy is a branching field of research but research in general (Mittelstraß, 2005). More and more disciplines are emerging, partly due to the required specialisation in order to be at the forefront of research. In addition to the growing number of disciplines, the boundaries between disciplines are blurred both by the instruments and equipment utilised, and by the research goals. Simultaneously, the connexion between social stakeholders and research is decreasing due to an increasing specialisation in the fields of research. Thus, the hurdle for societal stakeholders to grasp the relevance of research increases with specialisation. As a result, the outcome of a research study might not be accepted by society. This might particularly be a problem in fields where the research is carried out to solve a societal problem. These societal problems can be categorised as climate change, natural resource management (Osinski, 2021), water management (Dedeurwaerdere, 2013), sustainability (Dedeurwaerdere, 2013), air pollution, energy harvesting and storage as well as social injustice and migration (Pohl et al., 2017). To tackle these problems and guarantee a mutual acceptance among all stakeholders, transdisciplinary research (TD) is considered to be a very promising approach. The fundamental idea of transdisciplinary research is to include societal stakeholders during all phases of the research process. Joint solutions between societal and academic stakeholders are crucial for tomorrow's society. However, the simultaneous integration of highly specialised technologies and societal knowledge is still a challenge.

The following chapter illuminates the challenges and prospects of implementing transmission electron microscopy as a highly specialised technology in transdisciplinary research approaches to solve societal problems. Therefore, transdisciplinary definitions and approaches are explained, and the basic concept of transmission electron microscopy is introduced. After examining examples where TEM is applied in the context of societal questions and problems, arising challenges of TEM-based research in TD research projects are reviewed. In closing the prospects of TEM and TD are highlighted. Most of the findings are transferable to other research areas.

## 1 Transdisciplinary research

Transdisciplinary research is a possible means for tackling large societal questions, e.g. air pollution, energy harvesting and storage, as well as social injustice and migration. The concept of TD arose in the 1970s and was first described as research beyond disciplinary boundaries (Jahn, 2008; Nicolescu, 2014). This means that methods that are not limited to a certain discipline are implemented. This contrasts with multi- and interdisciplinary research, where the problem is solved in each discipline individually or through collaboration among disciplines (Stokols, 2006), meaning that all applied methods are still tied to their specific discipline. In the following years, the definition of TD was transformed, and a common approach to improve the methodology beyond disciplinarity was defined to include social stakeholders (Nicolescu, 2014). Therefore, the different definitions were also referred to as modes of transdisciplinary research. While in the first mode the transdisciplinarity is defined by research that is not located in any specific science discipline, the second mode also includes societal stakeholders in the research process (Stokols, 2006). The second mode and the way to include societal stakeholders in the research process has been discussed frequently in pertinent literature in recent years (Hall et al., 2012; Scholz, 2020; Miah et al., 2015). In the following, when using the term transdisciplinary TD, the second mode is addressed.

In general, the inclusion of societal stakeholders creates a high possibility for reducing the imbalance in power among different contributing stakeholder groups, which not only results in the incorporation of a broad spectrum of interests during the research but also facilitates a high degree of acceptance of the research outcome. In addition, transdisciplinary research also opens a door to the probability for new ideas on how to tackle a certain problem, since all the contributing actors have different views on the topic. Non-academic stakeholders have the responsibility to enlighten the academic stakeholders about what they know, think, and want to be studied (Maasen & Lieven, 2006). Thus, TD research can also be considered as mutual learning of scientists and societal stakeholders (Osinski, 2021). Therefore, the gains achieved by means of knowledge transfer are omnidirectional in an ideal scenario. This omnidirectionality is crucial during TD research. In TD research, the scientists and researchers must consider the power differences among the contributing stakeholder groups at all times (Stokols, 2006). In this case, the term "power" stands for the ability to discuss and negotiate (Osinski, 2021). For example, untrained and less well-educated people involved in the research progress might be influenced and biased by experts. In addition, experts might ignore the view and opinions of untrained stakeholders on the research topic. This would result in an undesirable direction for the research progress and might reduce the acceptance of the research outcome (Osinski, 2021). Moreover, the necessity for integrating interests and knowledge without a biased opinion of their quality, and the way of understanding and knowing needs to be aligned in order to produce socially robust knowledge (Scholz & Steiner, 2015). To overcome such barriers, long-term interactions and research help to build mutual trust among societal actors, policymakers, and scientists (Osinski, 2021). All stakeholders need to be embedded in the research process, preferably on a long-term basis.

Today, TD research with "environmental, environmental-economic and integrating" goals is already applied in many cases, and the applied methods to include all stakeholders vary among different research goals (Osinski, 2021). In most examples, the empowerment of disadvantaged groups is enormously increased, and the transdisciplinary research is not only beneficial when it comes to solving the problem but generates mutual learning space for all stakeholders as well. In addition, a subsequently lowered barrier for integrating different types of knowledge into problem-solving is faced (Miah et al., 2015).

Since there must be no bias among the participants in order to achieve a research outcome that is accepted by the participants, funding plays a crucial role in TD research. However, since TD research has, until today, been most likely funded by the government and research programs with clearly defined goals, researchers need to fulfil the expectations of the funding agent. Therefore, researchers are *ab initio* biased and not completely independent (Scholz, 2020). Funding in the form of sponsorships without any bias is more promising (Scholz, 2020) and should therefore be applied in TD research. This leads to another crucial point when applying TD approaches. Unless the research topic is completely restricted to the natural or engineering sciences, the outcome of the research is not easy to evaluate due to the inclusion of different perspectives and the fact that the object or social phenomenon under investigation is significantly presumptively value-laden as it probably depends on the preferences of the social stakeholder (Sprenger & Reiss, 2014) since many different perspectives and opinions shape the research result. And in some cases, it is not guaranteed that there *will* be any research outcome by applying TD methods.

As one can see, the concept of TD research is complicated to apply, and its evaluation is even more complicated. In fundamental research, the project is typically evaluated in a more or less binary sense, i.e. whether the proposed research goal is achieved or not. The outcome of TD research is multidimensional. In addition to the success or failure of the research project, one can add more aspects to the evaluation of the output of TD research: product-related and process-related aspects (Binder et al., 2015). The latter can, for example, be empowerment, integration of heterogeneous knowledge sources and the initial and final power differences among stakeholders.

Today's TD research projects are typically conducted to solve societal problems, and most of them only apply forms of interviews as participatory research. Thus, mutual learning is only partially achieved, (Scholz & Steiner, 2015) and acceptance by societal stakeholders is not guaranteed. In fundamental research questions, i.e. in disciplines such as physics, material science or chemistry, TD approaches are, to our knowledge, not considered. Although the research topic might be very specialised, acceptance by society is typically not rendered during the research process. This does not mean that every fundamental research process needs to be conducted transdisciplinarily; however, in some cases, where the outcome concerns the society in general or a specific subgroup of the society, the researchers might want to consider including societal stakeholders in the research process. Applying TD approaches in fundamental research, e.g. in TEM, might be useful, especially in the research fields of direct societal impact, such as energy storage or energy harvesting.

## 2 Transmission electron microscopy

After its invention in 1933 by Ernst Ruska and Max Knoll at the Technische Hochschule Berlin (Haguenau et al., 2003), the transmission electron microscope became an analytical tool in many disciplines and research areas, e.g., in the analysis of biological samples, structural and functional materials, micro- and nanostructures, and, more recently, in the observation of in-situ processes, i.e., live observation of a particular physical, chemical or biological reaction or process.

The transmission electron microscope works similarly to an optical microscope. Instead of using light, electrons forming a beam are used as a probe which is focused onto a specimen and magnified by magnetic lenses. The interpretation of an image obtained by a TEM was made possible by the discovery of wave-particle duality, i.e. the wavelength of moving particles, by Louis De Broglie in 1923. The wavelength of an electron accelerated at a voltage of 200 kV amounts to 2.508 pm ( m). This wavelength is 20 times smaller than the Bohr radius (Bohr, 1913) of the hydrogen atom (0.053 nm), the smallest atom within the periodic table of elements, and according to Abbe's theory, should allow for resolution far below typical atom distances. However, the first electron microscope only achieved a magnification of 12000 x with a resolution that was only marginally better than the resolution of an optical microscope due to the quality of the electron source and magnetic lenses. Therefore, much attention was paid to increasing the electron optics and beam quality, and, by the end of the previous century, it was possible to resolve features smaller than 0.2 nm.

Just as the human eye, a magnetic lens also shows image distortions arising from an imperfect lens. A human utilises glasses to sharpen the image. In transmission electron microscope lens aberration correctors are used. Based on calculations by Rose (Rose, 1990), these correctors were realised by Haider, Krivanek and Urban (Haider et al., 1998; Krivanek et al., 1999; Urban et al., 1999). Today, these correctors allow resolutions of less than 50 picometres (Erni et al., 2009), making it possible to look among atoms in a crystal and resolve structures about 50,000,000,000 times smaller than a human being. Since resolving structures on such short length scales is necessary to understand and optimise the structure of nanomaterials, Rose, Haider, Urban and Krivanek received the Kavli Prize in nanoscience in 2020 for their works (Kavli, 2020).

*Figure 1: a) TEM beam path. The electron beam emitted by the electron gun is subsequently shaped and directed by the condenser lens system. After transmission and interaction with the specimen, the electron wave is projected onto a camera by the objective, intermediate and projection lenses. A typical TEM bright-field micrograph is shown in b) in which a silicon single crystal is analysed. A typical STEM dark-field micrograph of the same specimen is shown in c). In both b) and c) a projection of the crystal structure is included by the yellow dots. It is necessary to note that only in STEM mode atomic column positions can be directly determined from the white dots as the signal is proportional to the projected atomic number of the analysed specimen area.*

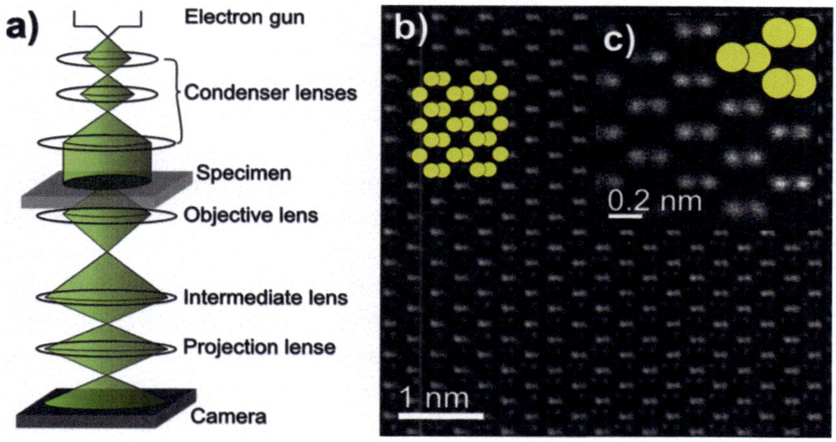


There are two major operation modes, TEM and STEM, supplemented by many different analytical methods which are especially designed for certain applications. Descriptions of most of the available methods are beyond the scope of this article; however, good literature can be found in (Williams & Carter, 2009; Tanaka, 2014; Fultz & Howe, 2012). Here, only the basic modes are explained briefly.

In TEM mode, where image acquisition is highly similar to that of a light microscope, a broad electron beam is incident on the sample and the microscopist captures an image of the electron wave after the interaction. As can be seen in Figure 1 a), the electron beam emitted by an electron gun and shaped by a set of condenser lenses transmits through and interacts with the specimen. The interaction of the electron beam with the specimen leads to a specimen exit wave forming an image in the image plane of the objective lens, which is further magnified by intermediate and projection lenses and finally projected onto an electron sensitive camera. In the past, this camera used a film that had to be developed like a photograph; today – as in photography – a silicon chip acts as a two-dimensional sensor and produces digital images. In Figure 1 b), a TEM image of a silicon specimen with a resolution smaller than the typical distance of atoms in the crystal is shown. It is necessary to note that bright contrasts inside the image do not resemble atomic column positions (stacking of atoms in beam direction) but result from periodic potentials inside the specimen.

In the other major mode of TEM operation, the electron beam is focused on a tiny spot and afterward scanned across the surface. In this so-called scanning transmission electron microscopy (STEM) mode, the image is constructed sequentially, which means pixel by pixel. Several contrast mechanisms, such as scattering and diffraction, occur within the specimen, and, by using special detectors and detector geometries, certain contrast mechanisms can be exploited, e.g., to visualise atoms and their ordering inside the specimen. Figure 1c) displays an image of a silicon crystal structure with a resolution much higher than the typical distance of atoms inside a crystal. This image is a so-called STEM dark-field image, in which the number of scattered electrons at each pixel is analysed. The image was captured from the same specimen as in Figure 1b). Scattering, in general, is a strongly localised process, which happens when the electrons of the incoming electron beam interact with the positively charged nucleus of an atom and its surrounding negative electrons. Thus, the bright spots inside the STEM dark-field (STEM-DF) image correspond to atoms. Since silicon is a crystal and crystals exhibit a highly periodic ordering of atoms, the specimen can be tilted in such a way that several atoms forming an atomic column are analysed in projection. This means for Figure 1 c) that each bright spot corresponds to several atoms (approximately 60) sitting on top of each other.

The specimen itself also influences the obtainable resolution, mainly by its thickness. If a thick specimen is analysed, the beam strongly interacts with the specimen and scattering leads to a smearing of image information. Therefore, specimen thicknesses are typically below 100 nm. Specimen preparation is therefore crucial and may lead to artefacts and a variation of structures later being analysed (Carenco et al., 2015). Thus, the operator needs to make assumptions about the structures at hand with caution. Typically, the operator also analyses only a few spots on the specimen but assumes they are representative for the complete specimen.

The acceleration voltage determines the kinetic energy and thus the wavelength of the electrons of the beam. Therefore, it does not only have an influence on the diffraction-limited resolution but must also be carefully chosen when any beam-sensitive material is analysed to avoid radiation damage. This applies mostly to biological and polymer specimens but also to some semiconductors. In addition, the number of electrons of the beam passing a certain area of the specimen in a specific time frame plays a critical role (Russo & Egerton, 2019). Water-containing specimens are likely to be destroyed in a vacuum due to hydrolysis and due to the fact that water evaporates. This drastically alters the structure of cells and further leads to wrong interpretations. To analyse cells or other biological structures, such structures must be vitrified if they contain water and must remain in the vitrified state throughout the analysis. Therefore, cryo-microscopy was invented in the 1960s. In combination with other techniques, cryo-microscopy allows the creation of atomistic models of virions, DNA, RNA and other polymers.

When the electron beam hits the specimen, it interacts with the atoms inside the specimen in several ways. Electrons can get scattered elastically (without the loss of electron energy) and inelastically (with loss of energy). Inelastic scattering may be based on a variety of interactions of the electrons with the specimen. For example, if an electron of the incident electron beam hits an electron from an inner electron shell of an atom, the electron might be kicked away from the atom due to the energy transferred during the collision. This leaves an empty spot for electrons which is energetically favourable for other electrons to take. When energetically weaker bound electrons take over these spots, the energy difference, which is, in addition, characteristic for the chemical element, is typically emitted as light in the x-ray range of the spectrum. The transmission electron microscope offers several ways to analyse this interaction. One of the common analytical techniques is energy-dispersive x-ray spectroscopy, in which a detector collects the x-rays emitted by the specimen. Since these emitted x-ray photons exhibit characteristic energies depending on the chemical element, EDX allows for elemental mapping. Another way to map chemical composition is the utilisation of electron energy loss-related techniques such as energy-filtered TEM and electron energy loss spectroscopy, because the afore-mentioned interaction is also measurable in the energy distribution of the electron beam after the specimen. The process, which leads to the emission of characteristic x-rays, results in characteristic energy losses of the beam electrons. When analysing the spatial occurrence of these characteristic energy losses, chemical maps can be calculated. Due to the high spectral resolution and beam stability in terms of energy, it is also possible to deduce the type of binding in a molecule, for example C-O and C=O. Thus, it is also possible to distinguish between different polymer species, which due to their chemical similarity, have a quite similar density and are hard to differentiate with other imaging methods, e.g. using a scanning electron microscope or an atomic force microscope (Bürger et al., 2020).

In addition to analytical techniques, which have been under development and were improved over the past decades, TEM tomography is an imaging technique which makes it possible to obtain a three-dimensional model through a series of two-dimensional images. The basic principle of tomography is also used in other fields, such as computer tomography scans in medicine. The combination of cryo-electron microscopy and tomography readily enables us to study of the structure of biological samples in three dimensions.

In times when nanostructures and devices become increasingly important in our daily lives, the transmission electron microscope is a necessary tool to study nanomaterial properties and develop sustainable materials and devices. The importance of TEM can also be observed by the establishment of transnational research projects, for example the EU-funded ESTEEM2, in which universities and research centres across Europe jointly offer their infrastructure and knowledge to research facilities that do not have a TEM at hand (Snoeck, 2017). As part of the ESTEEM2 project, 15 academic facilities and three companies from across Europe provided their microscopes and infrastructure from 2012 to 2016 to more than 500 researchers who successfully submitted a proposal to an independent committee (Snoeck, 2017).

## 3 Examples of applied TEM in the context of solving societal problems

The following are examples of applications where TEM has contributed an almost atomically small but fundamentally important piece for solving the puzzle of a societal problem. These examples will highlight the significance of electron microscopy.

Most electronic devices today, such as cell phones, central processing units of computers and televisions, are made up of various functional parts composed of nanometer-scale structures. Nanostructures play a significant role not only in electrical devices but also in different fields affecting societal issues, such as medicine, energy harvesting, and environmental issues (Carenco et al., 2015). As an illustration: nanostructures can be found in as different fields as biosensors or are used in cosmetics. Nanometer-sized particles can, for instance, act as catalysts to remove CO from exhaust gases due to their high surface-to-volume ratio (Nilsson Pingel et al., 2018; Schlicher et al., 2022). Figure 2 a) shows nanometer-sized iron oxide particles on an $Al_2O_3$ substrate. Since the contrast depends on the atomic number, the STEM dark-field image already gives evidence on particle size and distribution. This evidence is approved by the corresponding EDX maps of the iron, oxygen and aluminium. Many physical properties, such as the shape, morphology, chemical composition, and optical properties can be measured by TEM and its various analytical methods. Especially the precise control of the properties of nanostructures, which may sometimes only consist of a few hundred atoms or even only 20 atoms in diameter, is required, making the characterisation of such structures with atomic resolution necessary. Researchers (Nilsson Pingel et al., 2018) have shown that the catalytic activity of nanoparticles depends on the exact distance between atoms, i.e. the strain on the atomic level has an influence on the question of how much CO can be removed from exhaust gases. Yet another example: nanometer-sized particles in steel also play a role in the performance of tool steel tailored for applications such as spreaders in rescue services. For high-performance steel, the nanoparticles are utilised for grain refinement, improving the mechanical behaviour under stress and reducing the formation of cracks. In this case, TEM has helped to investigate the crystal structure and the relationship with the surrounding steel matrix to solve questions such as whether the nanoparticles show a systematic crystallographic relation to the matrix. In addition, TEM allows us to estimate the chemical composition inside the nanoparticle or at the interface with the steel matrix as can be seen in Figure 2 b), where an overlay of titanium, nitrogen, vanadium, and iron elemental maps is shown. These maps are obtained utilising the EDX elemental mapping analytical TEM technique, and the corresponding line profiles of the atomic percentage of nitrogen, vanadium, titanium and iron are depicted in Figure 2 c).

*Figure 2: a) STEM high-angle annular dark-field image of an $Al_2O_3$ particle covered with nanometer-sized iron oxide catalyst particle and corresponding EDX elemental maps of oxygen, aluminium, and iron. b) Overlay of nitrogen, titanium and iron EDX elemental maps of an area depicting a TiVN particle embedded in a steel matrix mostly composed of iron. c) line profile across the TiVN nanoparticle shown in b). d) high-resolution STEM HAADF image of the CF-ZnO whisker interface. The atomically sharp interconnection between ZnO and CF is visible.*

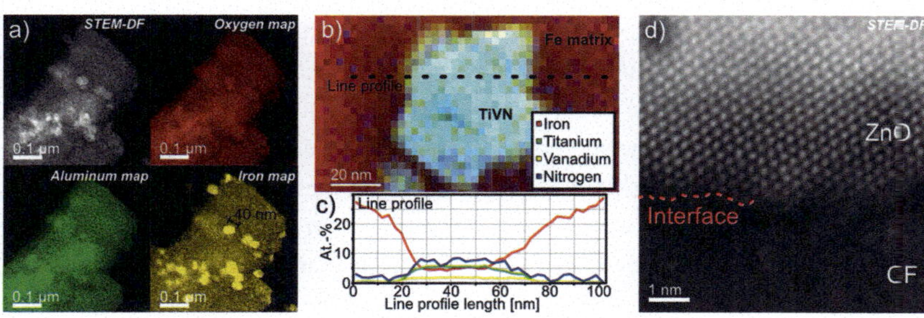


Not only the nanoworld but our world in general strongly depends on the characteristics of interfaces. In carbon-fibre (CF) reinforced materials used in the design of new light-weight vehicles, which are designated candidates for the reduction of the emission of greenhouse gases of vehicles, the interface between the CF and the surrounding matrix strongly influences the device's performance, e.g. the shear strength. To optimise the performance of the hybrid components, one possible optimisation method is the functionalization of the CF interface, e.g. by attaching whiskers to the CF or roughening the CF surface to promote better adhesion between the CF and the matrix. Figure 2 c) shows a STEM image of a CF interface with ZnO whiskers. Since in STEM-HAADF, the contrast depends on the projected number of atoms and their atomic number, it is observable that the ZnO interconnects with the CF and follows the roughness of the CF with atomic precision.

Transmission electron microscopy is a versatile tool both in material science and biology. It contributed during the research on the SARS-CoV-2 virions. SARS-CoV-2 is a virion from the corona-type virus. SARS-CoV-2 is less lethal than SARS-CoV-1 and MERS-CoV but more infectious (Stip et al., 2020). By January 2022 it had infected more than 338 million individuals with almost 5.57 million deaths. The impact of the corona virus on the body of infected persons, the mind of infected individuals and even not infected individuals – such as nurses (Fan et al., 2020) – and family members of infected persons, the economy and many other sectors is being researched. Even not infected individuals suffer psychologically from the corona crisis, reducing the personal interactions and changing their work-life balance (Stip et al., 2020). It is obvious that the SARS-CoV-2 has a major impact on our society. It concerns every single individuum on this planet, and therefore transdisciplinary approaches for pandemic forecasting and knowledge availability are needed or already under development (Popova et al., 2020). The goal of the development of vaccination and medication to relieve symptoms during the progression of the disease was an urgent quest. For the development of vaccines and medicines, various techniques are applied to decipher the inner structure and functioning of the SARS-CoV-2 virions. The applied techniques range from proteomic studies analysing the protein composition to structural investigations mainly by NMR, SAXS and X-ray diffraction (Robinson et al., 2007). In addition, TEM (in cryo-mode) is also applied for the inner structure. By exploiting various techniques of the afore-mentioned ones, the atomic structure and the ordering of polymeric chains inside a virus can be analysed. This information can then be condensed to a model of its structure. Thereby, it was found that the coronavirus is an RNA-based virus with one of the longest genomes known (Stip et al., 2020). But TEM is capable of more than just imaging the inner structure of the virions. It also facilitates the analysis of how the virions reproduce in the cell (Hopfer et al., 2021) by cryo-electron microscopy. Due to the shock freezing of the specimen, the cell-virion-interaction is a snapshot at a certain stage, allowing to conclude on the way of the virus during reproduction and its cytopathic effect (cell destruction and deformation arising from the reproduction) (Kim et al., 2020). Thanks to the manifold information on the coronavirus, researchers could develop a vaccine in a short period of time.

In times when energy generation and distribution are critical problems of humankind, new inventions concerning the harvesting and storage of energy which are safe to use and do not exhibit any risk of damage to the environment or single individuals are necessary. Due to their relatively low cost, long life, fast charging capabilities and high energy density, lithium-ion batteries are one of the promising ways to store energy (Sakuda, 2009). These batteries are already utilised in mobile devices like smartphones, laptops, electric cars and many others. Their layout consists of two different electrodes, which are used to store the lithium ions, an electrolyte and a separator membrane, separating both electrodes and allowing for the transport of lithium ions. The charge and discharge processes of lithium-ion batteries are based on the transport and incorporation of $Li^+$ ions into the electrode materials. Electrons from the lithium-ion containing electrode create a current towards the positive electrode over an external circuit during discharge. Simultaneously, $Li^+$ ions move across the electrolyte towards the other electrode and release energy due to the higher affinity of $Li^+$ towards the other electrode's material. In general, there are many lithium-ion battery layouts, which differ mainly in terms of materials for the electrodes and in the electrolyte. The latter is typically based on a flammable organic liquid or an inorganic solid. Especially the electrode materials and structures determine the battery's maximum capacity by the number of ions they can store. Therefore, it is crucial to incorporate lithium ions into the electrode materials, and intercalation, i.e. the incorporation of Li+ without drastic changes in the material structure, is desired. In this regard, transmission electron microscopy is a powerful tool for investigating the performance of such batteries on the nanometric scale and understanding the performance, gradual decrease in capacity and failure of lithium-ion batteries. Using in-situ TEM imaging, the charge-discharge-processes can be visualised. Applying in-situ TEM, chemical processes can be studied in real time during charge and discharge (Yuan et al., 2017). In in-situ TEM, due to the fast electronics and cameras of modern microscopes, videos of the process can be recorded at rates of several thousand images per second instead of a single image. In most cases, the preparation of a specimen that is thin enough to allow for sufficient electron transparency and the possibility to transfer the reaction occurring at one of the battery components into the microscope remains challenging. There are possible ways to overcome the challenges of specimen preparation owing to the numerous dedicated in-situ holders (Wu & Yao, 2015). In TEM studies, it was observed that the cathode is prone to structural changes during imperfect intercalation. Thus, transformation in crystallographic phases and changes in morphology, e.g., expansion, cracking or fracture of electrode materials, reduce the performance in terms of capacity and lead to a failure of batteries (Liu, 2011). Potential improvements are the changes in structure and composition of electrode material (Liu, 2011), e.g. by coating the electrode surface for protection (Chen et al., 2010) or by changing the morphology in order to minimise stress inside the electrode during intercalation (Chan et al., 2008; Huang, 2010). The optimisations mentioned need then to be rechecked with the TEM. In addition, there may be reactions that decompose the electrolyte and increase the battery resistance, which will ultimately increase heat generation during charging and discharging. Heat generation, in particular, is critical because when using an organic liquid electrolyte, the low-boiling electrolyte already evaporates at a temperature of 70 °C (Park et al., 2018). In addition, mostly oxygen-containing electrode materials that dissolve at temperatures between 150 °C and 250 °C and thus release oxygen are used (Park et al., 2018). This will then lead to further exothermic reactions and a thermal runaway of the device. The evaporation of the materials will lead to a pressure increase in the encapsulated battery cell. Conventional lithium-ion batteries with a flammable organic liquid electrolyte therefore have a high risk of explosion or fire (Wang et al., 2005) if a flammable atmosphere forms in a compartment of the battery cell due to a variety of causes, including charging or discharging too quickly (Park et al., 2018), manufacturing defects and mechanical damage (Baird et al., 2020). Using in-situ TEM, Sacci et al. have directly observed how Li ions assemble in tree-like geometries (dendrites) which poke through the separator membrane, leading to short-cuts between anode and cathode (Sacci et al., 2015). Such investigations are essential in order to find safe technical solutions and to minimise risks to which anyone could be exposed. Knowing the reasons for catastrophic failure is the first step to exclude risks and to make sure that new technologies are accepted by the public. In 2016, 2.5 million smartphones of a certain series had to be recalled by the manufacturer, and their use on aircrafts was prohibited after several incidents with overheating Li-ion batteries on board. Imagine the public opinion would turn against the use of Li-ion batteries, e.g. vehicles, because they might catch on fire on the road or in a parking garage; in that case there would be one important option fewer to reduce $CO_2$ emissions.

As we have seen in the afore-mentioned examples, TEM is an important technique for tackling the roots of many of the big societal problems related to pollution, health, safety, and technological development. Thus, it is obligatory to improve existing TEM techniques and invent new analytical methods to provide the society with techniques that can solve arising issues.

## 4 Challenges of incorporating TEM in TD research

Although TEM contributes to several research areas where major societal issues are solved, TEM is not yet extensively embedded in transdisciplinary research projects. In literature, the process of a TD research project is typically divided into three periods (or four periods as described by Hall et al. (2012)). In the first period, not only the problem is framed, but also the participating stakeholders are selected to form the TD research team. This first period is crucial for the success of the whole TD project. Social stakeholders and experts need to express their opinions and find a common language to allow for mutual understanding. Furthermore,

TD-based research projects often rely on previous results of fundamental research projects, especially in the first phase during project framing. In the second phase, all stakeholders work on their tasks, which were defined in the first phase. Although the whole project is declared to be a transdisciplinary project, it is not necessarily the case that every task needs to be worked on in a transdisciplinary manner. In some cases, interdisciplinary or even monodisciplinary realisations are unavoidable. The application of sophisticated methods like TEM requires the employment of their scientific standards to guarantee objective results. The dependence on fundamental research is therefore also a critical problem for transdisciplinary research, as the formulation and implementation of the research will be influenced by the results of the fundamental research. At the end of the second phase, knowledge defined by the goals framed in the first phase should be produced. This knowledge is then combined and merged in the third phase to form commonly accepted and integrated knowledge (Binder et al., 2015). The implementation of transdisciplinary approaches during all three phases is a difficult task not only for TD research with TEM but also for fundamental research in general. Especially the interplay of social stakeholders and experts from different scientific backgrounds and the integration of their specific knowledge and perspective into the research process is crucial. Thus, one of the significant challenges when applying TEM in TD research projects is the difference in knowledge among the TEM expert and the other stakeholders. Typically, a university student *(hier "student" passender als "colleague" oder "specialist" usw.)* would learn about TEM techniques if he or she specialised in the subject towards the end of a master's degree course, i.e. after about four years of studying physics and mathematics plus related subjects. It takes some knowledge of quantum mechanics and algebra to be able to understand how to interpret a TEM image correctly (as the examples of the TEM BF and STEM DF images in Figure 1 b) and c) show), even though much of this knowledge today is implemented in computer programmes available for this purpose. Of course, the simple use of a TEM can be learned by a technically trained person in a much shorter time of perhaps six months. During TD research, it cannot be expected that all contributors will undergo this instruction process to understand how a TEM works. Thus, the communication of knowledge and trust in the expertise and honesty in the TD partners are crucial for the success of the TD research process.

In addition to the knowledge gap of the stakeholders involved, the difference in objectivity and the discipline-specific definition of science when incorporating TEM or other (natural) sciences into TD research approaches are crucial. Objectivity, in general, is a term that is and continues to be heavily debated in philosophy and epistemology, and a more detailed explanation of different concepts of objectivity is far beyond the scope of this section. However, it is recognised that all views and deductions of results are subjective (Sprenger & Reiss, 2014). Therefore, at least in the natural sciences, results are measured against specific, recognised methods and standards of research to ensure that the results are negligibly influenced by a particular perspective, social background or personal interest of the researching scientist (Sprenger & Reiss, 2014). The dimension of social background is particularly noted in modern definitions of objectivity. As an example, Haraway's definition of situated knowledge, which stems from feminism, states that objectivity can only be achieved by considering the social background and the accompanying perspectives of the researcher (Haraway, 1995). Would this possibly mean that the microscopists significantly influence the results of their analysis because of their disciplinary and even social backgrounds (Barad, 2007)? As an example for the influence of disciplinary background, one could perhaps mention the determination of the specimen thickness, which is possible in the TEM using several methods based on different imaging modes, signals and theories. The determination of specimen thickness is, for instance, possible by using the EELS log-ratio method, which is based on the energy loss of electrons travelling through the specimen (Malis et al., 1988; Iakoubovskii et al., 2008; Egerton, 2011). It is also possible to use characteristic features of a convergent beam electron diffraction pattern that arise due to diffraction of electrons inside the specimen (Kossel & Möllenstedt, 1939; Kelly et al., 1975). Depending on the methods the microscopist or his or her community prefers, he or she will use the same for the measurement. Although the different methods are accepted as valid, the obtained specimen thickness for the different methods may differ slightly since its determination is based on different signals and theories. Scientists therefore indicate an accuracy with which a value was determined. If the method is applied correctly, the true value should lie within this measurement accuracy. Universally objective values can only be obtained if the value cannot be disproved by all previous and future measurement methods. Like physical constants, which are independent of time and universal in nature, scientific experiments and theories claim to be universally valid unless specified for explicit cases. As long as they apply the technique correctly, microscopists from different social and disciplinary backgrounds should therefore obtain the same results which are accepted as valid by their community. However, the acceptance of knowledge is not trivial in projects where disciplines related to scientific standards and methods are not congruent. In a TD project, in which societal stakeholders as well as scientists from sociology and natural sciences collaborate, this starts with the fact that in the social sciences, the objects of research – human beings – are themselves controlled by feelings and perspectives. Since TD research projects are ultimately about incorporating the perspectives and desires of society, which applies different measures and not the same scientific standards, into the research process, it is precisely the difference of objectivity that is a critical point. In addition, the contribution of societal stakeholders and social scientists to TEM investigations is, due to their different standards of (scientific) knowledge, difficult to imagine. A more in-depth elaboration of this issue is far beyond the scope of this section. However, since the aim of transdisciplinary research is generally to produce socially robust knowledge rather than scientifically correct knowledge (Rosendahl at al., 2015), we want to emphasise that just as a common language, common criteria for objectivity and epistemology must be found in transdisciplinary research to ensure the acceptance of all stakeholders and scientific accuracy of the research result.

Due to the multidisciplinarity of transmission electron microscopy, microscopists are based in various fields, like physics, biology, mechanical engineering, material science, chemistry or geology. During their studies, disciplinarity is strongly supported. Students of the above-mentioned courses typically do not learn transdisciplinary approaches, while interdisciplinarity is promoted more and more at universities. This is proven by the formation of interdisciplinary study programmes, like, for example, the material science courses combining physics, chemistry, and mechanical engineering. Due to disciplinarity, transdisciplinary topics are not included in curricula. Thus, TD methods are not explained or even trained during studies, raising the barrier to perform in TD projects at the later stage of the carrier. In addition, typically, only the transfer of knowledge within a specific discipline is part of the curriculum (e.g. a bachelor's defence), and ways to transfer knowledge when a significant knowledge gap needs to be overcome are usually not discussed. The openness to TD approaches and knowledge communication, which is a major part of the TD research, might also be helpful in other contexts, e.g. interdisciplinary or multidisciplinary research projects.

Sophisticated TEMs are mostly installed in modern facilities, typically in small rooms that are decoupled from floor vibrations and magnetic fields, i.e. the Earth's magnetic field and magnetic fields due to moving electrons in, for example, cars, busses, trains outside of the laboratory. Since the beam has to be stable with sub-atomic precision, any kind of instabilities typically reduce the possible resolution and influence the results. Thus, the TEM room has acoustically treated walls, and loud talking during measurements is disadvantageous. The machine is sensitive to various extraneous influences; therefore, unless the machine allows for remote control, typically only one operator works on the machine at a time. This makes TD approaches in which the presence of all stakeholders is favourable or needed during analysis difficult to perform. TEM microscopes typically are expensive machines in the range of several millions of euros and have large hourly operation costs. The application of TEM in a research project will be financed by research funding agencies only if the information expected to be gained by TEM cannot be obtained by simpler techniques. In addition, funding for a research project is typically only granted with a clearly defined goal. It is therefore necessary to include the social stakeholders in the framing phase of the research proposal.

## 5 Prospects of TEM and TD

The typical work of an electron microscopist is multi- or interdisciplinary because the operator of a TEM is not simply doing images of the specimen but analyses the specimen and, therefore, needs to understand the specimen structure; the research goal is to find the required answers. Often, TEM microscopists work in institutions where service measurements are carried out, and specimens range from a variety of disciplines. Therefore, the TEM specialist also takes part in framing the research question. As the specimens to be investigated come from various fields of science, electron microscopists typically do not reside in one discipline. Through its inter- and multidisciplinarity, the threshold for transdisciplinarity is lowered because TEM experts typically need to align their style of thought to the stakeholders, who want their specimens to be analysed. In other words, TEM experts must adjust the way of working, style of thought, and the way to communicate knowledge to one of their collaborating partners.

Scientific knowledge shapes the way we think as a society. It also affects the way the society and every single individual, policy maker or regional cluster, and other institutions act (Bonfadelli et al., 2017). Typically, knowledge is distributed via classic mass media channels, e.g. print media, radio or television (Bonfadelli et al., 2017). Scientific knowledge is spread by peer reviewed science journals which in the past were only accessible via subscribing libraries (e.g. at universities) or in a pay-per-article system and only recently have become increasingly freely available if published in "open-access" journals. The distribution of knowledge via the internet plays an increasing role in our society and reduces the power differences between experts and society due to the increasing availability of knowledge. Knowledge is no longer reserved to the experts at universities or other institutions (Bromme & Kienhues, 2014). It is essential in modern societies to communicate scientific knowledge due to the increasing societal challenges and implementation of high-tech products in daily life. The communication of knowledge is one of the key aspects of science. In science communities themselves, knowledge is distributed via the afore-mentioned publications and conferences. Topics that contribute to solving big societal issues are not only discussed within their disciplines but are also frequently discussed on all media channels mentioned above. Communication and discussion of science-related topics are typically conducted via online platforms and chat forums, in which people discuss the hot topics in the media or the topics they are interested in (Bonfadelli et al., 2017). When doing TEM analysis on a specimen, the camera image can be easily streamed via all video conference platforms. This streaming just requires a video capture card, which is able to capture the video output signal of the computer showing the live image viewed by the camera. This highly facilitates the interaction of societal stakeholders with TEM operators during the research process and not only during the phase of problem framing or during knowledge integration in transdisciplinary research processes. Compared to other techniques, TEM imaging can typically be done within a few hours or a day. This allows for live interaction and streaming during a complete specimen analysis session, thus enabling TD approaches. More importantly, since TEM shows images of the analysed structure, the power differences between the contributing stakeholders are lowered. Although the interpretation of the physics behind the contrast formation is not always straightforward, all stakeholders have an image in mind even if it might be misinterpreted. Images in science communication or even newspapers can have different uses. They can be used as a supportive illustration of the spoken word, be evidence for a certain fact or act as an eye-catcher. Images or videos can display and explain complex information in a way spoken text is never able to (Kessler et al., 2016). Thus, the barriers on a cognitive-epistemic and on the communication dimensions, which were defined by Jahn (Jahn, 2008), are drastically reduced, since researchers and societal stakeholders can talk about things both see. Since a TEM creates images, reports in magazines (which also allow comments by readers) can be utilised to enable interaction with society and increase acceptance by society. In some cases, TEM investigations are the only way to obtain the desired information, for instance if the data cannot be detected by the naked eye. The TEM micrograph then acts as the empirical evidence for a fact not available to any of the human senses (Lohoff, 2008). In addition to these points, the audience's attention is more likely drawn when images or videos are shown, and images are more likely to be remembered than words (Kessler et al., 2016). This increased remembrance also helps to increase the awareness on a certain topic, e.g. the corona virions. However, the insights societal stakeholders will gain when seeing TEM images highly depends on their background and education, since the TEM images obtained and their possible interpretation depend on the TEM method used (STEM dark-field images have a different contrast mechanism than TEM dark-field images), and missing knowledge might lead to a misinterpretation. To illustrate this, the brighter spots in an atomically resolved TEM bright-field image might be misinterpreted as atomic column positions, which is only the case for STEM dark-field images (Figure 1 b) and c)). The pure image itself could let the societal observer assume the reality and similarly forget the mechanisms which led to the contrast inside the image. This ultimately reinforces misinterpretation. Typically, during transdisciplinary research, both experts and other stakeholders have intense knowledge exchange making misinterpretations less likely. TEM operators are typically settlers (definition by Lettkemann, 2017), staying at their institutions for a long time, not jumping from institution to institution. Thus, contact with local societal stakeholders can be kept over a long time, helping to build mutual trust between societal actors, policymakers and scientists (Osinski, 2021).

## 6 Summary

Significant societal issues concerning environmental, medical, climate, and energy problems need to be solved, and the acceptance of the solution by society is of great importance. One promising way is transdisciplinary research, which includes societal stakeholders during the research projects. Through transdisciplinary approaches, all stakeholders, including the experts from academic fields, take part in problem framing and solving. Thus, not only acceptance in society is increased; however, TD also facilitates mutual learning, reduction of the knowledge gap among all stakeholders and the invention of new innovative transdisciplinary methods.

One of the methods presently applied in material science, biology, physics, chemistry, and mechanical engineering is transmission electron microscopy, which allows for investigation of the crystallographic structure, physical, and chemical properties of specimens with sub-atomic resolution supplemented by many analytical techniques. Examples are given that display the contribution of TEM to solving selected societal problems, like examinations of the corona virions, energy storage with lithium-ion batteries as well as the characterisation of materials for hybrid light-weight design and catalyst particles.

Applying transmission electron microscopy and other advanced characterisation techniques in a transdisciplinary context is not straightforward but also not impossible to achieve. Especially the objectivity and generality of the research outcome and the knowledge gap between participants are crucial issues. In addition, the direct interaction with societal stakeholders is complicated due to the sensitivity of the microscope to any extraneous influences, e.g. noise, magnetic fields and vibrations of the building. Training on the machine takes a long time and the acquisition of a physical background required for both; the appropriate application of the right TEM technique and the correct interpretation of data collected, is an even longer process. However, due to the typically multi- and interdisciplinary work of TEM specialists, the hurdle to align styles of thought to the ones of other stakeholders is drastically lower than for other techniques applied in disciplinary contexts. Furthermore, this hurdle is readily reduced since TEM images of the specimen are shown, which are often appealing to non-expert observers. Although the interpretation of contrasts is not straightforward, TEM experts and societal stakeholders are able to talk about what they see. This can be the starting point where societal stakeholders and microscopists exchange their knowledge, enhance mutual trust, start to do mutual investigations and find the fundamental puzzle pieces to solve substantial societal issues.

## References

Abbe, E. (1873). Beiträge zur Theorie des Mikroskops und der mikroskopischen Wahrnehmung. *Archiv für mikroskopische Anatomie* 9, 413-468. https://doi.org/10.1007/BF02956173

Baird, A. R., Archibald, E. J., Marr, K.C., & Ezekoye, O. A. (2020). Explosion hazards from lithium-ion battery vent gas. *Journal of Power Sources* 446, 227257. https://doi.org/10.1016/j.jpowsour.2019.227257

Barad, K. (2007). Agential Realism: How Material-Discursive Practices Matter. *Meeting the Universe Halfway.* Duke University Press. https://doi.org/10.1515/9780822388128-006

Bardell, D. (2004). The invention of the microscope. *Bios,* Vol. 75, Issue 2, 78-84.

Binder, C. R., Absenger-Helmli, I., & Schilling, T. (2015). The reality of transdisciplinarity: a framework-based self-reflection from science and practice leaders. *Sustainability Science* Vol. 10, 545-562. https://doi.org/10.1007/s11625-015-0328-2

Bohr, N. (1913). On the constitution of atoms and molecules. *The London, Edinburgh, and Dublin Philosophical Magazine and Journal of Science,* Vol. 26, Issue 151, 1-25. https://doi.org/10.1080/14786441308634955

Bonfadelli, H., Fähnrich, B., Lüthje, C., Milde, J., Rhomberg, M., & Schäfer, M.S. (2017). Das Forschungsfeld Wissenschaftskommunikation. In H. Bonfadelli, B. Fähnrich, C. Lüthje, J. Milde, M. Rhomberg, & M. Schäfer (Eds.) *Forschungsfeld Wissenschaftskommunikation* (pp. 3-14). Springer VS, Wiesbaden. https://doi.org/10.1007/978-3-658-12898-2_1

Bromme, R., & Kienhues, D. (2014). Wissenschaftsverständnis und Wissenschaftskommunikation. In Seidel T., & Krapp A. (Eds.). *Pädagogische Psychologie* (pp. 55-81), 6 Ed., Beltz.

Bürger, J., Kunnathully, V.S., Kool, D., Lindner, J.K.N., & Brassat, K. (2020). Characterisation of the PS-PMMA interfaces in microphase separated block copolymer thin films by analytical (S) TEM. *Nanomaterials* Vol. 10, 141. https://doi.org/10.3390/nano10010141

Carenco, S., Moldovan, S., Roiban, L., Florea, I., Portehault, D., Vallé, K., Belleville, P., Boissière, C., Rozes, L., Mézailles, N., Drillon, M., Sanchez, C., & Ersen, O. (2015). The core contribution of transmission electron microscopy to functional nanomaterials engineering. *Nanoscale* Vol. 8, Issue 3, 1260-1279. https://doi.org/10.1039/C5NR05460E

Chan, C. K., Peng, H., Liu, G., McIlwrath, K., Zhang, X. F., Huggins, R. A., & Cui, Y. (2008). High-performance lithium battery anodes using silicon nanowires. *Nature nanotechnology* Vol. 3, 31-35. https://doi.org/10.1038/nnano.2007.411

Chen, Z., Qin, Y., Amine, K., & Sun Y.-K. (2010). Role of surface coating on cathode materials for lithium-ion batteries. *Journal of materials chemistry,* Vol. 20, Issue 36, 7606-7612. https://doi.org/10.1039/C0JM00154F

Dedeurwaerdere, T. (2013). Transdisciplinary sustainability science at higher education institutions: science policy tools for incremental institutional change. *Sustainability* Vol. 5, Issue 9, 3783-3801. https://doi.org/10.3390/su5093783

Egerton, R. F. (2011). *Electron energy-loss spectroscopy in the electron microscope.* Springer New York. https://doi.org/10.1007/978-1-4419-9583-4

Erni, R., Rossell, M. D., Kisielowski, C., & Dahmen, U. (2009). Atomic-resolution imaging with a sub-50-pm electron probe. *Physical review letters,* Vol. 102, Issue 9, 096101. https://doi.org/10.1103/PhysRevLett.102.096101

Fan, J., Hu, K., Li, X., Jiang, Y., Zhou, X., Gou, X., & Li, X. (2020). A qualitative study of the vocational and psychological perceptions and issues of transdisciplinary nurses during the COVID-19 outbreak. *Aging (Albany NY),* Vol. 12, Issue 13, 12479-12492. https://doi.org/10.18632/aging.103533

Fultz, B., & Howe, J. M. (2012) *Transmission electron microscopy and diffractometry of materials.* Springer Berlin, Heidelberg. https://doi.org/10.1007/978-3-642-29761-8

Haguenau, F., Hawkes, P., Hutchison, J., Satiat–Jeunemaître, B., Simon, G., & Williams, D. (2003). Key events in the history of electron microscopy. *Microscopy and Microanalysis,* Vol. 9, Issue 2, 96-138. https://doi.org/10.1017/S1431927603030113

Haider, M., Uhlemann, S., Schwan, E., Rose, H., Kabius, B., & Urban, K. (1998). Electron microscopy image enhanced. *Nature,* Vol. 392, 768-769. https://doi.org/10.1038/33823

Hall, K. L., Vogel, A. L., Stipelman, B. A., Stokols, D., Morgan, G., & Gehlert, S. (2012). A four-phase model of transdisciplinary team-based research: goals, team processes, and strategies. *Translational behavioral medicine,* Vol. 2, Issue 4, 415-430. https://doi.org/10.1007/s13142-012-0167-y

Haraway, D. J. (1995). Situiertes Wissen: Die Wissenschaftsfrage im Feminismus und das Privileg einer partialen Perspektive. In E. Scheich (Eds.) *Vermittelte Weiblichkeit: feministische Wissenschafts- und Gesellschaftstheorie* (pp. 217-248), Hamburger Edition. ISBN: 3-930908-23-9

Hartridge, H. (1922). Visual acuity and the resolving power of the eye. *The Journal of physiology,* Vol. 57, Issue 1-2. https://doi.org/10.1113/jphysiol.1922.sp002042

Hofmann, D. M., Hofstaetter, A., Leiter, F., Zhou, H., Henecker, F., Meyer, B. K., Orlinskii, S. B., Schmidt, J., & Baranov, P. G. (2002). Hydrogen: a relevant shallow donor in zinc oxide. *Physical Review Letters,* Vol. 88, Issue 4, 045504. https://doi.org/10.1103/PhysRevLett.88.045504

Hopfer, H., Herzig, M. C., Gosert, R., Menter, T., Hench, J., Tzankov, A., Hirsch, H. H., Miller, S. E. (2020). Hunting coronavirus by transmission electron microscopy–a guide to SARS-CoV-2-associated ultrastructural pathology in COVID-19 tissues. *Histopathology, Vol.* 78, Issue 3, 358-370. https://doi.org/10.1111/his.14264

Huang, J. Y., Zhong, L., Wang, C. M., Sullivan, J. P., Xu, W., Zhang, L. Q., Mao, S. X., Hudak, N. S., Liu, X. H., Subramanian, A., Fan, H., Qi, L., Kushima A., & Li, J. (2010). In situ observation of the electrochemical lithiation of a single SnO2 nanowire electrode. *Science* Vol. 330, Issue 6010, 1515-1520. https://doi.org/10.1126/science.1195628

Iakoubovskii, K., Mitsuishi, K., Nakayama, Y., & Furuya, K. (2008). Thickness measurements with electron energy loss spectroscopy. *Microscopy research and technique,* Vol. 71, Issue 8, 626-631. https://doi.org/10.1002/jemt.20597

Jahn, T. (2008). Transdisciplinarity in the practice of research. In M. Bergmann, & E. Schramm (Eds.) (2008). *Transdisziplinäre Forschung. Integrative Forschungsprozesse verstehen und bewerten (pp. 21-37).* Campus Verlag.

Kavli (2020). The Kavli Prize, 07.04.2022, https://www.kavliprize.org/prizes/nanoscience/2020

Kelly, P. M., Jostsons, A., Blake, R. G., & Napier J. G. (1975). The determination of foil thickness by scanning transmission electron microscopy. *Physica status solidi (a),* Vol. 31, Issue 2, 771-780. https://doi.org/10.1002/pssa.2210310251

Kessler, S. H., Reifegerste, D. & Guenther, L. (2016). Die Evidenzkraft von Bildern in der Wissenschaftskommunikation. In G. Ruhrmann, S. H. Kessler, & L. Guenther (Eds.) *Wissenschaftskommunikation zwischen Risiko und (Un)Sicherheit (pp. 170-192).* ISBN: 978-3-86962-196-8

Kim, J.-M., Chung, Y.-S., Jo, H. J., Lee, N.-J., Kim, M. S., Woo, S. H., Park, S., Kim, J. W., Kim, H. M., & Han, M.-G. (2020). Identification of coronavirus isolated from a patient in Korea with COVID-19. *Osong public health and research perspectives,* Vol. 11, Issue 1, 3-7. https://doi.org/10.24171/j.phrp.2020.11.1.02

Knoll, M., & Ruska. E. (1932a). Beitrag zur geometrischen Elektronenoptik. I. *Annalen der Physik,* Vol. 404, Issue 5, 607-640. https://doi.org/10.1002/andp.19324040506

Knoll, M., & Ruska. E. (1932b). Das Elektronenmikroskop. *Zeitschrift für Physik,* Vol. 78, 318-339. https://doi.org/10.1007/BF01342199

Kossel, W., & Möllenstedt, G. (1939). Elektroneninterferenzen im konvergenten Bündel. *Annalen der Physik,* Vol. 428, Issue 2, 113-140. https://doi.org/10.1002/andp.19394280204

Krivanek, O. L., Dellby, N., & Lupini, A. R. (1999). Towards sub-Å electron beams. *Ultramicroscopy,* Vol. 78, Issue 1-4, 1-11. https://doi.org/10.1016/S0304-3991(99)00013-3

Kubli, F. (1970). Louis de Broglie und die Entdeckung der Materiewellen. *Archive for History of Exact Sciences,* Vol. 7, Issue 1, 26-68. https://doi.org/10.1007/BF00328784

Lettkemann, E. (2017). Nomads and settlers in the research-technology regime: The case of transmission electron microscopy. *Social Science Information,* Vol. 56, Issue 3, 393-415. https://doi.org/10.1177/0539018417719396

Liu, X. H., & Huang, J. Y. (2011). In situ TEM electrochemistry of anode materials in lithium ion batteries. Energy & Environmental Science, Vol. 4, Issue 10, 3844-3860. https://doi.org/10.1039/C1EE01918J

Lohoff, M. (2008). *Wissenschaft im Bild: performative Aspekte des Bildes in Prozessen wissenschaftlicher Erkenntnisgewinnung und -vermittlung.* No. RWTH-CONV-112492. Fakultät für Architektur, Dissertation. http://publications.rwth-aachen.de/record/49924/files/Lohoff_Markus.pdf

Maasen, S., & Lieven, O. (2006). Transdisciplinarity: a new mode of governing science? *Science and Public Policy,* Vol. 33, Issue 6, 399-410. https://doi.org/10.3152/147154306781778803

Malis, T., Cheng, S. C., & Egerton, R. F. (1988). EELS log-ratio technique for specimen-thickness measurement in the TEM. *Journal of electron microscopy technique,* Vol. 8, Issue 2, 193-200. https://doi.org/10.1002/jemt.1060080206

Marcovich, A., & Shinn, T. (2017). How scientific research instruments change: A century of Nobel Prize physics instrumentation. *Social Science Information,* Vol. 56, Issue 3, 348-374. https://doi.org/10.1177/0539018417709099

Miah, J. H., Griffiths, A., McNeill, R., Poonaji, I., Martin, R., Morse, S., Yang, A., & Sadhukhan, J. (2015). A small-scale transdisciplinary process to maximising the energy efficiency of food factories: insights and recommendations from the development of a novel heat integration framework. *Sustainability Science,* Vol. 10, Issue 4, 621-637. https://doi.org/10.1007/s11625-015-0331-7

Mittelstraß, J. (2005). Methodische Transdisziplinarität. *TATuP-Zeitschrift für Technikfolgenabschätzung in Theorie und Praxis,* Vol. 14, Issue 2, 18-23. https://doi.org/10.14512/tatup.14.2.18

Nicolescu, B. (2014). Methodology of Transdisciplinarity. *World Futures,* Vol. 70, Issue 3-4, 186-199. https://doi.org/10.1080/02604027.2014.934631

Nobel Media (2022). Full text of Alfred Nobel´s Will. Available online at https://www.nobelprize.org/alfred-nobel/full-text-of-alfred-nobels-will-2/, checked on 11/18/2022.

Osinski, A. (2021). Towards a Critical Sustainability Science? Participation of Disadvantaged Actors and Power Relations in Transdisciplinary Research. *Sustainability,* Vol. 13, Issue 3, 1266. https://doi.org/10.3390/su13031266

Park, Y. J., Kim, M. K., Kim, H. S., & Lee, B. M. (2018). Risk assessment of lithium-ion battery explosion: chemical leakages. *Journal of Toxicology and Environmental Health,* Part B, Vol. 21, Issue 6-8, 370-381. https://doi.org/10.1080/10937404.2019.1601815

Nilsson Pingel, T., Jørgensen, M., Yankovich, A. B., Grönbeck, H., & Olsson, E. (2018). Influence of atomic site-specific strain on catalytic activity of supported nanoparticles. *Nature communications,* Vol. 9, Issue 1, 1-9. https://doi.org/10.1038/s41467-018-05055-1

Pohl, C., Krütli, P., & Stauffacher, M. (2017). Ten reflective steps for rendering research societally relevant. *GAIA-Ecological Perspectives for Science and Society*, Vol. 26, Issue 1, 43-51. https://doi.org/10.14512/gaia.26.1.10

Popova, M., Stryzhak, O., Mintser, O., & Novogrudska, R. (2020). Medical Transdisciplinary Cluster Development for Multivariable COVID-19 Epidemiological Situation Modeling. *Proceedings of 2020 IEEE International Conference on Bioinformatics and Biomedicine (BIBM) (pp. 1662-1667)*. https://doi.org/10.1109/BIBM49941.2020.9313204

Sprenger, J. M., & Reiss, J. (2014). Scientific Objectivity. In E. Zalta (Ed.) *Stanford Encyclopedia of Philosophy* (2014 ed.) http://plato.stanford.edu/entries/scientific-objectivity/

Robinson, C. V., Sali, A., & Baumeister, W. (2007). The molecular sociology of the cell. *Nature*, Vol. 450, 973-982. https://doi.org/10.1038/nature06523

Rose, H. (1990). Outline of a spherically corrected semiaplanatic medium-voltage transmission electron microscope." *Optik*, Vol. 85, Issue 1, 19-24.

Rosendahl, J., Zanella, M. A., Rist, S., & Weigelt, J. (2015). Scientists' situated knowledge: strong objectivity in transdisciplinarity. *Futures*, Vol. 65, 17-27. https://doi.org/10.1016/j.futures.2014.10.011

Russo, C. J., & Egerton R. F. (2019). Damage in electron cryomicroscopy: Lessons from biology for materials science. *MRS Bulletin*, Vol. 44, Issue 12, 935-941. https://doi.org/10.1557/mrs.2019.284

Sacci, R. L., Black, J. M., Balke, N., Dudney, N, J., More, K. L., & Unocic, R. R. (2015). Nanoscale imaging of fundamental Li battery chemistry: solid-electrolyte interphase formation and preferential growth of lithium metal nanoclusters. *Nano letters*, Vol. 15, Issue 3, 2011-2018. https://doi.org/10.1021/nl5048626

Schlicher, S., Prinz, N., Bürger, J., Omlor, A., Singer, C., Zobel, M., Schoch, R., Lindner, J. K. N., Schünemann, V., Kureti, S., & Bauer, M. (2022). Quality or Quantity? How Structural Parameters Affect Catalytic Activity of Iron Oxides for CO Oxidation. *Catalysts*, Vol. 12, Issue 6, 675. https://doi.org/10.3390/catal12060675

Scholz, R. W., & Steiner, G. (2015). Transdisciplinarity at the crossroads. *Sustainability Science*, Vol. 10, Issue 4, 521-526. https://doi.org/10.1007/s11625-015-0338-0

Scholz, R. W. (2020). Transdisciplinarity: science for and with society in light of the university's roles and functions." *Sustainability science*, Vol. 15, Issue 4, 1033-1049. https://doi.org/10.1007/s11625-020-00794-x

Snoeck, E. (2017). ESTEEM-2, Enabling Science and Technology through European Electron Microscopy, FP7. *Impact* 2017(3), 74-76.

Stip, E., Rizvi, T. A., Mustafa, F., Javaid, S., Aburuz, S., Ahmed, N. N., Abdel Aziz, K., Arnone, D., Subbarayan, A., Al Mugaddam, F., & Khan, G. (2020). The Large Action of Chlorpromazine: Translational and Transdisciplinary Considerations in the Face of COVID-19. *Frontiers in pharmacology*, Vol. 11, 577678. https://doi.org/10.3389/fphar.2020.577678

Stokols, D. (2006). Toward a science of transdisciplinary action research. *American journal of community psychology*, Vol. 38, Issue 1, 63-77. https://doi.org/10.1007/s10464-006-9060-5

Tanaka, N. (Ed.) (2014). *Scanning transmission electron microscopy of nanomaterials: basics of imaging and analysis*. Imperial College Press. https://doi.org/10.1142/p807

Urban, K., Kabius, B., Haider, M., & Rose, H. (1999). A way to higher resolution: spherical-aberration correction in a 200 kV transmission electron microscope. *Microscopy*, Vol. 48, Issue 6, 821-826. https://doi.org/10.1093/oxfordjournals.jmicro.a023753

Wang, Q., Sun, J., & Chu, G. (2005). Lithium ion battery fire and explosion. *Fire Safety Science*, Vol. 8, 375-382. https://doi.org/10.3801/IAFSS.FSS.8-375

Williams, D. B., & Carter, C. B. (2009). *Transmission Electron Microscopy*. 2. Ed., Springer New York. https://doi.org/10.1007/978-0-387-76501-3

Wu, F., & Yao, N. (2015). Advances in sealed liquid cells for in-situ TEM electrochemial investigation of lithium-ion battery. *Nano Energy*, Vol. 11, 196-210. https://doi.org/10.1016/j.nanoen.2014.11.004

Yuan, Y., Amine, K., Lu, J., & Shahbazian-Yassar, R. (2017). Understanding materials challenges for rechargeable ion batteries with in-situ transmission electron microscopy. *Nature Communications*, Vol. 8, 15806. https://doi.org/10.1038/ncomms15806

# Case Study II: Application of Transdisciplinarity in the Context of Sustainable Product Development

*Alexander Henkes, Alexander Klingebiel, Lakshmi Anusha Innem, Maximilian Richters, Najmeh Filvan Torkaman, Philipp Hesse, Swetlana Schweizer, Thomas Borgert, Elmar Moritzer, Ilona Horwath, Iris Gräßler, Rolf Mahnken, Werner Homberg, Wolfgang Bremser*

## 1 Introduction and state of the art

### 1.1 Sustainability

> "If you want creativity, take a zero off your budget. If you want sustainability, take off two zeros." – Jaime Lerner

Even prior to the COVID-19 pandemic, global problems, such as climate change, land degradation, water scarcity, and environmental exploitation, have risen dramatically at an alarming rate. Environmental issues, such as carbon emissions, air pollution, the depletion of the ozone layer, climate change, etc., have raised significant concerns for countries, groups, and organisations. Due to the pandemic, we have been facing a lengthy health crisis that had a significant impact on practically every aspect of business operations. Hence, the outbreak of the novel Coronavirus drastically shifted the landscape of sustainable consumption.

Sustainability is no longer just "nice to have", we need to do something to counteract current developments. The term sustainable development means "meeting our own needs without compromising the ability of future generations to meet their own needs" (World Commission on Environment and Development,1987). It is a transdisciplinary endeavour to provide insights that involve in or relate to two or more different areas of study of the human world, from business to technology to environment and social sciences. Nowadays, sustainability and environmental awareness prioritise the reduction of carbon emissions and the discover and development of future technologies. One of the newest subjects one can study attempts to bridge social science with civic engineering and environmental science with future technology. We can balance our natural environment and ecological health with sustainability while driving innovation and without compromising our way of life. While most people associate it with the environment, sustainability can be explored in various contexts, including economic development and social responsibility.

Sustainability aims to improve the quality of life, protect our ecosystem, and preserve natural resources for future generations. A green and sustainable approach is beneficial to the company; it also maximises the long-term benefits of an ecological mindset. Practising sustainability ensures that we make ethical choices that provide everyone with a safe and liveable future. Being committed to sustainable products will reduce our carbon footprints and the number of toxins released into the environment, making it safe. Sustainable actions make the entire world better to live in and provide clean and healthier conditions. (World Commission on Environment and Development,1987)

Sustainable development is the need to consider "the three pillars": society, the economy and the environment. These three pillars are informally referred to as people, planet, and profits. True sustainability can be achieved by balancing all three pillars in equal harmony. "Circular economy (CE) and Transparency" are the strategies to achieve true sustainability to tackle urgent environmental deterioration and resource scarcity. The 3Rs, "Reduce, Re-Use and Recycle", is a well-known concept in resource efficiency that helps us "return× materials and resources to a product's life cycle, ensuring that we use less energy and produce less waste/ pollution and emissions. For a more circular approach, the 3R concept shows a few "R" s: "Refuse×, "Rethink×, "Reduce×, "Re-Use×, "Repair", "Refurbish", "Remanufacture", "Repurpose", "Recycle" and "Recover" explained in the next chapter. (Strange & Bayley, 2008; Heshmati, 2015; Srinivas, 2022; Okorie et al., 2018)

Adopting sustainable materials as alternatives to contemporary materials will be an environmentally benign manufacturing process. Wood Plastic Composite (WPC), Polylactic Acid (PLA), Polypropylene (PP), etc., contribute positively to all three pillars of sustainability. We recycle for sustainability and contribute to our economic wealth, happiness, and well-being.

## 1.2 Sustainable product life cycle

Nowadays, companies must fulfil customer needs while bearing a high social responsibility (Brüggemann et al., 2018). Customers are increasingly interested in sustainable products and services (Isaksson & Eckert, 2020). For sustainable products, relevant aspects of ecology, economy and social issues have to be considered in product development (Raabe et al., 2019). Concepts to ensure sustainable engineering of products are Cradle-to-Cradle (McDonough & Braungart, 2002), reduction of waste in production and the Circular Economy (Ellen MacArthur Foundation, 2013). These concepts aim to return materials to the economic system in order to close material cycles after use of the product. The central idea of the Circular Economy is to achieve economic growth primarily by recycled materials and only secondarily by additional materials (Ellen MacArthur Foundation, 2013).

The Circular Economy influences product and material life cycles and engineering approaches. The product concept and initial design of a product and its features must be investigated explicitly with regard their influence on the Circular Economy and the End-of-Life (Pahl et al., 2007). This results in actions that have a major effect on protecting limited natural resources. In addition, the design determines how well materials can be treated in subsequent processes. In this way, the design influences quality and cost of the second product life (Cruz Sanchez et al., 2020).

The circular economy strategies are oriented towards the behaviour of products, assemblies and Parts in relation to the ecosystem (product life phase, process, technology, etc.) in order to achieve company's goals (Schuh and Klappert, 2011). Strategies for the circular design of products are described in the 9R framework (Okorie et al., 2018). The framework comprises ten approaches, starting with R0 (Refuse) (Figure 1). Each of the strategies aiming at circular economy is to be considered in product design. The approaches are not explicitly formulated for one branch of industry but are generic and can be applied to any application. The strategies apply to as many disciplines as possible. Implementing the 9R framework strategies is a subjective interpretation and creative implementation of the engineer.

In literature, engineering guidelines address proven product designs and strategies (Ellen MacArthur Foundation, 2013). One example for design guidelines is Design for X (DfX) an interdisciplinary knowledge system, which addresses social, ecological and economical sustainability (Bender and Gericke, 2021). The X represents technologies, processes and product life phases (Ponn and Lindemann, 2011). These concretely formulated engineering guidelines support designers in realising the initial product concept.

The strategies of the 9R framework address different phases along product life. Different life cycle models are presented in literature that describe the product life in terms of time. Different types of market life cycles are listed in the pertinent literature (Geyer, 1976); the technical product life cycle (VDI 2221), the intrinsic product life cycle (Eigner et al., 2014; Gräßler & Pottebaum, 2021) and technology life cycles (Ford & Ryan, 1981; Tiefel, 2008; Tiefel, 2007; Ehrlenspiel & Meerkamm, 2013). The generic Product Life Cycle (gPLC) (Figure 2) by Gräßler and Pottebaum focuses on engineering, mechatronic and cyber-physical systems considering the core contents of the literature. The gPLC also enables circular economy using for explanation.

After the product has passed the phases "strategic planning", "engineering", "realisation", "operation/service delivery" and "decommissioning", materials (green arrows) are returned to the previous phases. Likewise, a small part of ma-

*Figure 1: The 9R Framework of the Circular Economy for Product Engineering, according to (Council for the Environment and Infrastructure (Rli), 2015; Potting et al., 2017)*

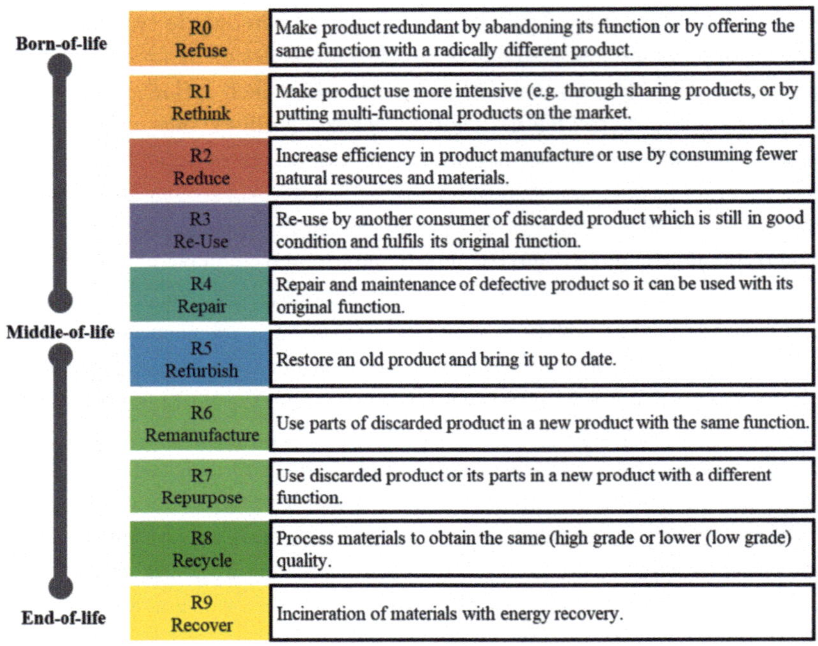


terials in the "realisation" phase is fed back into itself and the "engineering" phase. Recycling of materials is the foundation for the economic growth of the Circular Economy (Ellen MacArthur Foundation, 2013). The different phases build on each other and are arranged in a structured way over the product life cycle. A product or the materials can pass through the phases repeatedly or by setback (Potting et al., 2017). The phases represent area-specific influences. The influences affect the product and form the initial state of a subsequent phase.

On the right side of the gPLC, the information circularity is visualised. The fed-back information provides the basis for optimising absolute supply chains and engineering new products. An exemplary technology for implementing information circularity is the digital twin.

The gPLC has the following characteristics: intrinsic, circular, holistic, generic and adaptive. The intrinsic characteristic addresses value creation for businesses, consumers and users. Circularity also integrates the return of materials and information fundamental to the product life cycle. In the holistic model, single and multidisciplinary engineering projects are considered. Corresponding engineering methodologies ((VDI 2221; VDI 2206) etc.) can be embedded in the model depending on the of industry. Due to its generic property, the gPLC can be applied

*Figure 2: generic Product Life Cycle model (Gräßler & Pottebaum 2021, p. 13)*

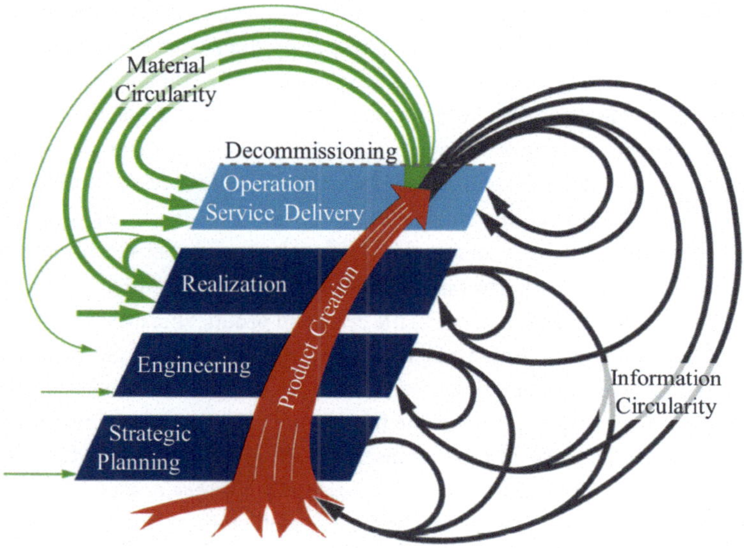


to a large variety of products from different industry sectors. The model can be adapted to different applications and allows individual adjustments to represent product classes and instances better. In addition, it considers distinguishable inputs, phases and flows. The unique feature of the product life cycle in direct comparison to the product life cycle model is that material and product instance data are fed back. The materials and product instance data serve product creation as a basis for developing new products.

To fully map the phases of the product and the materials that are involved, the life cycles of the materials and production must be combined. The combination facilitates a detailed view, which is decisive for the design of the products. This makes it easier to implement the needs of the end-of-life processes in the products and components. The product life is thus accessible to the designer and is considered subjectively in the design.

In addition to the product life cycle, different detailed material life cycles are noted in the pertinent literature. Each class of material is described by an individual life cycle. Basically, it is possible to look at materials via their specific extraction (Raabe et al., 2019). These representations facilitate a detailed description of the extraction process and are the basis for a life cycle assessment according to (DIN EN ISO 14040). In addition to material extraction models, some models describe material and product quality reduction per lifecycle (Ishii et al., 1994). These material life cycle models are supplemented by feedback on production and product use phases (Regenfelder & Ebelt, 2012).

Other models in the pertinent literature do not differentiate between the material and product life cycle but focus on the product. The material life cycles are combined in a product as a material cycle (Jawaihr et al., 2005; Herrmann, 2010). For example, mechatronic and cyber-physical products consist of material composites, including rare earth elements (Abdelbasir et al., 2018).

The materials are bound in the product and pass through the life cycle of the product instance until it reaches the end-of-life phase. The materials are separated from the product in the end-of-life phase, sorted and processed for renewed industrial use. The separation, sorting and treatment processes take place in treatment companies. The environmental influences become an active influence in the middle-of-life phase and affect materials implemented in product.

Figure 3 shows how the material life cycle and product life cycles interact with each other. In the beginning there is the material life cycle, whose materials are extracted from nature and processed for industrial use. The materials obtained from nature are thus made available for the prevailing economic model and are integrated into life cycle of product instance. The product instance describes the actual object, machine or immaterial goods, such as a service (Stark et al., 2020). After the product instance has reached the end of its life cycle, the materials are recovered. The recovery takes place in the "multi-material recycle cycle". If one of the materials in the multi-material cycle reaches the end of its life, it is recycled for energy or disposed of.

The product instance with multi-material lives through life phases and is exposed to environmental influences. After the product user defines the product instance as waste (Europäisches Parlament, 2008), the product is fed into the multi-material recycling cycle. The material cycle is distinguished from the product instance life cycle, as the focus is on the recovery of materials. The initially developed function fulfilment of the instance is subordinate to material recovery. The treatment process aims at recovering many materials as possible from products and making them usable again for the economic model at hand, while at the same time keeping material loss to a minimum. This circularity continues according to the repeating pattern.

In order to combine the material life cycle, the product life cycle and strategies of the Circular Economy, an integrated life cycle model is presented. For a generic view, the different materials are considered as a multi-material cycle. If the product and the material flow are considered as a system, repeating patterns can be identified (Herrmann, 2010). The sequence and the relationships of the repeating phases are identical in each cycle.

The Circular Economy strategies are formulated from the perspective of the product. Therefore, the perspective does not address the individual material, but encompasses the materials included in the product. According to the multitude of materials within the product, the term multi-material cycle is implemented.

*Figure 3: Dependencies between the multi-material life and the product life*

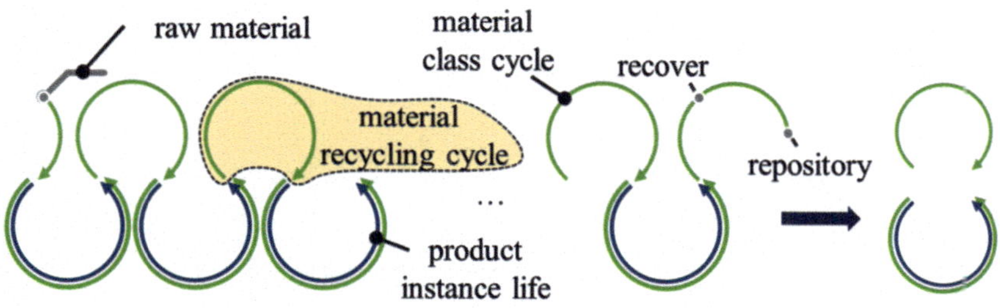


The multi-material recycling cycle, together with the life cycle of product instance, forms the repeating cycle in Figure 4.

The phases of the product life cycle – "strategic planning", "engineering", "realisation", "operation" and "decommissioning" – are taken from the gPLC model (Gräßler & Pottebaum 2021). The gPLC model considers all product classes, disciplines and requirements holistically and generally. These characteristics are suitable for combining with the material life cycle, as different product classes and disciplines integrate different material inputs.

The phases of the multi-material cycle are derived from the models according to Dyckhoff (2000), Ellen MacArthur Foundation (2013) and Pan & Li (2016). In the "Collection" phase, end-of-life products of the product users are combined in waste stream. The waste stream consists of the sum of end-of-life product instances directed toward waste treatment (Gräßler & Pottebaum, 2021). In sorting, the product instances are identified, grouped according to product class, and forwarded. The waste stream is divided into several parallel streams of different product classes. Sorting can take place in several stages. After the product classes have been identified, they are further treated according to the class. In case of material recovery, materials are separated from products in the "decomposition/disassembly" stage. This can be done by mechanical crushing or manual disassembly. After the materials have been separated and are available in pure form, they are prepared in the "preparation" phase. Preparation means that the materials are processed in a suitable way for the industry. For example, the plastic injection moulding process requires granulates to ensure trouble-free production. Finally, the materials are measured in the "evaluation" phase. This means that the physical properties are examined. The physical properties are necessary for development of new products. The product´s performance in the phases of the multi-material cycle is predetermined in the engineering phase (Kriwet et al., 1995).

When a product instance is in the last phase of its life, this is collected through local infrastructure. In addition, waste is generated in the "realisation" and "operation" phases, which are also assigned to the cycle. Subsequently, the materials

*Figure 4: Product and Multi-Material Life Cycle, according to (Gräßler & Hesse, 2021)*

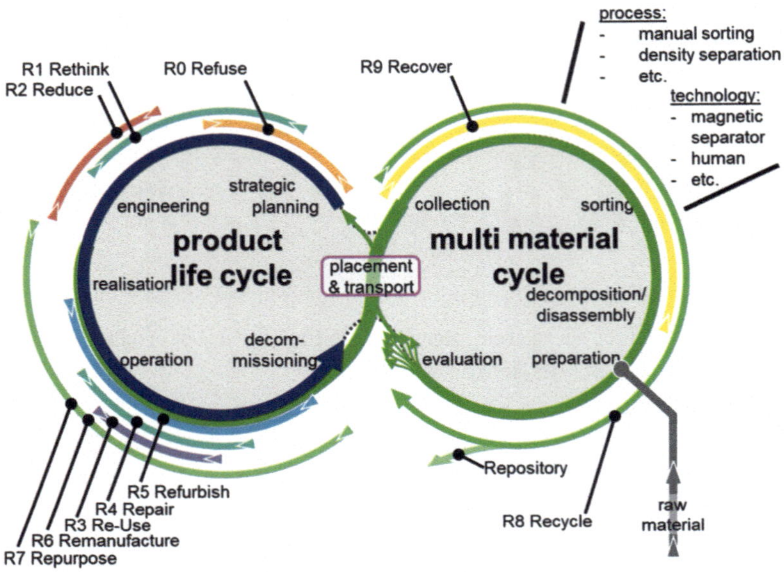


are sorted and transferred to the appropriate treatment plants. The product instances are disassembled in the treatment plants by systematically dismantling the elements or mechanically crushing them. The separated material is brought together and processed in a suitable way for industrial use. The final step is the measurement of the physical product properties. The product properties enable manufacturing companies to select the materials for their new products.

With the help of named lifecycle phases, it is possible to assign the strategies to the CE, represented by the 9R framework. The strategies of the 9R framework are positioned around the material and product lifecycle. According to Okorie et al., 2018; Klenk et al., 2019; Ellen MacArthur Foundation, 2013, the positioning results from the description.

The strategies do not address a point of time within the life of a product instance but refer to a period and life cycle. The product instance can, for example, be refurbished and re-used by the previous user or another user. It becomes apparent that the strategies fully encompass the model of the integrated lifecycle model. In the product and multi-material life cycle, after the strategies have been classified, the life cycle phase-specific stakeholders, processes and technologies are analysed. Figure 4 shows an example of the "sorting" phase. Manual sorting and density sorting can be identified as processes, and magnetic separators and humans can be identified as technologies. These elements form an ecosystem in which the product is embedded. The ecosystem describes the product environment, which changes with the life phase. As the ecosystem changes, the product is confronted with different requirements and influences that need to be thought through in advance during product engineering.

## 1.3 Natural fibre-reinforced plastics

The recycling of materials is often at the expense of mechanical properties. To achieve similar mechanical properties, such as tensile strength and modulus of elasticity by using recycling plastics, fibre reinforcement is conceivable. Glass, carbon, aramid or natural fibres are predominantly used as reinforcing fibres. To achieve a reinforcing effect, the fibre must have a greater stiffness (Young's modulus) or tensile strength compared to the matrix material. Due to their outstanding specific properties at comparatively low density compared with metallic materials, fibre-reinforced plastics (FRP) have significantly contributed to weight reduction in the automotive sector. Depending on the type and function of individual components in the automotive sector, subcomponents can be replaced by hybrid construction and metallic components by pure substitution with an FRP. Furthermore, applications for bicycles, such as bicycle stands or gearshifts, are conceivable. (Stewart, 2011)

The portfolio of fibre-reinforced plastics ranges from short-fibre reinforcement (<< 4.5 mm fibre length) to extended fibre reinforcement (4.5 - 50 mm) to continuous fibre-reinforced plastics, in which the fibre length roughly corresponds to the component length. Despite their low density, continuous fibre-reinforced plastics have mechanical properties that compete with aluminium materials. This can be shown if material-specific properties are standardised to the density, and the specific properties are considered. Here it can be seen, particularly in terms of tensile strength, that glass- and carbon-fibre-reinforced plastics have clear advantages for lightweight construction (Breuer, 1997). In the future, fibre-reinforced plastics will continue to play an essential role in weight reduction and maximisation of the car range and during e-mobilisation.

In divergence to the contribution to weight reduction in the automotive sector, there is a high energy consumption involved in the production of fibres (glass, aramid, carbon) and fibre-reinforced plastics. The production of glass fibres requires 3.6 MJ/kg for melting the glass (e.g. an injection moulding machine needs 2,1 MJ/kg for a product). For this purpose, the glass batch is melted in electric furnaces using electrical energy. The molten glass is then spun into fibres via nozzles (Teschner, 2013).

The most familiar representative of continuous fibre-reinforced plastics is the organic sheet. To produce organic sheets, the glass fibres are first woven in bundles to form woven fabrics; then the fabric is soaked in a thermoplastic matrix system. A double-belt press is used to press the organic sheets together to produce a preform. The organic sheet is heated in a press and then formed using a defined force to generate a component. (Breuer, 1997) To produce short glass-fibre-reinforced plastics, previously shredded glass fibres are compounded into thermoplastic matrix material, usually polypropylene (PP) or polyamide (PA), by a twin-screw extruder. A glass-fibre-reinforced granulate is then produced, which can be processed in the injection moulding process. The good mechanical properties of glass-fibre-reinforced plastics are in divergence to their recyclability. After just a few recycling cycles, the achievable strength decreases sharply due to fibre shortening. As soon as the required fibre length is reached, the force introduction into the fibre can only take place insufficiently. (Evens et al., 2019)

An option for increasing the recyclability of injection moulded articles is using wood fibres as reinforcing fibres. In the study of fibre-reinforced compounds, Evens et al. (2019) showed that although wood fibres, like glass fibres, tend to degrade in fibre length when recycled in the injection moulding process, the test specimens do not have a significant decrease in mechanical properties as a function of the recycling step. Within the scope of the investigations, test specimens were produced from PP-based compounds with 20-wt-% fibre content (glass fibre, carbon fibre, flax fibre) and from an unreinforced compound. The test specimens were shredded, and the material was then injection-moulded again to form test specimens. The test specimens were subjected to a tensile test, three-point bending test, and impact strength test to determine the relevant mechanical properties. Then the fibre size distribution was determined as a function of the recycling step. Evens et al. (2019) were able to show that after only two recycling cycles, the tensile strength decreased by about 25% for glass-fibre-reinforced polypropylene and 20% for carbon-fibre-reinforced polypropylene. Flax-fibre-reinforced polypropylene showed no significant change in tensile strength in this range. After ten recycling cycles, tensile strength decreased by 50% of the initial value for glass-fibre-reinforced polypropylene and 25% for carbon-fibre-reinforced polypropylene. The investigations of the three-point bending test showed similar findings in this respect. Regarding impact strength, the flax-fibre-reinforced and carbon-fibre-reinforced polypropylene showed an increase of about 50% after ten recycling cycles. In contrast, the impact strength of the glass-fibre-reinforced polypropylene had a decrease of 50% with respect to the initial value (Evens et al., 2019).

The findings of Evens et al. (2019) imply an enormous recycling potential for the use of natural-fibre- or wood-fibre-reinforced plastics. This potential can be applied to end products at the end of the product life cycle and especially to rejects (sprue systems, defective articles). In this context, material costs can be saved, and the consumption of fossil resources is reduced. Considering the use of renewable raw materials, the consumption of fossil resources can be further minimised. In the extrusion of wood-plastic composites (WPC), fibre contents of 90-wt-% and WPC injection moulding up to 50-wt-% can be realised very quickly. This allows

50 - 90-wt-% of the plastic matrix to be saved. In connexion with the excellent recyclability and the use of renewable raw materials, the $CO_2$ backpack of injection-moulded articles can be significantly reduced, especially in non-decor areas in the automotive sector. On the other hand, it must be noted, especially in the application of WPC, that advantages in mechanical properties offset the advantages in terms of sustainability and recyclability. The reinforcing effect of wood fibres is significantly lower, compared to glass- or carbon fibre-reinforced plastics; therefore, WPC is not suitable for every application. However, this problem can be countered with the increased use of materials if production and assembly make this possible and the weight saving is not strongly affected. Furthermore, there are other technological challenges to be solved in the process of natural-fibre-reinforced plastics. Drying before processing is essential for the material due to moisture absorption. Residual moisture can lead to corrosion, especially in low-alloy injection moulds (Steidl et al., 2018). In addition, the filling and flow behaviour of WPC melts is not trivial, and segregation phenomena cannot be ruled out at high-flow path lengths (Schröder, 2013).

When selecting the matrix material, it should be noted that wood fibres start to decompose at a temperature of 200 °C and above. Therefore, only a few polymers are suitable matrix materials as these often have a processing temperature above 200 °C. In the European market, the most important representative is polypropylene (PP), and in the United States it is polyethylene (PE). Other plastics used for wood-fibre reinforcement are polyvinyl chloride (PVC) and polystyrene (PS). However, their share of the market is negligible. Another challenge in the selection of starting components is fibre-matrix adhesion. Most matrix materials used (PP, PE) are non-polar. Wood fibres, however, are polar because of their complex chemical structure. Due to this discrepancy in polarity, satisfactory bonding of the fibre to the matrix does not occur. This leads to insufficient force transfer from matrix to fibre, and a reinforcing effect of the fibres cannot be fully achieved. This is remedied with coupling agents, which are additives up to 5-wt-%. The best-known representative of this additive group is maleic anhydride (MAH), but silanes or isocyanates are also suitable for increasing fibre-matrix bonding. Another possibility is the selection of a polar-matrix material. For this purpose and to open new markets for wood-fibre reinforcement, the wood-fibre reinforcement of thermoplastic polyurethanes (TPU) is being advanced. TPU belongs to the material class of thermoplastic elastomers (TPE), which can impress with their thermoplastic processing and elastomeric properties. TPEs can be produced either as polymer blends, in which rubber particles are dispersed in a thermoplastic matrix, or as copolymers. The chain structure is composed of alternating hard and soft segments in copolymers. In the case of TPU, which serves as the matrix for wood-fibre reinforcement, the molecular chain consists of urethane as the hard segment and ester or ether as the soft segment. The advantage of recyclability is given due to the molecular structure analogous to thermoplastics and implies good recyclability. Simple applications are handles for bicycles, anti-slip components in the furniture industry or plastic wheels.

## 1.4 Production of aluminium profiles

As already described for wood-fibre-reinforced plastics, efforts to develop innovative material concepts to improve the properties of a wide range of products are steadily increasing. At the same time, a rethink is taking place in the industrial environment toward energy- and material-efficient manufacturing processes that integrate the processes into a circular economy. The emissions generated in the transport area are also to be reduced through consistent lightweight construction of vehicles and the associated reduction in unloaded weight. These previously named areas are all conditioned by the production and use of semi-finished aluminium products. A major advantage of aluminium as a construction material in a variety of applications is a significantly lower density of $\rho_{Al} = 2.7\ g/cm^3$ compared with steel $\rho_{St} = 7.9\ g/cm^3$. When using aluminium profiles and components, the unloaded weight of the vehicle can be reduced and thus also the emissions generated during use. Aluminium is also increasingly used in the construction sector due to its low density, combined with high strength, favourable workability, and good natural corrosion protection. Regardless of the application, different process and method strategies exist in the production of aluminium components.

The following explanations are limited to an exemplary description of the most diverse possibilities and process chains to produce semi-finished products from a wide variety of aluminium alloys. However, it is generally possible to apply the processes described to sheets or other products. The primary production process of aluminium ingots is one of the most energy-intensive and resource-intensive processes compared to other construction materials. It is based on mining bauxite ore in large mines and subsequent transport for further processing. With the addition of water and anodes, 1 kg of aluminium is obtained in ingot form from 5.1 kg of bauxite ore. However, the production process also produces rejects such as red mud, which must be disposed of at great expense to prevent contamination of the environment. Due to the dependence of the energy required for the process of the energy mix used at each site, it is impossible to give an all-encompassing average value for the energy required for the primary production of one kilogramme of aluminium. Considering that 40% of the electrical energy is obtained from hydropower plants and 60% from coal-fired power plants, the energy input to produce one kilogramme of primary aluminium is 191.9 MJ (Schwarz, 2004). One way of improving this energy balance and generally reducing the emissions generated in the entire primary production process is to obtain electrical energy from alternative energy sources. However, since the location of primary aluminium production has shifted significantly in recent years, an opposite trend is currently taking place. Most of the world's primary aluminium production has shifted to China (Boin et al., 2004; Soo et al., 2018). To satisfy the huge demand for electrical energy, the share of coal-fired power plants in China has increased to more than 60% (Cooper & Allwood, 2012). Therefore, the energy balance of primary aluminium production has deteriorated in recent years. More emissions are generated per kilogramme of aluminium produced.

One way of reducing energy consumption in production of a kilogramme of aluminium in ingot form is smelting metallurgical recycling of rejects or scrap. These rejects are (often) returned to the raw material cycle at the end of the life of the original purpose. The melt metallurgical recycling process is also described in the pertinent literature as the secondary production process. Here, only a small amount of the primary resources is required, but primarily aluminium scrap is collected, sorted, cleaned and subsequently fed to the smelting furnace. The scrap is melted and alloyed into "as-new" aluminium ingots. In the area of feeding the different types of scrap to the secondary production process, a distinction is made between the terms of new scrap and old scrap. The term "new scrap" refers to the surplus material produced during the manufacture of aluminium production until it is sold. Examples of this are chips or stamping residues. Old scrap is obtained from products after a workpiece has been manufactured and used. The effort of the recycling process is lower for new scrap due to grade purity and lower contamination. The energy consumption of secondary aluminium production is lower by an order of magnitude compared to primary production. However, there is a dependence on the composition of the scrap used as well as the need for alloying and other influencing factors. An average value of the energy demand is given as 17.7 MJ/kg aluminium (~ 9 % required for the primary manufacturing process) (Schwarz, 2004). Despite the significantly improved energy efficiency, some disadvantages remain. For each ton of recycled aluminium, 300 to 500 kg of salt slag and up to 35 kg of filter dust are produced. The salt slag has an environmentally hazardous potential due to its high salt content and must be processed and disposed of at great expense (Boin et al., 2004).

As described above, both the primary and secondary aluminium manufacturing processes are used to produce an aluminium ingot. This cannot be used in the cast form and is further processed using downstream manufacturing processes. To produce semi-finished aluminium products (e.g., tubes, profiles), the hot forming process of extrusion is often used. The aluminium ingot is heated to 450 °C to improve processability. The aluminium ingot is then pressed through an individual shaping opening to produce a semi-finished product with the desired geometry. Due to the temporal as well as the spatial distance between the casting of the aluminium ingot (primary as well as secondary), it is usually already completely cooled down and must therefore be reheated before processing by extrusion. Additional thermal energy must be introduced into the process. Despite the enormous improvement in energy efficiency and the greatly reduced impact on the environment, secondary aluminium production is not a universal solution. There is not enough aluminium in circulation or recycled for a complete switch to secondary aluminium production (Soo et al., 2018; Cooper & Allwood, 2012).

To continuously improve the entire manufacturing process of semi-finished aluminium products, extensive investigations into alternative recycling processes have been carried out in recent years. One term frequently used for these (alternative) recycling processes is solid-state recycling. In a typical solid-state recycling process, the scrap to be recycled is not heated to the melting point of 680 °C applicable to aluminium but is plasticised and processed below this temperature. The significantly lower amount of heat to be introduced represents one of the greatest advantages of the solid-state recycling processes over the melting metallurgical approach. From a thermodynamic point of view, the material only needs to be heated to about 300 - 500 °C, and correspondingly less energy needs to be introduced into the process (Wideroe & Welo, 2013; Güley, 2014). This accounts for the significantly improved energy efficiency present for most solid-state recycling processes. Another advantage that many solid-state recycling processes have is that the process step of plasticising as well as the production of the semi-finished product geometry takes place in one step. An example of such an approach is the extrusion of pre-compacted ingots of aluminium chips using a conventional extrusion press. When using a die system that requires a high degree of forming the material, mechanical properties comparable to those of conventionally produced semi-finished products can be produced (Tekkaya et al., 2012). Due to the many possible applications and the high energy input of aluminium production, an improvement in the environmental balance for aluminium can be generated by improving current recycling strategies.

## 1.5 Interfacial design for catalytic recycling of carbon-fibre-reinforced thermoset polymers (CFRPs)

CFRPs, as an engineered composite, have attracted major attention due to the combination of unique properties like a high degree of rigidity, thermal stability, resistance to corrosion, electrical conductivity, also light weight and low density. These features have caused its worldwide usage in a variety of industries and applications, such as aerospace, automobiles, sports equipment, wind power generation, construction and so on. Following by new targets for lower $CO_2$ emissions and the need for light-weighting in different kinds of structures and products, the global demand for composites is projected to continue to grow at a compound annual growth rate (CAGR) of approximately 6%, with the total market increasing from $26 billion in 2018 to $41.4 billion in 2025. (Meng et al., 2018)

The high demand of CFRPs for different purposes in industry sectors presents major environmental challenges in wastes, such as off-cuts generated during composite manufacturing (as much as 40%) and end-of-life CFRP products. The global CFRP waste is projected to increase to 20 KT annually by 2025. With around 6000–8000 commercial aircraft reaching their end-of-life by 2030 (McConnell, 2010), there is a clear and critical demand for developing and organizing economically-sustainable waste management and recycling techniques and processes for CFRPs.

This steady growth of global demand for CFRP in both established and new sectors has also created challenges for recycling and managing waste. The demand for CFRPs has tripled from 2010 to 2020 and is expected to surpass 190 KT by the year 2035 (Pickering & Turner, 2014; Meng et al., 2017; Mishnaevsky et al., 2017).

The production of carbon fibres is a process that consumes around 198–595 MJ/kg (Meng et al., 2018). As a result, the energy consumed by the production of carbon fibres is approximately 10 times higher than that of other synthetic fibres, such as glass fibres. Thus, recovery techniques for waste carbon fibres can enormously reduce their potential environmental impact. As data in the pertinent literature shows, 38.4 MJ/kg is consumed to recycle CFRP by a chemical method (Meng et al., 2017), which is close to 10–30% of the total energy required to manufacture virgin fibres. CFRP recycling is often controlled by the properties of the polymer matrix. Currently, thermoset polymers (e.g., epoxy and unsaturated polyester) are predominantly used as a matrix for CFRPs, representing around 80% of polymer matrix composites (Mishnaevsky et al., 2017). Thermoset polymers undergo a chemical change when cured with low-fracture energy. Another main characteristic of thermoset polymers is high resistance to solvents and low strain to failure (Baker et al., 2004). Besides good fibre-wetting property and formability into complex shapes, these properties have led to the widespread use of thermoset matrixes in CFRP composites (Baker et al., 2004). However, the irreversible cross-linked structure of cured thermoset polymers leads to significant difficulties in the recovery of the fibres and the thermosetting polymer, since they, once cured, cannot be melted, remoulded, reprocessed, or re-crosslinked into solid polymers (Wang et al., 2013).

The global CFRP market is classified according to composite manufacturing methods. The conventional prepreg and lay-up processing are still the most widely used routes for manufacturing products in aerospace and sport (40%) applications (Vita et al., 2019).

Thermoset composites can be recycled by three different methods: (1) chemical recycling refers to processes like pyrolysis in which the material is heated in an oxygen-free environment to produce one or more recoverable substances; (2) in particle recycling, the thermoset composite is mechanically milled into particles to be used as a filler in new plastic or composite applications as a replacement for calcium carbonate or talc, and (3) energy recycling refers to the possibility of incinerating the material to recover energy from its organic portion. Like thermoset composites, thermoplastic composites can also be recycled by chemical or energy methods as described above. In addition, thermoplastic composites can also be recycled by grinding, followed by reprocessing by means of several techniques, such as injection moulding.

There are six potential waste treatment routes for CFRP: landfill, incineration, mechanical, pyrolysis, fluidised bed and chemical recycling processes. For all recycling processes, collected CFRP waste materials are transported to materials disposal facilities for shredding and separation before waste treatment.

## 1.6 Continuum mechanics in material simulation

During the development of technical products, materials and information, their results play an important role. In the end, every technical product consists of a material and frequently a combination of different ones. The choice of a specific combination has a huge impact on the behaviour as well as the environmental impact of the product. For example, building a bicycle from wood, metal, or polymers leads to different responses in different situations (driving through rain, a crash, etc.), but also to different approaches of manufacturing (wood is plant-based, steel is made of iron ore, obtained from mining, polymers mostly rely on oil). To be able to use a specific class of materials, such as sustainable bio-grade WPC, precise knowledge of their behaviour is needed. This excerpt provides ideas that have been detailed in standard works such as Mahnken (2011), (2016), (2019), Gross et al. (2009).

The choice of material for a certain product is influenced by the material's properties to resist loadings, which occur in the life cycle of the product. Every loading induces a reaction of the material in the form of deformation (if one stretches a rubber band, it will largely deform) and internal forces. The internal forces are mostly hidden from us if they are low, but if they get too high, permanent deformations remain and/or fracture can occur, leading to catastrophic failure of the product (e.g., a car crash). The number of internal forces which can be resisted is a characteristic of every material and needs to be obtained through experiments. The actual state of internal forces, also called stresses, can be calculated and depend on the geometry of the product. By smartly choosing the geometry (e.g., thickness, radii, etc.), the stresses can be distributed over large areas, avoiding peaks, which could lead to potential areas of failure. A smart distribution can economise material, as high-stress areas are often compensated for by large amounts of material ("if something repeatedly breaks, make it thicker"). The area of engineering dedicated to the analysis of stresses is called engineering mechanics.

Engineering can be considered the physics part of mechanical engineering. According to Maxwell, "Physics is the natural science that studies matter, its motion and behaviour through space and time, and the related entities of energy and force." While modern physics is mostly concerned with subatomic phenomena, engineers are interested in the behaviour of macroscopic ("real world") effects. More precisely, the "continuum mechanics" branch of physics is concerned with materials modelled as a continuous mass rather than particles, typically on scales from 100 nanometers upwards. The entities of interest are the relationships among force, matter, and motion. The assumption of a continuous body greatly simplifies calculations of these quantities, and hundreds of years of engineering accomplishments have proven the effectiveness of this approach (exceptions confirm the rule).

Forces acting on structures from the outside induce inner forces inside them. These inner forces, or stresses, define the ratio of forces acting on small material surfaces. In the simplest case, the case of a rod with a constant radius over its length under uniaxial loading, the formula of stress is given by: stress equals force to cross-section area.

The larger the external force, the larger the stress. The larger the cross-section area the force is acting on, the smaller the stress, as the force distributes over a larger area. Unfortunately, this simple law only remains true for the rod with a constant radius. Just by altering the radius at some point of the rod, disturbs the flow of force through it, which leads to increased stress locally. For simple geometries, like rods, beams, shells and plates, formulas are known to calculate the outgoing stresses by hand. For more complex structures, computer methods, often expensive and long-lasting, must be applied.

Besides stresses, absolute deformation of the structure and relative displacements are of interest. The absolute deformation is defined by displacements, which gives a number to the amount of deflection of a part. So-called strains describe the relative deformation of two neighbouring points. Strains and displacements are related to each other and can be calculated, if one or the other is given. Between stresses and strains, there exists the so-called constitutive relation, which is defined by a material law. For a given stress field, the corresponding deformation can then be calculated or vice versa.

These material laws are very important to capture the behaviour of real-world structures and materials in a simulation environment. Consequently, many sophisticated material laws were invented. Often, these need to be calibrated by experiments.

Although continuum mechanics studies fluids as well, the main concern of this text is solids. A solid material can withstand several load cases, namely pressure, stretching and shearing. If the material response, e.g., the deformation, is the same for all possible loading directions, the material is said to be isotropic. This is the case for most homogeneous materials, such as steel. If the material response is different in only one direction but the same in all the others, it is called transversely isotropic. The general case is anisotropic behaviour, which is different for all loading cases. The direction-dependent material response strongly depends on the microstructure of the material. Long-fibre-reinforced plastics have a pronounced transversely isotropic behaviour, whereas short-fibre-reinforced plastics with randomly dispersed fibre can be described as isotropic.

A further distinction must be made with respect to the stress magnitude. For small stress levels, the material will deform and return to its original state after relief. This behaviour is called elastic. If the stress exerts a certain point, called the yield limit, permanent deformations remain. This is called plastification. Plasticity is mostly considered in manufacturing processes, whereas the elastic part is interesting for general structural engineering, where permanent deformations need to be avoided.

The characteristic modes of behaviour of materials are mathematically described by material laws, which couple deformations and stresses. The key features of these laws are so-called material parameters. The more complex the material behaviour, e.g., fully anisotropic, the more material parameters are needed to describe the response for all possible loading states. These parameters must be obtained by experiments, like tensile and shear tests.

An engineer can manipulate the response of a structure by choosing its shape and material accordingly. In the case of structural elements, the key is to design a part in such a way that the stresses don't exert the specific yielding point of the material. If certain stresses are too high, the structure needs to be sturdier, the material must be added, or a different material must be chosen.

If the choice of material is restricted, the safest method of avoiding high stresses, which could lead to the failure of the structure, is to add more material – this will, of course, result in higher mass and material consumption. Often a lack of knowledge or expertise in stress analysis leads to such a safe, but inefficient approach of structural engineering. By smartly exploiting direction-dependent behaviour, stress analysis and stress-driven design, the material can be saved.

To go one step further, the optimal distribution of stresses in a structure can aid as a first principal design decision baseline by using techniques such as topology optimisation. Here, the first design is chosen by means of a computer-generated structure, considering only boundary conditions like building space, loading, and fixation. Then the optimal design is found by minimising the material needed while fulfilling conditions such as maximally allowed stress or displacement.

More complexity to material simulations is added by including the effects of recycling processes on material response. Not only the microstructure of, e.g., fibre-reinforced materials is altered due to shredding or heat treatment, but also the material parameters are modified. For example, polymers show a degradation effect after several cycles of melting and reprocessing. A better knowledge of the effect of recycling leads to a better understanding of the behaviour of structural elements made of recycled materials, which leads to more acceptance and usage of such materials.

In summary, the better an engineer knows the stress distribution inside a product, the less material is needed because stress peaks can be avoided where bulk material would be needed to bypass failure. A lack of knowledge forces the engineer to consider additional material in certain product areas for safety purposes. Furthermore, uncommon materials or recycled materials can only be used in engineering contexts if their behaviour is predictable, calling for tailored calculation methods in such cases.

## 2 Industry project

To clarify the process and also the challenges of interdisciplinary and transdisciplinary work, an example of collaboration between an industrial partner and scientists from different disciplines is discussed in this section. For this purpose, the possible optimisation potentials in terms of sustainability are shown on the basis of a bicycle stand (Turrix stand). The Turrix considered in this work is already established on the market and is manufactured by injection moulding from a thermoplastic with glass fibre content. The material used is made from fossil raw materials. Disposal at the end of life takes place via household waste; so there is no re-use of either the structure or the material. A recycling process that has been established in this context is thermal recycling.

This project shows how a positive benefit for the environment can already be achieved with small changes in the choice of materials. It also investigates how further positive effects can be achieved through constructive design with the use of lightweight construction principles.

First, the actual state of the material (glass-fibre-reinforced polypropylene) as well as the current production process are recorded. Alternative materials are shown and compared with each other in terms of mechanical properties and sustainability. Furthermore, the finite element method is used to determine the stress distribution and the lightweight design potentials. Based on this information, suggestions for improvement and design optimisation potentials can be identified. These have a positive effect on the strength of the product and reduce the amount of material to be used. Finally, the future perspectives regarding the changed geometry and areas of application as well as the changed material are shown.

To give the reader a better insight into the communication channels and processes during the entire project, these are also described. A central component here is the communication as well as the interaction of all participants in networks of industry, trade and research partners. Hereby, the great potentials that arise from interdisciplinary and transdisciplinary communication and cooperation are to be demonstrated on the basis of a real industrial project.

## 2.1 Cooperation

The industrial partner in this project is the manufacturer of the Turrix, Hebie GmbH & Co. KG. The foundation of Hebie was set on 21 January 1868, and bicycle elements have been part of the company's product range since 1905. Hebie has existed by name since 1925 and is an acronym for **He**mmelskamp (founder's name) and **Bie**lefeld (location). Today, in 2021, Hebie is a company with 60 employees. The company is well versed in steel, aluminium, and plastic processing. The product range includes important accessories for operating a bicycle. The company manufactures bicycle stands, spray mudguards, transport containers, and other add-on parts. As a guiding principle, Hebie addresses aspects of Corporate Social Responsibility (CSR). Hebie focuses on a humane working environment and considers measures to counter the scarcity of resources as a responsibility towards future generations. To sensitise its employees for a sustainable way of life, Hebie supports employees to travel by bicycle. Among other things, Hebie offers its employees well-placed parking facilities and showers to make the journey as pleasant as possible.

For the Turrix, proven materials and production methods were used, as the company already has expertise and experience in this area. Materials made from renewable raw materials are for the most part still in the development process. The knowledge about many of these materials and about the manufacturing conditions is often already available, but the transfer from research to the broad range of industrial products is not as fast. Many manufacturers are uncertain about using unknown materials, which are usually more expensive than the already established materials. The higher price also often deters customers from buying. These uncertainties can be eliminated through targeted education.

Researchers always focus on scientific and technological challenges and questions. Scientists want to find out how the world works and how the physical and chemical relationships can be used optimally for the prosperity and development of society. It is precisely this link to society and the needs of individuals or groups of people that is not easy and requires separate consideration. Among other things, communication channels between society's actors and scientists must be developed and used extensively because only through communication at the same level can new and innovative approaches to society's problems be generated.

This is exactly the challenge the authors of this paper faced at the beginning of their research. The first challenge was to develop solutions for recycling issues in a new, interdisciplinary team. At this stage, structures had to be developed for common understanding and joint working among the researchers from different disciplines. In addition, social actors were involved in defining the issues to be investigated. Networking among researchers from different disciplines is comparatively easy, e.g., through papers and conferences. Networking with industry, politics and associations/organisations/networks, on the other hand, is more complicated. Only rarely are the wishes of the other actors for the future known. Often, these are only insignificant or even non-existent. Or the willingness to work on innovations is not given. In addition, transdisciplinary research collaboration is especially challenging when it comes to engineering topics (Horwath et al., 2018). Thus, the search for suitable partners often turns out to be tedious and elaborate.

A common, clearly defined goal is a must for successful collaboration. An obvious definition is best worked out together with partners. In addition, a prevailing vision and commitment must already exist. Finding suitable partners in network organisations with similar interests is a proven strategy. In a network, a major theme already exists. The members are interested in issues in this area and are usually willing to actively participate in projects. For our main topic of recycling, we have been in contact with some networks. The events/workshops organised in these networks provided important initial input for the authors' work, as the composition of the participants included representatives from different fields of recycling. In order to create an overview of the field of recycling, all the players involved need to explain the challenges from their point of view. Besides the recycling companies themselves, there are the raw material producers, the product and process developers, the legislators. The waste must not only be collected and sorted but also appropriately processed so that what was supposed to be garbage becomes a usable material again. It is the duty of the product developers to ensure the recyclability of the product already in the development phase and to provide already recycled materials for new products. Legislators must create legal requirements, such as mandatory labelling for materials, or recycling quotas.

To get a more specific input, a "thought school" with the topic "Sustainable and responsible engineering" was organised. The event concept consisting of two specific workshops and a keynote lecture has proven to be very effective for transdisciplinary research as well as for the dialogue between science and society. Other research institutions, industry representatives, network representatives, Scientists for Future, Ingenieure ohne Grenzen (Engineers without Borders), and interested members of the public participated. In a productive collaboration, significant issues concerning sustainability in technology were identified. Among other things, the use of renewable or recycled materials was discussed. The advantages of these materials were emphasised, but the challenges and prohibitions in their use were also addressed. After intensive discussions with the network representatives, it was also possible to identify industrial partners with the respective product groups for further research. In this way, a reliable industrial partner was found in a company from the region.

During the project, one typical problem within transdisciplinary research is communication and integration of different points of view, styles of thought and bases of knowledge (Jahn et al., 2012; Pohl et al., 2017). Here, not only the different experts from the university had to contribute to the outcome, but also the company and its different departments. A huge difference in acceptance of, for example, bio-grade materials, such as WPC, was observed among them. Whereas the marketing department was euphoric about the possibilities of sustainable engineering, the manufacturing department was sceptical. Additionally, communication with experts from the company was tunnelled through a single individual, which led to a delay in information flow. This was, of course, amplified by the global pandemic situation. Clear documentation of the needs of every single contributor included in the project helped to make everybody's interest visible and to identify suitable subgroups for tackling specific problems. Also, motivated management helped everyone to stay on track and to keep the project's goals clearly defined while staying within the schedule.

## 2.2 The Turrix stand

The conventional version of the bicycle stand to be optimised is made of a glass-fibre reinforced polypropylene with a fibre content of 30-Ma-%. The stand is constructed from three components: standing foot, stand, bracket(s) (Figure 5).

The standing foot is connected to the stand by a plug-in system and secures the stand against a tilting moment when loaded. To be able to illustrate different frame sizes and shapes, the brackets can also be attached at different distances via a plug-in system. With a weight of about 1100 g, the bike stand can be taken on a huge number of bike tours and is very well suited for MTB and road bikes, which are often specified without a fixed stand on the wheel. The suspension of the tire makes it easy to work on the rear wheel or adjust the gearshift because the crank and the wheel can rotate freely. Furthermore, two bike racks can act as wall fixtures so that the bike can be stored in a space-saving way. The high load capacity of approx. 12 kg as a floor stand or 20 kg as a wall mount was achieved through rib structures in the component design.

*Figure 5: bicycle stand - Turrix*

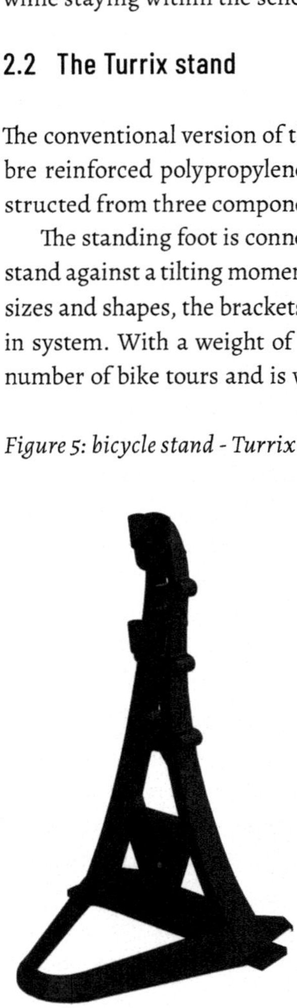

## 2.3 Materials

The need for new, innovative and sustainable materials is great. Increasing mechanical properties should be combined with an increasingly sustainable manufacturing and recycling process. Composite materials are one material class that has the potential to comply with these requirements.

A composite material can be defined as a combination of two or more materials that results in better properties than those of the individual components used alone (Campbell, 2010). Composite materials are classified according to their content, i.e., base material and filler material. The base material, which binds or holds the filler material in structures, is termed as a matrix or a binder material, while filler material is present in the form of sheets, fragments, particles, fibres or whiskers of natural or synthetic materials. In terms of sustainability aspects, the binder material as well as the filler material can be replaced with more environmentally friendly materials (La Mantia, 2011). Besides more environmentally friendly binder materials, especially the filler material shows great potential to produce more sustainable composites. (Alireza, 2008)

Composites can be classified into three main categories based on the different filler materials used (Altenbach et al., 2004). Besides the sheet-moulded as well as the particle-reinforced composites there is a third class which is based on fibre-reinforced composites. These fibre-reinforced composites show interesting mechanical behaviour which is reflected in the used fibre material as well as in the length of the used fibre.

Composites with long-fibre reinforcements are termed as continuous fibre reinforcement composites, while composites with short-fibre reinforcements are called discontinuous fibre reinforcement composites. The orientation of the fibres in the matrix material is also an important parameter for the mechanical properties.

The material of the used fibre has also an influence. On the one hand composite materials contain fibres of glass, carbon, basalt, and aramid in the dispersed phase. These fibres were conventionally used in the matrix structure of fibre-reinforced polymer (FRP) composite materials.

On the other hand, there is a second class of composites based on natural fibre content. These natural fibre polymer composites (NFPCs) have potential applications in modern industry, as researchers currently are directed towards the development of materials with low environmental impact due to stringent environmental laws. There are numerous fibres available for composite materials, and they are primarily categorised as natural or synthetic fibres.

## Synthetic Fibres:

Technical fibres produced by chemical synthesis are named synthetic fibres and further classified as organic or inorganic based on their content. The use of synthetic fibres in composite materials offers the opportunity to produce components with great stiffness. For different application areas there are several synthetic fibres available. (Sathishkumar et al., 2014; Friedrich, 2017)

Glass fibres (GFs) are most widely used among all the synthetic fibres as they offer excellent strength and durability, thermal stability, resistance to impact, chemical, friction, and wearing properties. For applications where the highest stiffness is needed, carbon fibres are used instead of glass fibres. The used carbon fibres are about 5–10 micrometers in diameter and composed mostly of carbon atoms. Carbon fibres have several advantages other than that already mentioned, such as high tensile strength, low weight, high chemical resistance, high temperature tolerance, and low thermal expansion. There are many more synthetic fibres, which are produced from different materials, like polyacrylonitrile- (PAN-), polyethylene terephthalate- (PET) or polypropylene fibres (PP-F) (Unterweger et al., 2013; Friedrich, 2017)

However, there are some disadvantages when using synthetic fibres in composite materials. The machining of glass fibre-reinforced polymers (GFRPs) is relatively slow, challenging, and shows reduced tool life while working on conventional machining systems (Prakash & Laxminarayana, 2019). Moreover, there is a great problem when it comes to the bad environmental aspect of synthetic fibres. GFs have the disadvantage that they cannot be simply reused at the end of life.

### Natural fibres:

As a consequence of the environmental and energy issues based on the unpalatable recycling potential of synthetic fibres and in terms of growing sustainability aspects, the use of natural fibres in composite materials is desirable. Natural fibre-reinforced polymer (NFRPs) composites have a high potential for producing new composite materials that have great renewability, sustainability and availability-aspects. Also, the good accessibility of natural fibre material leads to lower costs when it comes to manufacturing these materials. (Gangil et al., 2020)

Composites made of NF reinforcements seem to show diverse properties with respect to synthetic fibres, such as reduced weight, cost, toxicity, environmental pollution, and recyclability. These economic and environmental benefits of NF composites make them superior to synthetic fibre-reinforced composites for modern applications (Nair & Joseph, 2014)

There are many different materials which can be used as natural fibre materials: wood, hemp, flax. Conventional plastics and also bioplastics such as **poly-lactic acid (PLA)** can be used as a matrix. PLA is one of the most promising bioplastics because of its attractive mechanical properties, low emission of greenhouse gases, low amount of energy used for production, biodegradability and high industrial production capacity.

Wood-Plastic Composite (WPC) is the term that refers to any number of composites that contain wood (wood flour, wood fibre) and either thermoset or thermoplastic polymers. Adding fibres rather than flour increases mechanical properties such as strength, stiffness. Thermosets are plastics that, once cured, cannot be remelted by heating, such as epoxies and phenolics. Thermoplastics are plastics that can be repeatedly melted, such as polyethylene, polypropylene, and polyvinyl chloride (PVC). (Rowell, 2013; Jacobson et al., 2002)

These composites also contain additives that are added in small amounts to affect processing and performance, such as coupling agents, light stabilisers, pigments, lubricants, fungicides, and foaming agents. Since the wood component of a wood-thermoplastic composite is hydrophilic and the plastic is hydrophobic, a compatibiliser is often used to improve the interfacial bonding of the two different phases. One of the most common compatibilisers used today is a maleic anhydride grafted polypropylene (MAPP). Because of the limited thermal stability of wood, it was believed initially that only thermoplastics that melt or can be processed at temperatures below 200°C could be used in WPCs, and currently that is the practice. Most WPCs are made with polyethylene, both recycled and virgin. However, WPCs made with wood-polypropylene are typically used in automotive applications and consumer products. (Yuan et al., 2008; Mapleston, 2001)

*Table 1 Selected mechanical properties of fibre materials (Sears et al., 2001; Caulfield et al., 2001; Kuo et al., 2009)*

| **Plastic/Composite** | **Tensile Strength (MPa)** | **Bending Strength (MPa)** | **Tensile Young's modulus (GPa)** | **Bending Young's modulus (GPa)** |
|---|---|---|---|---|
| PA-6+33% Glass fibre | 111 | 146 | 8.0 | 7.5 |
| PP+33% Wood flour | 33 | 49 | 3.4 | 3.2 |
| PA-6+33% Hardwood fibre | 86 | 121 | 5.7 | 5.9 |
| PA-6+33% Softwood fibre | 81 | 113 | 5.3 | 5.5 |

Table 1 shows the mechanical properties of composites with glass fibre and renewable fibres. Depending on the type of renewable fibre used, WPC can achieve up to 80 % of the properties of GFRP. From a technical point of view, a substitution of materials can be carried out in many applications. Composites with glass fibres consist entirely of fossil raw materials and cannot always be fully recycled. By substituting glass fibres with fibres from renewable materials, 33% of the material is already replaced by a sustainable material. The positive effect this has on our environment is enormous.

## 2.4 Manufacturing

Injection moulding machines are used to manufacture such fibre-reinforced plastic components. In principle, injection moulding machines consist of a plasticising unit and a mould bed with a mould. In the plasticising unit, a screw conveyor melts the material by thermal energy input and friction. Mass temperatures of

200-300 °C are used for injection moulding a 30-wt% glass-fibre-reinforced plastic, so that a sufficiently low-viscosity melt is present in the screw antechamber. For injection moulding of 30-wt% wood-fibre-reinforced plastics, a much lower temperature is used. To protect the material and fibres, an increasing temperature profile is set from the feed to the nozzles. The maximum temperature of 200 °C should not be exceeded under any circumstances, as the wood fibres and their constituents begin to decompose above a temperature of 200 °C.

Against a back pressure, which can be set to a defined value, the material is conveyed by the rotary motion of the screw into the screw antechamber. The increasing volume of material in the screw forechamber causes the screw to be successively pressed against the conveying direction of the screw. The back pressure represents the resistance to this translational movement and ensures that the melt in the screw antechamber develops a high thermal melt homogeneity under pressure. This is essential for the filling process and ensures the reproducible production of injection-moulded components. Fibre degradation occurs in the metering phase due to fibre-fibre, fibre-melt and fibre-cylinder wall interaction. Fibre degradation depends on machine parameters such as barrel and screw geometry and process parameters such as speed (Moritzer & Bürenhaus, 2021). Furthermore, the properties of the polymer and fibre used are decisive. Generally, longer fibres in the final component imply higher strengths. In science, the term "critical fibre length" is often used. If the fibre length falls short of this value, no reinforcing effect can be achieved by the fibre (Evens et al., 2019).

Although wood fibres are very flexible, they tend to degrade in length, just like glass fibres. Furthermore, the mechanical properties are reduced by thermal decomposition due to high-temperature exposure of the fibre. Due to this fact, the barrel temperature, as well as the residence time in the plasticising unit, are crucial for successful injection moulding. In addition, residual water in wood-fibre-reinforced compounds affects the mechanical properties of the injection-moulded articles and the surface properties (streaking). (Radovanovic, 2007)

To generate a reproducible part quality, pre-drying of the compound at 90 °C for at least four hours is necessary.

After the temperature-controlled mould is closed, the injection unit moves to the sprue bushing of the mould so that the nozzle is flush with the sprue. The melt is then injected into the cavity of the mould by the forward movement of the screw. The speed of the screw's forward motion, which corresponds to the injection volume flow, can be set in a defined manner. Here it is possible, especially for demanding geometrical components, to set the injection speed as a step profile (ex. 22 - 240 mm/s) so that the moulding cavity is filled in a few seconds (ex. 4 -5 s).

The holding pressure phase begins as soon as the cavity is filled volumetrically. During the holding pressure phase, melt flows into the cavity at a defined pressure level to compensate for the shrinkage caused by cooling. As soon as the sealing point, which reflects the freezing of the sprue, is reached, residual cooling time begins (approx. 40 s). During this time, the dosing phase for the next cycle begins. Once the part has cooled, the mould opens, and the part is removed from the cavity by the forward motion of the ejector. In the case of the bicycle stand, the rib structure is a special feature and has a significant influence on the high load. Rib structures form an undercut in the injection moulding process, making simple demoulding impossible. Smaller undercuts can be easily realised by forced demoulding. A large undercut can only be realised by sliders, which release the undercut when the mould is opened.

Comparing the two basic starting materials, good sustainability aspects can be identified for the wood-fibre-reinforced Turrix. The reinforcing material used is a renewable material that has converted $CO_2$ into oxygen via photosynthesis during its lifetime. The production of glass fibres and glass-fibre-reinforced plastics requires more energy than wood and wood-fibre-reinforced plastics, which results in advantages in terms of the carbon footprint.

In the current development of fibre-reinforced components, the use of the product at the end of its life also plays a major role. At the end of the product life at least, recycling the material should be the premise. Separation of the matrix from the fibre, which corresponds to feedstock recycling, is possible for wood-fibre-reinforced plastics and glass-fibre-reinforced plastics. However, this is only possible with a high energy input, and mechanical recycling should be preferred. In terms of this, wood-fibre-reinforced plastics also have an advantage here. Glass fibres tend to degrade during recycling so that the fibre length is reduced below the critical fibre length. As a result, the force from the matrix to the fibre can no longer be transferred properly and the mechanical properties decrease. Wood-fibre-reinforced plastics also tend to degrade in length, but the reduction in mechanical properties is smaller compared to glass-fibre-reinforced plastics. This can be explained in the presence of a coupling agent by the increased true surface area of the wood fibres. As a result, the wettable surface is significantly higher; therefore the force can be better transferred into the fibre.

## 2.5 Results of technical development

The present design by the original Turrix was not engineered with optimal stress distribution or lightweight principles in mind. Therefore, we suggested that hidden potential with respect to weight reduction and material saving could be present.

To investigate these claims, the part had to undergo a state-of-the-art stress analysis with the help of the finite element method to determine its status quo. Luckily, the original construction (computer-aided design – CAD) data was available, which saved time that otherwise would have been spent on digitalising the geometry. Unfortunately, but as expected, the CAD files were partially corrupt-

*Figure 6: The repaired construction of the Turrix*

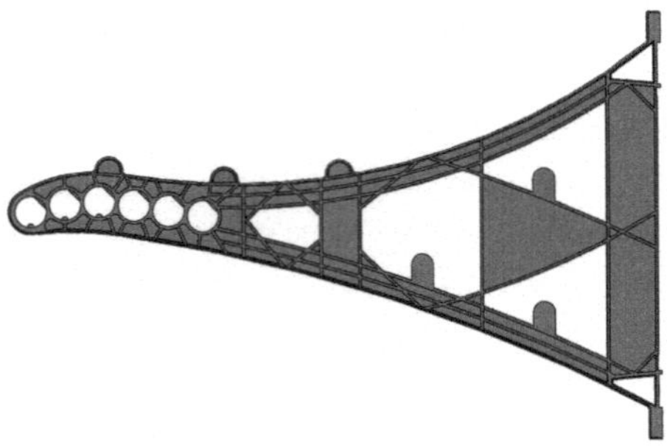

ed. This is often the case when the designer working with a CAD programme does not interact with a calculation engineer working in a simulation (finite elements method – FEM) programme. Due to different companies involved in these programmes, the interchangeability is not always straightforward and relies on a close interaction among professionals. Often a lack of attention paid to details in geometry creation, which does not interfere with the designer's work, leads to problems during the calculation stage for the FEM specialist. The first step is, therefore, to repair the problematic areas of the part to obtain a clean CAD file suitable for FEM calculations (Figure 6). This process can take days or even weeks, depending on the number of errors. It could have been avoided by working hand in hand from the first day on.

After this initial step, the so-called mesh generation stage follows. As the physics of complex shapes prohibits simple formulae for displacement, strains and stresses, a different approach must be taken. In FEM, complex geometry is divided into many small, simple geometric shapes, often cubes or tetrahedra, for which the solution can be obtained locally. By calculating the response of these small, simple geometric parts and adding them together, an approximate solution for the original part can be obtained. The process of dividing the large part into smaller parts is called meshing. The finer the mesh containing cubes or tetrahedra, the lower the approximation error. Unfortunately, the computational effort to calculate these many solutions also rises. To find an appropriate size for the mesh, a so-called convergence study must be carried out. Here, a coarse mesh is used to obtain the first solutions. Then, the mesh is refined step by step, whereas, for each refinement stage, the results will change. The finer the mesh gets, the smaller these changes will be until so-called convergence sets in, which means the change of two refinement stages is smaller than the desired precision. The resulting mesh is a compromise between accuracy and computational effort.

The next step is the analysis itself. Here, the appropriate boundary conditions must be applied, i.e., fixations and loadings. This step, although technically trivial, has arguably the highest impact on the outcome of the analysis. It is often difficult to replicate all possible loading situations of the real-world part within the simulation environment. In the case of the Turrix, the load case was predefined by Hebie, consisting of a typical problem in the lifetime of the product. The stand is fixed on a wall while carrying a bicycle in conjunction with another Turrix. The maximum load

*Figure 7: Displacement of the Turrix from GFRP*

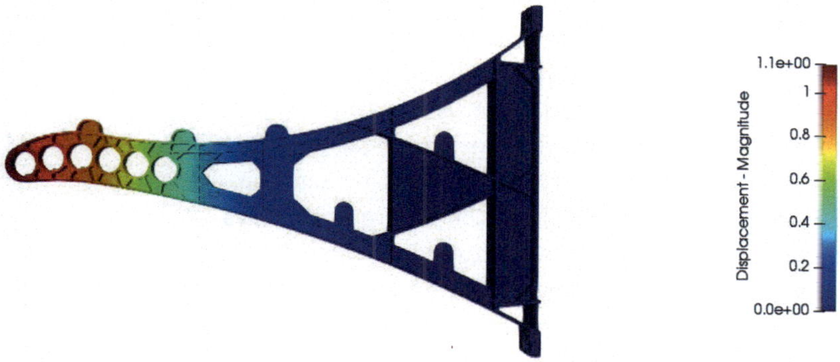


for this situation is 20 kg, which means that a 40 kg bicycle would be placed above both stands. This loading situation is reasonable. A typical bicycle has a much lower weight, but uncertainty with respect to many factors, including the ones explained above, justifies this loading assumption. By utilising higher loads than usually expected, a safety margin is introduced. After the definition of the boundary conditions, the computer will take care of the calculation process.

Once the calculations are finished, the engineer will be able to investigate the solutions of displacement, strain, and stress fields. Care must be taken to track errors made during boundary condition applications, such as downward bending of the structure while bending upwards due to an upwards directed load. Another common error is an interchange of units, e.g., tons instead of kg, etc. In the context of small deformations and linear elastic material behaviour, the maximum displacement must not be too large in order to avoid errors induced by the theory. As a rule of thumb, the maximum displacement should not exceed 5 % of the cross-section depth. The allowed displacement is calculated by the simple formula length of the part times 0.05. For different materials, the maximum displacement will differ, as stiffer material does not deform as much as a weaker one. Therefore, the displacement can be compared for the materials under consideration. In the case of the original material, a glass-fibre-reinforced plastic (GFRP), the maximum displacement is around 0.7 mm (Figure 7).

Arguably, the most critical part of the analysis is the resulting stress fields. The stress field should be continuous without having large jumps from one element of the mesh to another. If large jumps are present, the mesh is locally too coarse and needs to be refined. As mentioned in chapter 1.6, the stresses only depend on the geometry and the external loading. Thus, using different materials, the resulting stresses are the same. The only difference is the maximal stress a specific material can withstand. To compare different materials, first, the maximal equivalent tensile stress must be identified from the simulation. Then, the yield limits from the materials under consideration can be compared to that value. Generally, the maximal equivalent stress should be lower than the yield limit, including a safety factor of around 1.5 – 2 for structures that are not directly related to human safety. If the current structure is within this range for a certain material, this material can be regarded as appropriate for the construction. In the case of the original material mentioned above, the maximum v. Mises equivalent stress is 6.28 MPa, whereas the yield limit is 77 MPa. Therefore, the safety margin is up to ten times the yield limit, which is very high. One can argue that much material can be saved, as only a safety margin of two is needed. Additionally, the stress distribution is inhomogeneous, resulting in parts with high stresses and parts with low stresses (Figure 8). As described in chapter 1.6, this means that the structure is not optimal and possesses optimisation potential.

*Figure 8: Stress distribution in the Turrix*

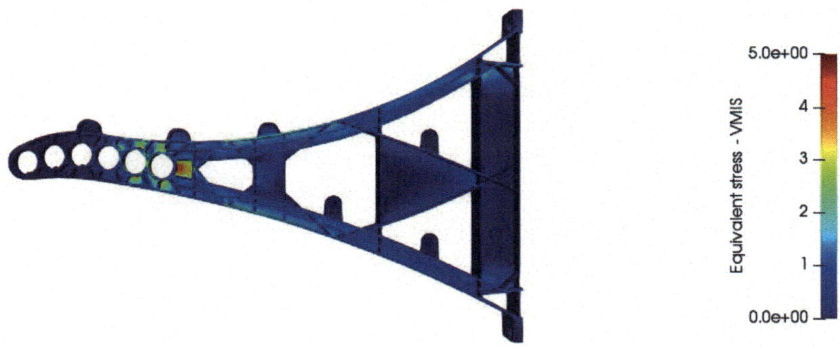


It was shown that the current design of the Turrix stand is far from optimal with respect to stress distribution and lightweight design potential. Now, an alternative design is found by means of topology optimisation, introduced in chapter 1.6.

The overall goal is to yield a more homogeneous stress distribution in the structure to avoid stress peaks and, therefore to use the structure to full capacity. Then the present material should be replaced by a more environmentally friendly one, in order to reduce the amount of plastic used in the original product. The decision, which material to use, will be based on a life-cycle assessment.

For topology optimisation, different design spaces were chosen to restrict the design. Functional parts, as well as design parts, were taken as predefined, such as the holes in the front part of the structure. The loading surface where the bicycle is placed should also remain. Additionally, the fixation structure on the backside is fixed. One possible design space (green) is shown in Figure 9.

After several optimisations and re-analysis, four designs were identified as feasible. They were investigated in more detail by first reconstructing the raw optimisation results using CAD software. The obtained designs were then analysed. The fourth design (Figure 10) had the best performance with respect to peak equivalent stress, displacement, and weight reduction. The resulting design is much simpler and straightforward, avoiding small details, which also makes it more workable for the manufacturing process. The stress magnitude lies around 10 MPa, which makes the design open for a wide range of possible material choices. The displacement and stress field can be seen in Figure 11.

*Figure 9: Design space of Turrix*

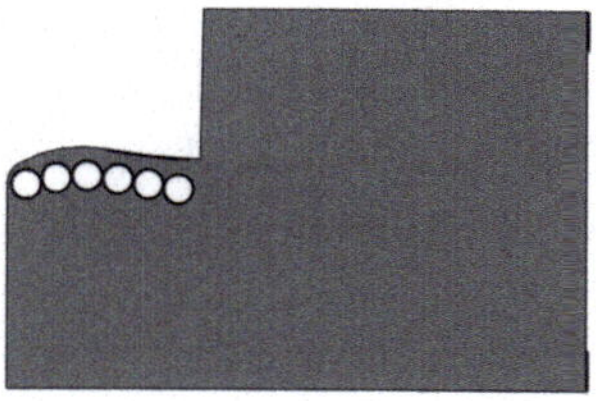

*Figure 10: left: Optimised design space; right: Design of a modified Turrix*

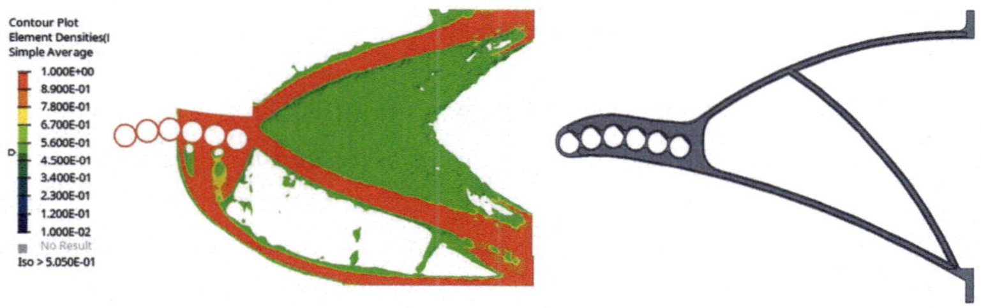


*Figure 11: Displacement (left) and stress (right) field in an optimised Turrix*

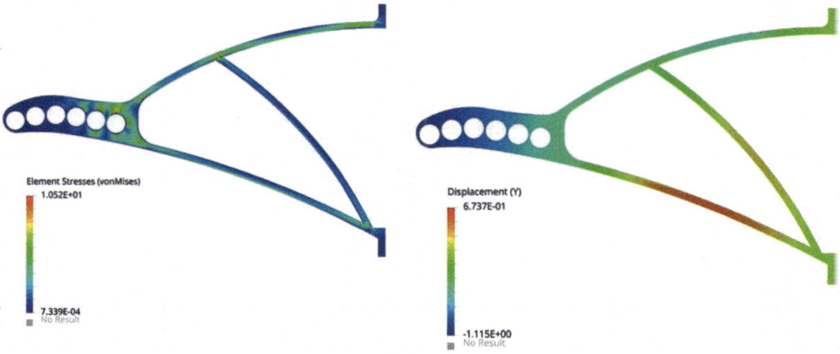


Compared to the original Turrix, the volume of the optimised bicycle stand has been reduced by about 50%. This means that half of the used plastic could have been saved by using an optimised geometry. This great potential for saving materials can contribute to reducing the impact on the environment.

To choose a material, not only mechanical metrics like displacements or stresses, but also environmental considerations should play a role in order to create a sustainable and economical design. A life cycle assessment (LCA) is a structured analysis of a product to determine its impact on the environment. The scope of the LCA depends on the objective of the investigation. A $CO_2$ balance is conceivable for recording the emissions in production, product use, and the product's end of life.

## 2.6 Implementation of the Life Cycle Assessment

By applying a Life Cycle Assessment (LCA), the influence of applied measures on the $CO_2$ balance of the Turrix is to be investigated in order to be able to assess whether an implementation of the measures is advisable. In the first step, objectives and scope of the LCA are defined. The second step involves drawing up the life cycle inventory. Here it is defined where the boundaries of consideration are drawn and what is included in the life cycle inventory. After the life cycle inventory has been drawn up, the impact assessment of optimisations is carried out. The fourth and last step of the LCA is the evaluation of steps carried out in advance.

### Definition of objectives and scope of investigation

In this section, objectives and scope of the LCA are defined. The product to be examined is the Turrix. Two variants of the Turrix are to be examined. On the one hand, the original Turrix of the Hebie company and on the other hand, the optimised Turrix variant T4, which is the result of the topology optimisation.

The aim of this study is to analyse to what extent the $CO_2$ emissions could be reduced by measures. The first part of the study deals with the $CO_2$ emission saving potential carried out by reducing volume by means of the topology optimisation. The second part looks at the extent to which emissions can be reduced by replacing the material. For this purpose, the previously used material PP GF30 is replaced by a WPC. The main focus is on the extraction of materials and their recyclability. Objectives and the scope of the LCA are thus defined. In the following section, the life cycle inventory of the LCA is sketched.

### Establishing the life cycle inventory

When preparing a life cycle inventory, it is defined which sections of the product's life cycle are to be considered. For the LCA to be carried out, two sections – raw material extraction and recycling – are to be considered. Areas such as use of product are not considered, as no $CO_2$ emissions occur there. The areas considered are highlighted in Figure 12.

*Figure 12: System environment of manufacturing (DIN EN ISO 14040)*

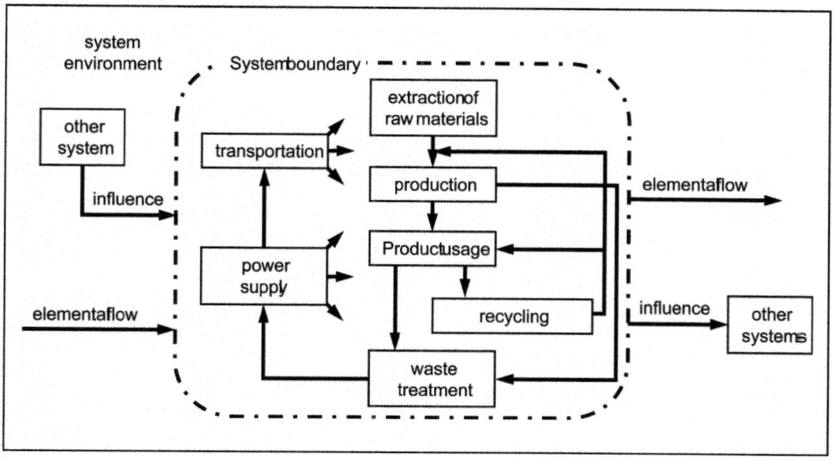


The process step "extraction of raw materials" is understood to be the complete process chain from the extraction of raw material to the finished granulate or fibre material. The parameter that is used for subsequent evaluation is $CO_2$ emissions that are emitted during the production of material.

Two materials were used, the PP GF30 originally used for the Turrix and WPC (PP WF30). Both materials use polypropylene as matrix material. Polypropylene is based on petrochemical raw materials; this has good recycling properties and is therefore also suitable for the desired recyclability. The fibre material in PP GF30 consists of glass and has poor recycling properties. In WPC, these glass fibres are replaced by wood fibres, which can be recycled. The recyclability of the two materials is discussed separately later in this section. The $CO_2$ emissions that are used to produce the individual materials are shown in Table 2.

*Table 2: CO2 emissions of individual components (Corbière-Nicollier et al., 2001; Vanderreydt et al., 2021)*

| **Component** | **$CO_2$ [kg $CO_2$ / kg m]** |
|---|---|
| Polypropylene (PP) | 1.9 |
| Wood fibre | 1.8 |
| Glass fibre | 2.1 |

As can be seen in Table 2, $CO_2$ emissions caused by the wood fibres are lower than those caused by conventionally produced glass fibre. The $CO_2$ emissions generated during further processing of the materials PP GF30 and WPC are assumed to be identical, since only fibre material is exchanged. For this reason, $CO_2$ emissions for compounding, pelletising and processing are not listed in detail. A process model with material and energy flows for the production of the two materials can be seen in Figure 13. The system considered for the subsequent balance calculation is also delimited in the figure.

*Figure 13: Simplified process model for the production of fibre composites*

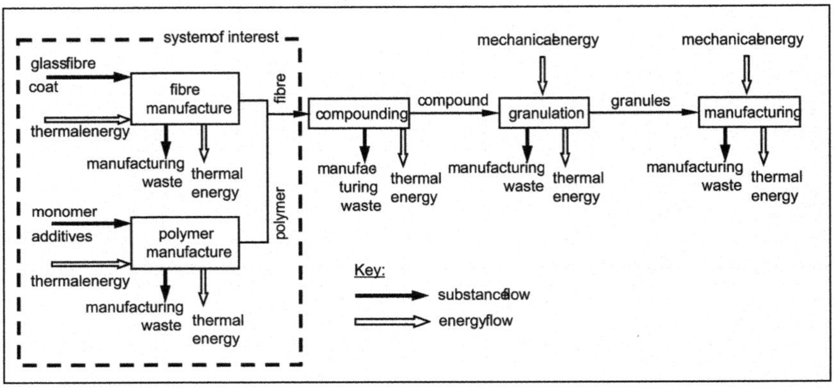


The $CO_2$ emissions for the production of raw materials have been considered; now the focus is turned to the recycling of materials and whether materials can be returned to the value chain.

The recycling of PP GF30 into the value chain is difficult. One problem with recycling is the separation of the glass fibres from matrix material. It is not possible to re-use the material for injection moulding processes. However, it is possible to recycle PP GF30 for other applications after it has been shredded. The crushed material can be added to cement production, for example. However, the aim of this study is to completely recycle material used for production of the Turrix and thus to form a closed material cycle. One possibility to realise this is the substitution of the fibre material with wood fibres. This makes it possible to completely recycle the material by shredding it and then processing it into granulate that is suitable for injection moulding. The advantage is that a closed material cycle can be established. A disadvantage of using recycled WPC is that wood fibres are damaged by the mechanical shredding of the component to be recycled and the thermal stresses in the injection moulding process. Figure 14 shows the percentage of fibre lengths for different recycling cycles.

*Figure 14: Reduction of fibre length with the recycling cycle*

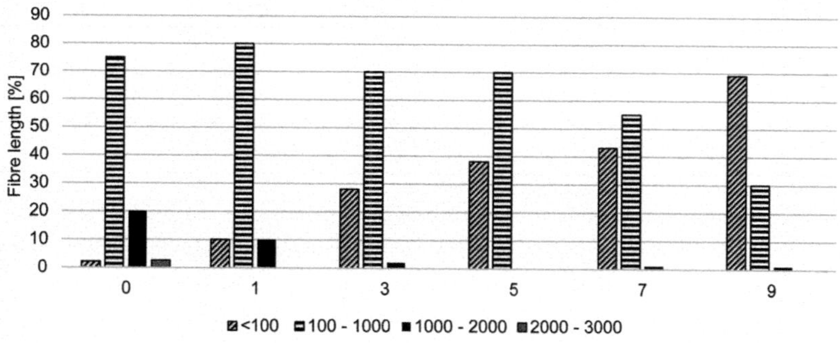


Figure 14 shows that the fibre length decreases with an increasing number of cycles. The reduction in fibre length is accompanied by a decrease in mechanical properties of WPC. In the following diagramme, which is shown in Figure 15, the decrease in tensile strength over the recycling cycles is depicted.

*Figure 15: Reduction of the tensile strength with the recycling cycles*

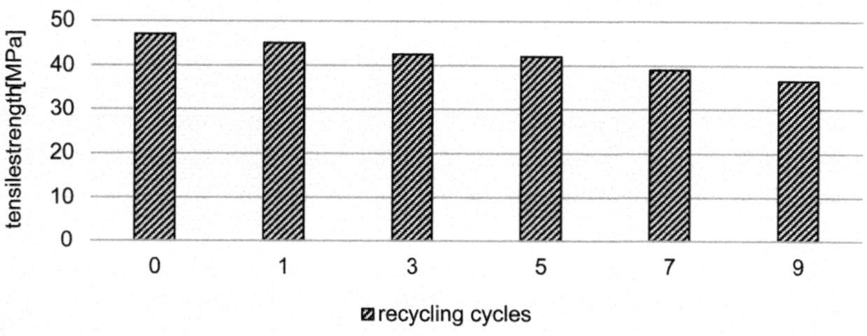


As shown in the diagramme, the tensile strength of WPC decreases by approx. 20% after 9 recycling cycles; whether this decrease is acceptable must be considered individually according to the underlying application of the product. When considering recycling cycles, it must also be taken into account that this does not take place entirely without the emission of $CO_2$. However, these emissions are significantly lower than the emissions that occur when the individual raw materials are newly extracted. A comparison of emissions per recycling cycle with the emissions for the new extraction of the raw materials is shown in Table 3.

*Table 3: Presentation of $CO_2$ emissions per recycling cycle*

| Material | $CO_2$ [kg $CO_2$ / kg m] |
|---|---|
| Polypropylene (PP) | 1.9 |
| Wood fibre | 1.8 |
| WPC recycled (PPWF30) | 1.15 |

The comparison shows that emissions can be significantly reduced by using recycled material. This assumption is mathematically proven in the following section.

## Impact assessment

This section examines the potential $CO_2$ emission savings resulting from optimisations. For $CO_2$ emissions, reference value for evaluation is formed by calculating $CO_2$ emissions generated for the production of materials needed to manufacture a Turrix. The volume of Turrix variants is multiplied by the density of the respective materials. The calculation of $CO_2$ emissions for a Turrix is calculated according to equation 5.1 (Tchana Toffe et al., 2019).

$$CO_{2,T} = \frac{CO_{2,Mat.}}{kg} \cdot m_T \qquad 5.1$$

The quantity $CO_{2,Mat.kg}$ describes how much $CO_2$ per kilogramme is emitted to produce one kilogramme of material used. Equation 5.2 (Tchana Toffe et al., 2019) shows how this quantity is calculated.

$$\frac{CO_{2,Mat.}}{kg} = 0{,}7 \cdot CO_{2,PP} + 0{,}3 \cdot CO_{2,fibre} \qquad 5.2$$

The values for $CO_{2,PP}$ and $CO_{2,fibre}$ can be found in Table 3. The pre-factors are formed by the percentage of the respective material in later composite material (70% PP/ 30% fibre content). The mass used in equation 5.1 represents the mass of the Turrix to be tested. This is calculated according to equation 5.3 (Tchana Toffe et al., 2019).

$$m_t = (0{,}7 \cdot \rho_{PP} + 0{,}3\,\rho_{fibre}) \cdot V_T \qquad 5.3$$

The pre-factors also refer to the percentage weight of individual raw materials in the subsequent composite material. The volume $V_T$ is taken from Table 4. In order to obtain a compact equation, 5.2 and 5.3 are inserted into equation 5.1, so that the following expression for equation 5.1 is formed.

$$CO_{2,T}=(0{,}7\cdot CO_{2,PP}+0{,}3\cdot CO_{2,fibre})\cdot(0{,}7\cdot \rho_{PP}+0{,}3\cdot \rho_{fibre})\cdot V_T \qquad 5.4$$

With the help of equation 5.4 (Tchana Toffe et al., 2019) it is possible to calculate the $CO_2$ emissions that arise during the production of material.

## Reduction through topology optimisation

Now that the calculation method has been presented, it will be calculated how high the saving potential of $CO_2$ emissions is through topology optimisation. To determine this, $CO_2$ emissions (equation 5.1) for Turrix 0 and for Turrix 4 are calculated and listed in the following Table 4.

*Table 4: Potential savings in $CO_2$ emissions through topology optimisation*

| Turrix- Variant | $CO_2$ - Emission [kg $CO_2$ / kg m] | Reduction $CO_2$ - Emission [%] |
|---|---|---|
| Turrix 0 | 2.14 | - |
| Turrix 4 | 1.03 | 52 |

The result shows that a reduction in emissions of 52 % can be achieved by optimising the topology.

## Reduction through substitution of the fibre material

Equation 5.1 is used to calculate how high the reduction in $CO_2$ emissions is by substituting the fibre material. The calculation was carried out with the volume of for both materials in order to be able to subsequently state the reduction in emissions in percent. The result of the calculation is shown in Table 5.

*Table 5: Potential reduction in CO2 emissions through the substitution of fibre material*

| Turrix- Variant | $CO_2$ - Emission [kg $CO_2$ / kg m] | Reduction $CO_2$ - Emission [%] |
|---|---|---|
| Turrix 0 PP GF30 | 2.14 | - |
| Turrix 0 WPC | 1.54 | 28 |

The results show that a reduction in $CO_2$ emissions of 28% can be achieved through the use of WPC.

## Combination of the two approaches

A reduction in $CO_2$ emissions could be achieved through each of the individual approaches. As the investigation has shown, it is also possible to switch to WPC for the Turrix 4 with regard to the mechanical properties, which could further increase the reduction of emissions. Table 6 below lists the respective reductions that could be achieved by combining the two previous approaches.

*Table 6: Potential savings in $CO_2$ emissions through a combination of topology optimisation and substitution of fibre material*

| Turrix- Variant | $CO_2$ - Emission [kg $CO_2$ / kg m] | Reduction $CO_2$ - Emission [%] |
|---|---|---|
| Turrix 0 PP GF30 | 2.14 | - |
| Turrix 4 WPC | 0.74 | 65 |

The result shows that a combination of two approaches can reduce $CO_2$ emissions by 65 %.

## Effect of the recyclability of WPC on $CO_2$ - balance sheet

A significant advantage of WPC over PP GF30 is the complete recyclability of the material, which allows a closed material cycle to be realised. This not only saves resources, but also considerably reduces $CO_2$ emissions. The calculation of emissions per Turrix, taking the recycling cycles into account, can be carried out by using equation 5.5 (Tchana Toffe et al., 2019).

$$CO_{2,T}=\left(\left(0{,}7\cdot CO_{2,pp}+0{,}3\cdot CO_{2,fibre}\right)+CO_{2,Rec.}\cdot n_{cyc.}\right)\cdot\left(0{,}7\cdot \rho_{PP}+0{,}3\cdot \rho_{fibre}\right)\cdot V_T \quad 5.5$$

In equation 5.5, represents the number of cycles performed and $CO_{2,Rec.}$ represents the $CO_2$ emissions generated for recycling the material. For the study, a recycling cycle is considered. The reference value for calculations to be carried out is $CO_2$ emissions emitted by Turrix 0 with material PP GF30. This value is compared with the results of the Turrix 0 WPC and the Turrix 4 WPC, whereby the material is fully recycled. The results of this calculation can be found in Table 7.

*Table 7: Influence of recycled material*

| **Turrix- Variant** | **$CO_2$ - Emission [kg $CO_2$ / kg m]** | **Reduction $CO_2$ - Emission [%]** |
|---|---|---|
| Turrix 0 PP GF30 | 4.27 | - |
| Turrix 0 | 2.49 | 42 |
| Turrix 4 WPC | 1.20 | 72 |

The results presented clearly show that the use of a fully recyclable WPC can significantly reduce $CO_2$ emissions per Turrix. After individual calculations have been carried out, the results will be evaluated in the next section.

## Evaluation

In this section, the results obtained in the section Impact assessment are evaluated and interpreted. In addition, the limitations that need to be taken into account when interpreting the results are discussed. It was investigated whether a reduction of $CO_2$ emissions that arise during raw material extraction can be realised by optimising the topology and substituting the fibre material. Four calculations were carried out, and the results are compared in Table 8 below.

*Table 8: Comparison of results*

| Turrix- Variant | $CO_2$ - Emission **[kg $CO_2$ / kg m]** | **Reduction $CO_2$ - Emission [%]** |
|---|---|---|
| Turrix 0 PP GF30 (comparative value) | 2.14 | - |
| Reduction through topology optimisation | 1.03 | 52 |
| Reduction through substitution of fibre material | 1.54 | 28 |
| Reduction combination | 0.74 | 65 |
| Reduction through recycling of material | 2.49 | 42 |

The results show that two factors have a strong influence. The first factor is the reduction in volume due to the topology optimisation that has been carried out. The result shows that the high material savings potential also reduces $CO_2$ emissions. The second factor is the recyclability of WPC, which results in a circular economy of material. The positive effect of the substitution of the material only comes about through the high savings potential that results from the recyclability of material. This is shown in the 4th calculation, where two life cycles of the Turrix were considered. By completely recycling the material, a reduction in $CO_2$ emissions of 42 % was achieved.

When interpreting the results, however, it should be taken into account that data for $CO_2$ emissions were not collected by the authors themselves. For this data, external reference books and studies were used by conducting comparable studies. In addition, there are deviations between individual values depending on the study.

In conclusion, it can be said that the life cycle assessment carried out has shown that a reduction in $CO_2$ emissions through the measures applied is promising.

### Outlook

This study investigated whether $CO_2$ emissions of a component can be reduced by optimising its topology and switching to a sustainable material. The topology optimisation carried out offers the greatest potential for reducing $CO_2$ emissions. Through this, the volume of the Turrix could be reduced by 52 %, with almost the same mechanical properties. The calculation carried out in this chapter, which was carried out within the framework of Life Cycle Assessment, showed that a reduction in $CO_2$ emissions of 52 % is possible with regard to the material used. The second optimisation approach consists of a substitution of the material by replacing the used PP GF30 by a WPC; thus, a reduction of emissions by 28 % could be achieved. A combination of the two approaches results in a 65 % reduction in emissions. The main advantage of using WPC is that it is fully recyclable, and thus a closed material cycle is possible. By using fully recycled WPC, $CO_2$ emissions can be reduced by 42 % over two product life cycles; if the material is recycled more than once, this value scales up linearly. Both optimisation approaches investigated in this thesis were successful. They offer the possibility for significantly reducing $CO_2$ emissions of the Turrix and are therefore recommended.

For the implementation of results, further precautions have to be taken, which are not included in the scope of this thesis. One is to adapt the design of the Turrix to the injection moulding process used for the production. This includes, for example, draft angles, adapting radii or modelling the attachment of the foot. Another point that needs to be investigated is how the reduction of the fibre material through recycling cycles leads to a reduction of the mechanical properties.

## 2.7 Summary and future perspectives

Companies show an interest in sustainable responsibility and strive to operate sustainably within the scope of their possibilities. The cooperation with the companies Hebie GmbH & Co. KG has successfully demonstrated that previously used material can be replaced by a counterpart that has a lower $CO_2$ balance. Polypropylene with 30 % glass fibre-reinforced (PP GF30) was replaced by a wood-plastic compound (WPC). Within the process of changing of the material, the idea of sustainable material has been positively received, as business performance and sales show. The representative effect towards society is in the foreground.

The challenge in substitution towards sustainable materials lies in the production of moulded plastic parts. Moulds are usually designed together with the material, with the aim of ensuring an optimal process window for specific plastic: the larger the process window, the more trouble-free the production of moulded parts. Material-specific warpage and shrinkage effects have an impact on demoulding behaviour and on the surfaces of products. In addition, tools for the use of WPC must be pretreated accordingly, as material leads to oxidation on the surface of the moulding tool. In addition, personnel are sceptical towards new materials as they have not yet gained any experience with it, and this leads to many rejects at the beginning of the introduction.

In summary, it can be said that the substitution of material was successfully implemented. Through topological optimisation of the moulded part, the volume could be reduced by approx. 50 %. For the implementation of new geometry, it is necessary to develop and manufacture a new moulding tool. The resulting expenditure of monetary means is justified by the number of pieces to be produced. The monetary expenditure must be amortised through material savings.

Despite the constant growth in technology and knowledge, future manufacturing of products faces significant challenges. Two examples of this are the provision of resources, which are only available in limited quantities, and the constant supply of electrical energy to the production facilities. To deal with these two issues, it is also necessary to optimise the products currently being manufactured in terms of material efficiency. One possibility for implementing this is the load-oriented topological optimisation of the components. As in the industrial project described above, the product requirements can and must be precisely defined and the components optimised so that no unnecessary material has to be used. This step can take place during a new product design or, as in the case described here, in the course of ongoing production. The customers will increase their understanding under the aspects of improving products in terms of sustainability. At the same time, the acceptance of imperfections in terms of appearance as well as variation in handicraft and artistically created products will also increase (Isaksson & Eckert, 2020).

Due to the improved mechanical properties through the application of hybrid materials, their use will also increase in the future. In the application and processing of these hybrid materials, it is necessary to bring together the expertise of a wide range of specialist groups so as to be able to exploit the full potential. Interdisciplinary and transdisciplinary working groups must be formed not only in the material-related and processing-related specialist areas, but also in cooperation with other working areas assigned to the product life cycle in order to improve the properties and the sustainability of the products produced. As shown in the example described here, the continuous review of products that are successful on the market also represents a sensible step towards resource efficiency and meeting future challenges.

# 3 Promising research topics

As described above, sustainability can be pursued in all areas of life and stages of the product life cycle. Energy-intensive or finite materials can be replaced by renewable ones. Methods for mass reduction and thus material reduction are developed and used. Alternative processing and manufacturing methods are being implemented. Some of these developments are presented in more detail in this chapter.

## 3.1 Interdependency study of design guidelines

### Product engineering

Goal of sustainable product engineering is to find a solution for a given task that needs a technical solving and constraints of strategic planning. During solution finding, time, costs and quality have to be taken into account. The task is formulated by relevant stakeholder requirements and is to be solved in compliance with these. To transform the given requirements into solution, activities synthesis and analysis are iterated. The model in Figure 16 illustrates this accordingly. Developed partial solutions are synthesised and analysed to ensure functionality, economic efficiency and sustainability. (Ehrlenspiel & Meerkamm, 2013)

*Figure 16: Iterative product development process (VDI 2221)*

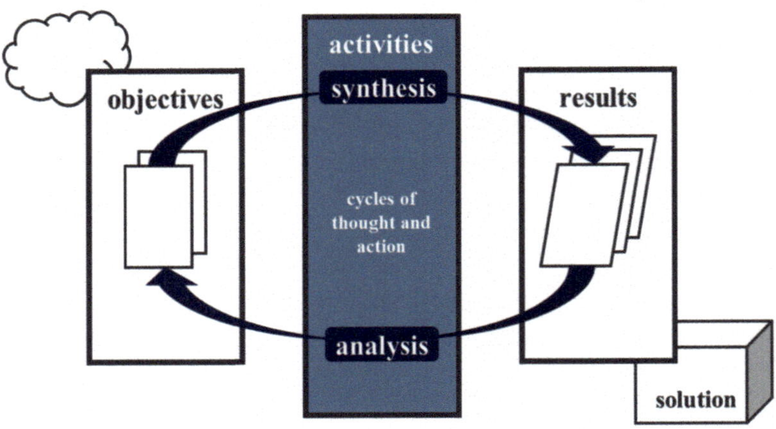


The first Procedure for systematically engineering for a specific product was given by Redtenbacher (1863). Further methodologies in literature consider and cover technical innovations and disciplines (Bender & Gericke, 2021; Pahl et al., 2007; Cross, 2000; van Kleef et al., 2005). Technical innovation is exemplified by cyber-physical systems, which are to be regarded as an interdisciplinary technology (Gräßler et la. 2018). Mechanical engineering (Bender & Gericke, 2021), electrical engineering and electronics (Gajski & Kuhn, 1983; Lienig, 2006) and software engineering (Boehm, 1988) are described as disciplines. Figure 17 shows exemplary product engineering methodologies in chronological order and classifies them into cross-disciplinary, integrated, abstract and discipline-specific approaches. The methods of Wögerbauer (1943) and Hansen (1968) lay the foundation of today's technical methodology. The methodology according to Roth, "Designing with Design Catalogues" (Roth, 2000), and Pahl and Beitz, "Engineering and Design Process" (Pahl & Beitz, 1977), were derived from these methodologies. These in turn form the basis for first version of VDI 2221, "Methodology for the Development and Design of Technical Systems and Products". One of today's most relevant development methodologies is VDI 2206, "Development of mechatronic and cyber-physical systems", from 2021. VDI 2206 is characterised by its interdisciplinarity (Gräßler et al. 2016). The V-Modell contains the new main feature list for mechatronic and cyber-physical systems (Gräßler et al. 2018) and serves as an interdisciplinary model in systems engineering (Gräßler & Yang 2016).

*Figure 17: Overview of existing product development methodologies*

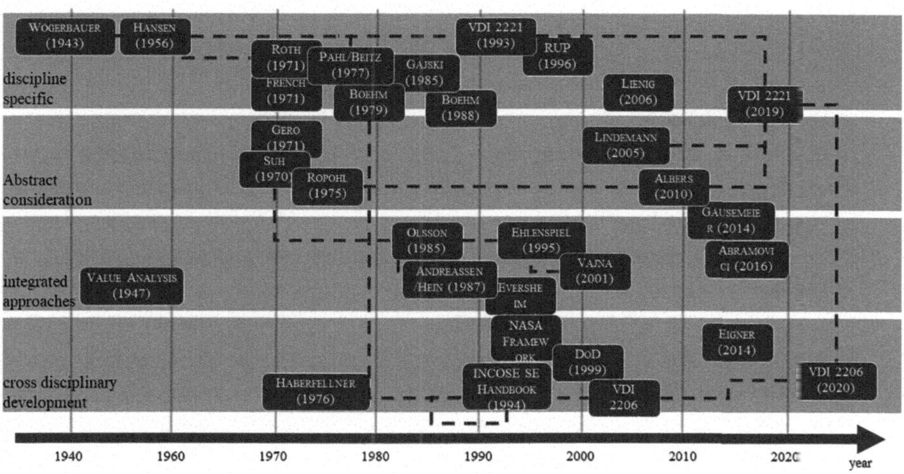


## Structured Product Engineering

In principle, the procedure within the methods of the discipline of mechanics can be described abstractly by phases: task clarification, conceptual design, embodiment design and detail desgin (Bender & Gericke, 2021; Cross, 2000). As the phases progress and the order given increases, so does the detail of product. In Figure 18, the phases are juxtaposed with artefacts and solution space. The solution space contains the set of all possible solutions to solve the problem (Ponn & Lindemann, 2011). It should be noted that the modelling process is preceded by strategic product planning, which includes the use of scenario techniques (Gräßler et al. 2017a).

*Figure 18: Modelling a Technical System, based on (Ehrlenspiel & Meerkamm, 2013)*

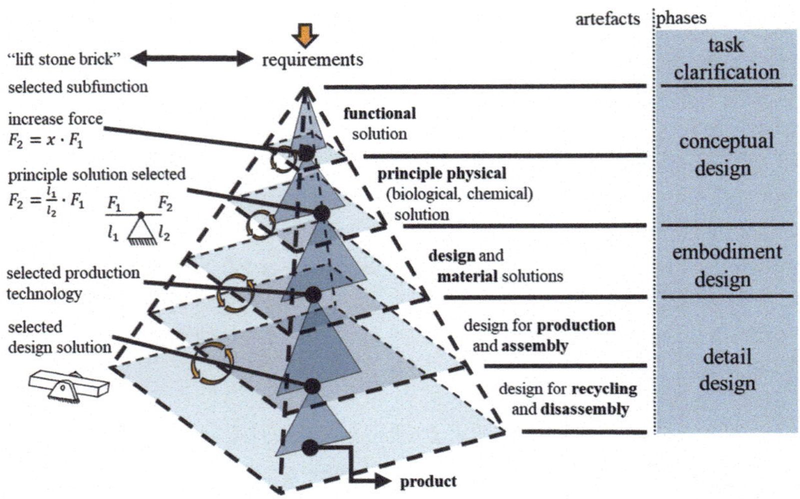


## Task Clarification

In the first phase, task clarification, the boundary conditions are defined according to which the material product is designed. All internal and external information are collected and linked to task. This includes, above all, collection of stakeholder requirements and documentation of requirements in the requirements list. For requirements elicitation, VDI 2206 also contains the main feature list, which is enriched with information on mechatronic and cyber-physical systems (Gräßler et al. 2018). The requirements list lays the foundation for central artefact for designing and evaluating the product. It should be noted that changes to requirements can occur during product engineering (Gräßler et al. 2020). These changes with accompanying propagation effects must be taken into account.

## Conceptual Design

In conceptual design, solution alternatives are developed and differentiated and further elaborated under technical and economic criteria. In conceptual design, the basic solution is developed, defined and documented through the artefacts: "combinations of working principles through morphology", "functional hierarchy" and "functional structure". This step is fundamental for realisation of products. The working principle represents the solution idea for an elementary function and thus the requirements at first concrete level (Bender & Gericke, 2021). The combination of working principles and evaluations leads to solution alternatives (Cross, 2000). Subsequently, criteria are needed to evaluate the solution alternatives. The evaluation serves to identify the best possible solution alternatives for further engineering processes. Based on the list of requirements, criteria for decision-making are formulated (Breiing & Knosala, 1997). The criteria must be consistent with corresponding quality criteria to form the basis for a decision. Criteria must be free of contradictions and must not overlap (Breiing & Knosala, 1997). After identification of target-oriented solution alternatives, these are prototypically realised in order to evaluate the implementation of certain functions. A prototypical realisation can take the form of software or hardware (Vajna et al., 2018). Based on prototypical realisation, the final solution alternative can be identified and further detailed. The solution alternative is translated into a three-dimensional technical geometry (Steinhilper & Rieg, 2012).

### Embodiment Design

During embodiment Design, geometry, surfaces, dimensions, materials, etc. are determined so that product parts can be realised in production (Pahl et al., 2007). It is important that recycling is thought through afterwards. The identified product architecture, working principles and the working surfaces are transformed into possible forms - the shape structure. Software programmes such as Computer Aided Design (CAD) are used for this (Bender & Gericke, 2021). These represent the components and interfaces and their properties. The necessary components and interfaces are thus described geometrically in the partial model.

### Detail Design

Final in detail Design, the characteristics of the identified solution alternative are formalised finaly and thus documented. The documentation makes the selected alternative solution, which can now be called a "solution concept", accessible for the production processes and recycling. The formalisation includes: Shape, properties, surface finish, individual parts, specified materials, verification of manufacturing feasibility as well as calculated costs at current time. In the detail design, the production and recycling technologies are determined and the geometry of the product parts are matched to the production technologies. For example, depending on geometry and material, draft angles must be provided for the injection moulding process in realisation.

In product engineering, human-centric design is carried out for cyber-physical production systems, among other things (Gräßler & Pöhler 2019). Cyber-physical systems are intelligent systems that are used in decentralised production concepts (Gräßler & Pöhler 2018). This enables the decoupling of product and production development processes, as cyber-physical production systems react flexibly (Gräßler et al. 2017b). The designer must consider a variety of disciplines, product environments, interacting systems and stakeholders in the modelling of the product. The consideration of all perspectives for inevitably compromise solutions in the modelling. The background is that possible properties are required in perspectives that in turn lead to challenges in others. In order to be able to consider these perspectives at all, the designer is given design guidelines.

### Design guidelines in Engineering

Product engineering is a process in which characteristics of the product are manifested physically or digitally. It is located in *concept design, embodiment design* and *detail design*. In this process, the creativity of engineers determines the product shape (geometry, material, surface roughness). A distinction is made between strategic and operative designing (VDI 2223). Strategic design refers to a general design procedure that can be applied to a large number of product classes (VDI 2223). In contrast to strategic design, operational design details the design process and adapts it to the individual tasks of the design. The operational design is carried out depending on the result and the findings and adapts the strategic design to product class the regarded (VDI 2223). In these processes, engineers have to fulfil a multitude of requirements and boundary conditions in order to develop the product for the product life (Kriwet et al., 1995). In order for the engineer to be able to implement design decisions, design guidelines are given. These design notes have already proven themselves in design tasks and offer a low risk in integrating a relevant function. Engineering guidelines are of interest to a wider range of users as they formalise and make available knowledge (VDI 2223). The use of engineering guidelines reduces the effort and the design risk in engineering. Design notes are divided into the categories basic rules, design principles and

*Figure 19: Design notes in product engineering, according to (Freund, 2018)*

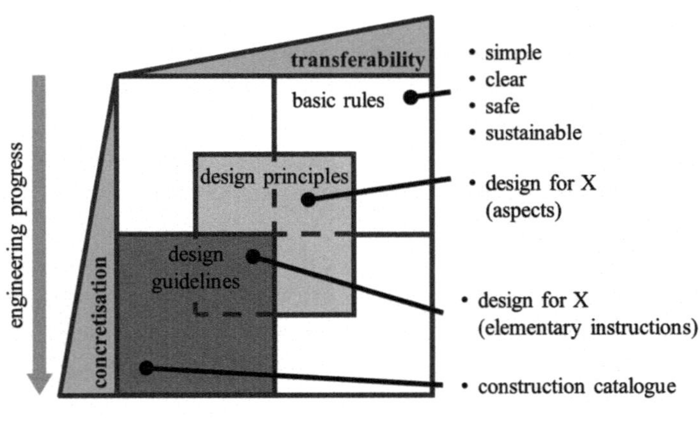

design guidelines (Freund 2018). The three categories of design guidelines differ in the concretisation of the formalisation and in the transferability to different cases, see Figure 19.

*The Basic Rules*
of design comprise *simple*, *clear* and *safe*. These ensure a product that is sustainable for humans and the environment and can be applied to the product type without restrictions (Steinhilper & Rieg, 2012; Bender & Gericke, 2021). Among others, technical feasibility and cost-effective realisation of the product should be clearly addressed. One example is the Poka Yoke method, which allows interfaces between system elements to be designed in such a way that they can only be positively joined via one possible positioning (Kirchner & Neudörfer, 2021).

*Design principles*
support engineers in taking selected restriction into account, e.g. a functionally reliable or cost-effective design, taking special values, such as transmission of forces, thermal influences on a product, and electromagnetic compatibility. Principles do not claim to be exhaustive but evoke associations for engineers. One of the best-known sets of design principles is the Design for X. Design for X is a knowledge system and contains tested approaches. The X represents restrictions resulting from of different product life phases, processes or technologies. Engineers apply the Design for X system in several phases of product engineering. The knowledge system is used to record the characteristics to be designed that lead to certain product properties. Accordingly, a required property can be implemented reproducibly in different products. (VDI 2223). The guidelines of Design for X can be differentiated into different levels of detail. Faerber distinguishes between aspects and elementary instructions in Design for X (Faerber et al. 2008). The elementary instructions describe basic instructions and specify concrete features and feature characteristics.

*Design guidelines*
depend on the required product class and the discipline (mechanics, electrical engineering, information technology, etc.). They are applicable to a product under certain conditions, e.g. geared towards the selected manufacturing process. For example, in case of plastic moulded parts, material-related and geometry-related draft angles must be considered. Draft angles ensure that the moulded part can be removed from the negative of the injection moulding tool. The specific angles value for a material is noted in design guideline.

When applying design notes, trade-offs have to be made (Bender & Gericke, 2021). These trade-offs lead to conflicts in the solution alternative, which the engineer must take into account. Conflicts among design notes are not directly apparent. BAUER examines conflicts of design notes and comes to the conclusion that a clear statement about the conflict can only be made with the product (Bauer, 2003). If system elements are joined by means of a small positive connexion in order to save weight in terms of lightweight construction, this connexion cannot be clearly separated at the end of the service life and leads to material contamination and loss. Soo et al. describe this using a riveted joint. The product is shredded in end-of-life and broken into fragments that are larger than the rivet joint. Accordingly, the fragment consists of three materials: substrate 1, substrate 2 and the rivet. Soo et al. refer to such design implementations as "fixes that fail" (Soo et al., 2018).

## Interdependencies of design guidelines

In order to support engineers in the selection of engineering guidelines, design guidelines of the DfX knowledge system are compared below and examined for inconsistencies. First of all, design guidelines are collected from the pertinent literature. For the identification and documentation within a database, the procedure according to Freund (2018) is applied (see Figure 20). The procedure integrates the need to standardise the wording. In this work, the technical wording according to Roth is used (Roth 2000). For the comparison, the design guidelines are compared

*Figure 20: Procedure for identifying engineering guidelines in literature, according to (Freund, 2018)*

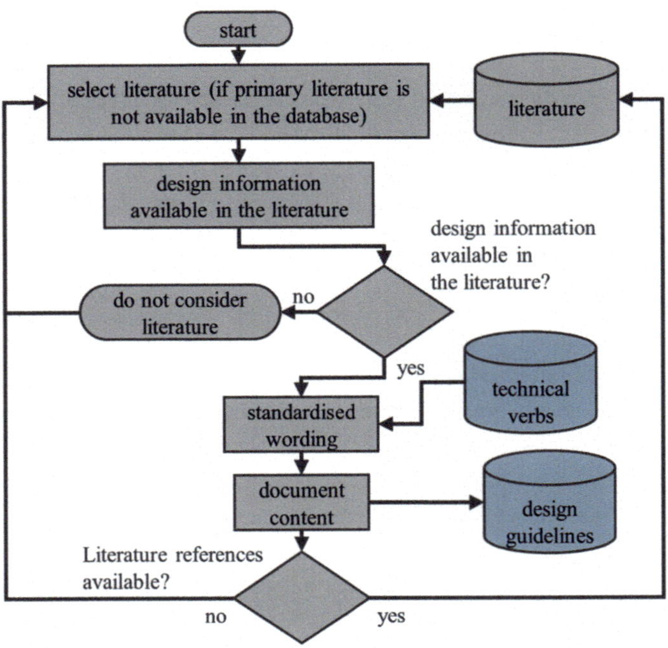

and the interdependencies are marked: independent (grey), supporting (green) and contradictory (red) (Breiing & Knosala, 1997). The interdependencies are assessed by interpreting the formalised description in the pertinent literature.

For the identification of the design guidelines, the pertinent literature was first searched according to MACHI and MCEVOY (Machi & McEvoy, 2016). The identified literature was then examined for available design guidelines. If no design guideline can be identified in the literature, the next literature is examined. Then it is determined whether the design guideline originates from primary literature or is referenced. If the design guideline is taken from another source, this is used and examined according to the previous procedure. Once a design guideline has been identified, it is integrated into a database.

The identified design guidelines are compared in a relation test matrix (Breiing & Knosala, 1997) and assessed via a pairwise comparison (Bender & Gericke, 2021). For the assessment of the design guidelines, the pairwise comparison is used by 4 experts of the "light efficient mobil" research college. The results are then discussed and consolidated in the consortium. Finally, the result of the assessment is summarised in Table 9.

Table 9 lists and compares DfX principles to give product engineers an overview of interacting DfX principles. The listed DfX principles are subordinate to the design note "Design for cost" and can be compared with each other accordingly. The interactions between DfX principles can be independent of (grey), supportive of (green) or contradictory to (red) each other, which influences the design implementation in products (Bauer, 2003). If there is a conflict between two guidelines, the product engineer will have to make a compromise on the basis of the product. In doing so, the features and their characteristics are changed, properties are weakened or design references as well as functions are excluded. The compromise is influenced by the strategic planning and the product (Bauer, 2003).

The identified dependencies, supports and inconsistencies give engineers a first orientation in the application of these guidelines. The extension of the matrix to include further engineering guidelines and assessment of interdependencies is conceivable. A detailed assessment of the engineering guidelines has the potential to reduce iterations through the formation of more goal-oriented compromise solutions.

For the application of the table, inexperienced designers were given a task and had to design a brewing unit for a fully automatic coffee machine. As a starting point, the inexperienced engineers were given the list of requirements and a list of engineering guidelines. The list of engineering guidelines detailed the design notes from Table 9.

After the first engineering activity, the inexperienced engineers were able to identify conflicts in the design notes with the help of Table 9. Considering the possible conflicts, the engineers designed the brewing unit as an assembly. Due to the identified conflict between the design guideline *Design for lightweight* and *Design*

*Table 9: Design notes under the Design for Profit hierarchy according to (Bauer, 2003)*

| **Design** | **References** | additive manufacturing | assembly | automated assembly | cost | disassembly |
|---|---|---|---|---|---|---|
| additive manufacturing | (Lachmayer et al. 2020) | | | | | |
| assembly | (Boothroyd et al. 2010) | | | | | |
| automated assembly | (Synes and Welo 2015) | | | | | |
| cost | (Mörtl and Schmied 2015) | | | | | |
| disassembly | (Fiksl and Wapman 1994; Capelli et al. 2007) | | | | | |
| | | | | | | |
| energy conservation | (Arnette et al. 2014) | | | | | |
| gluing | (Habenicht 2016; Bender and Gericke 2021) | | | | | |
| lifecycle | (Sy and Mascle 2011) | | | | | |
| life extraction | (Fiksl and Wapman 1994) | | | | | |
| lightweight | (Klein 2013) | | | | | |
| logistics | (Arnette et al. 2014; Dowlatshahi 1996) | | | | | |
| maintainability | (Mulder et al. 2012) | | | | | |
| manufacturing | (Arnette et al. 2014; Boothroyd et al. 2010; Kuo et al.) | | | | | |
| mass customization | (Gräßler 2004; Tseng et al. 2017) | | | | | |
| modularity | (Krause and Gebhardt 2018; Arnette et al. 2014) | | | | | |
| procurement | (Arnette et al. 2014; Pulkkinen et al. 2012) | | | | | |
| quality | (HUBKA 1992) | | | | | |
| reliability | (Mulder et al. 2012) | | | | | |
| reverse logistics | (Rogers and Tibben-Lembke 2001) | | | | | |
| robustness | (Freund et al. 2017) | | | | | |
| serviceability | (Chiu and Kremer) | | | | | |
| supportability | (Mulder et al. 2012) | | | | | |
| variety | (Kipp and Krause 2008) | | | | | |
| welding | (Habenicht 2016; Bender and Gericke 2021) | | | | | |

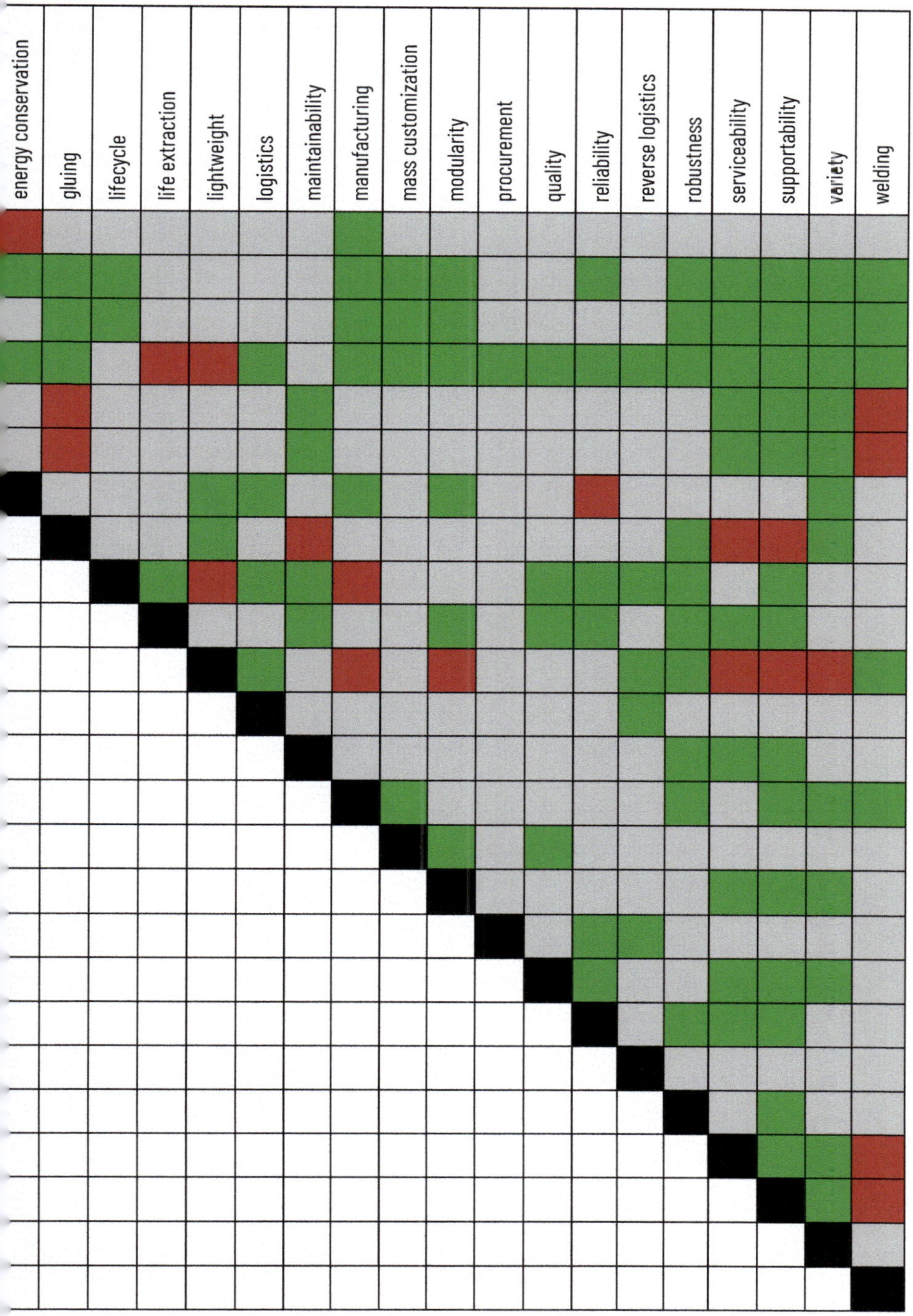
energy conservation
gluing
lifecycle
life extraction
lightweight
logistics
maintainability
manufacturing
mass customization
modularity
procurement
quality
reliability
reverse logistics
robustness
serviceability
supportability
variety
welding

*for serviceability*, the engineers decided against the integral design and in favour of a differential design. This ensured serviceability or repair of the brewing unit. Lightweight construction was taken into account by saving as much material as possible. Accordingly, the design guideline *Design for welding* has also been excluded. Welding represents an irreversible connexion, which can be beneficial for lightweight construction but is not in the spirit of *Design for Disassembly*. However, the *Design for Disassembly* guideline supports the *Design for Serviceability*, which is why its use was prioritised.

### 3.2 Preparation and characterisation of wood-plastic composites with a matrix of thermoplastic polyurethanes to produce a wood-WPC composite structure

In product design, fibre-reinforced plastics are often used to gather good mechanical properties and lightweight design. To integrate the ecological and sustainable aspects, engineers could use wood fibres instead of carbon or glass fibres. Wood-fibre-reinforced or wood-fibre-filled plastics (wood-plastic composites – WPC) are almost exclusively limited to thermoplastics. The most frequently used matrix materials are polyolefins polyethylene (PE) and polypropylene (PP), followed by polystyrene (PS) and polyvinyl chloride (PVC). WPC can be processed cost-effectively and with superior physicochemical properties compared to pure material and offer advantages over inorganically reinforced plastics in terms of sustainability and recyclability. In contrast, there are polarity differences between fibre (polar) and matrix (non-polar) and low process temperature due to fibre decomposition. In this context, thermoplastic polyurethanes (TPU) show great potential. These are polar and can be processed in ranges below the decomposition temperature of the fibres. Another advantage of TPU is the ease of processing with mechanical properties like elastomers. Using this matrix material, the application portfolio of WPC can be expanded in hand grips of bicycle, casters, anti-slip components in the furniture industry or similar industries, so that more WPC materials are used and the acceptance of sustainable materials increases. Especially with respect to hand grips, casters, and anti-slip components, good abrasion behaviour is a decisive factor for longevity.

In this project, wood-fibre-filled compounds based on an ester-based and ether-based TPU matrix material are first characterised for their properties with respect to thermodynamics and rheology. This is followed by a comprehensive analysis of processing in the injection moulding process and the influence of aging on the mechanical properties. In this context, the recycling approach is also pursued, and potentials are identified in this respect. Finally, a wood-WPC structure for the furniture industry will be produced as a demonstrator part, with special consideration of the separation of the individual components after the end of the product life. Based on the following, more detailed focal points of this project, further market potentials for WPC materials can be developed, the acceptance of WPC in society can be increased, and a contribution to sustainability can be made.

The production of compounds for investigations in the injection moulding process was realised with a co-rotating twin-screw extruder. Using the screw set-up shown in Figure 21, the material was compounded with fibre contents of 20-50 wt-%. Initially, the TPU is melted by the effect of temperature and by the kneading blocks (blue) present in the screw configuration (Figure 21). To ensure melting, a return element (red) is provided before the wood is fed in via a side feeder.

*Figure 21: Screw configuration for compounding wood-filled TPU (Moritzer & Richters, 2021)*

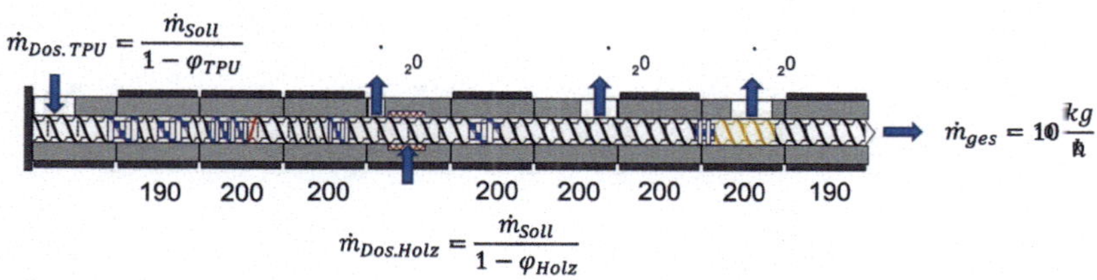


Since the wood and the TPU are hygroscopic, the metered mass flow must be adjusted as a function of the wood or TPU moisture content ($\phi_i$). The moisture present evaporates under the existing high temperatures and is removed by means of two atmospheric degassing. At the end of the twin-screw extruder, residual water vapour is degassed by means of vacuum degassing. A screw element with a high specific surface area (yellow) is installed for this purpose so that the residual moisture evaporates completely.

For pelletising the plastic at the end of the twin-screw extruder, hot die-cutting of the melt in an underwater pelletiser has proven effective. In the hot die-cutting process, the plastic is fed through a die plate and cut off by a rotating knife. The pellets are cooled by a stream of water and fed into a cyclone for drying. To generate reproducible results in the injection moulding process, further drying was necessary. Due to the hygroscopic material behaviour of the materials and high porosity, especially for higher filled compounds (≥40 wt-%), increased water absorption of the compounds is essential. This knowledge was gained immediately after the pelletising process and led to further investigations on the hygroscopic material behaviour of the pellets (Figure 22).

*Figure 22: Top: Water absorption as a function of time (left) and fibre content (right) for a wood-fibre-reinforced ether-based TPU; Bottom: SEM images for 20-wt-% and 50-wt-% filled compound. (Moritzer & Richters, 2021)*

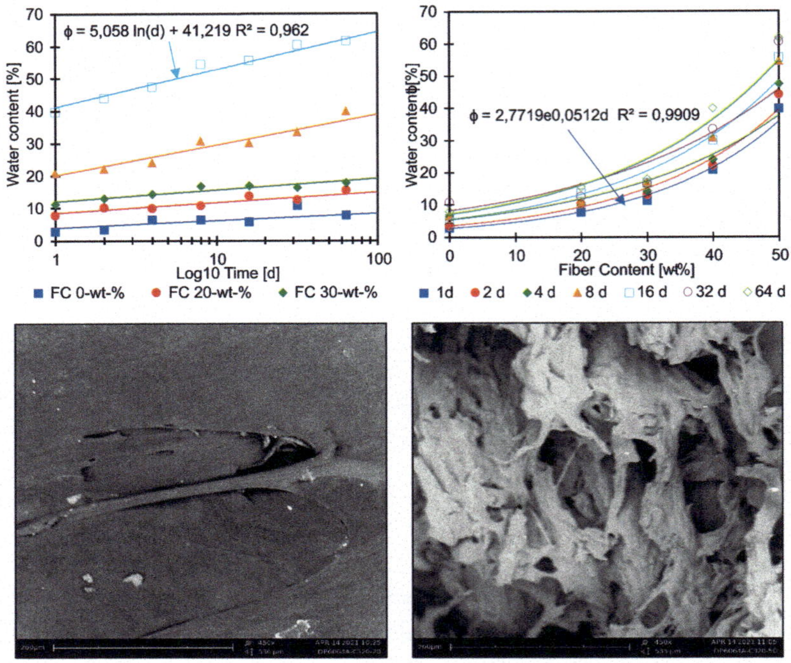


Scanning electron microscopy (SEM) images also demonstrated the porosity described above. Due to the elastic material behaviour, a compression and compaction of the material for higher filled materials is not present. Due to the high surface of the granules, the strong water absorption behaviour and the high-water content can be justified (Figure 22, top left, FC 50-wt%). Based on the findings from the material characterisation, the injection moulding process of wood-filled TPU was investigated using statistical design of experiment (DoE). It was found that temperature control is the main influence on mechanical properties. As the temperature increases, the melt has a lower viscosity, and more material can be injected into the cavity, but the decomposition of the fibres is higher. This decomposition results in reduced tensile strength at higher specimen mass (Figure 23). This finding is contrary to the correlation behaviour of tensile strength and mass.

*Figure 23: Tensile strength as a function of specimen weight (left) (Moritzer & Richters, 2021) and tensile strength, Young's modulus and elongation as a function of fibre content (ether-based matrix material).*

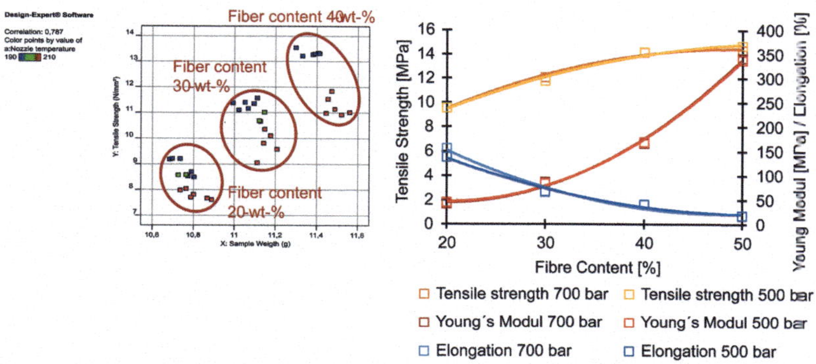


Furthermore, a reinforcing effect with increasing fibre content can be seen. The holding pressure, such as the mould temperature, has no significant influence on the mechanical properties in this case, whereas the rotational speed when metering the material and the injection speed is significant.

The investigation of the aging behaviour of the materials is indispensable for a later application, e.g., as a multi-component structure. In particular, the proven water absorption of the compounds due to the hygroscopic properties of the starting materials represents a starting point for further investigation topics, which are addressed in this project. The matrix material is susceptible to hydrolytic degradation mechanisms due to its molecular chain structure. Here, especially the urethane group or the ester group represents a starting point for degradation. The ether group is more stable against a hydrolytic attack, which is reflected experimentally in the results. To accelerate hydrolysis, a temperature window of 50 - 80 °C and a maximum storage time of 14 days were chosen as boundary conditions. As a function of time and temperature, a significant decrease in mechanical properties, such as tensile strength, can be detected which correlates with the measured residual moisture. The increased water content at high temperatures can be explained by the temperature dependence of the diffusion coefficient. The water content after 14 days is clearly below the detected values in the test series on the water absorption behaviour of granules. This supports the justification of the increased water absorption by the porous structure and the resulting high surface. In the injection moulding process, the test specimens are strongly compacted by the holding pressure after injection so that there is no longer any pore structure. Furthermore, there are only a few fibres on the surface, which are also strongly compacted.

*Figure 24: Decrease in tensile strength (left) and water content of test specimens (right) as a function of the storage conditions in distilled water*

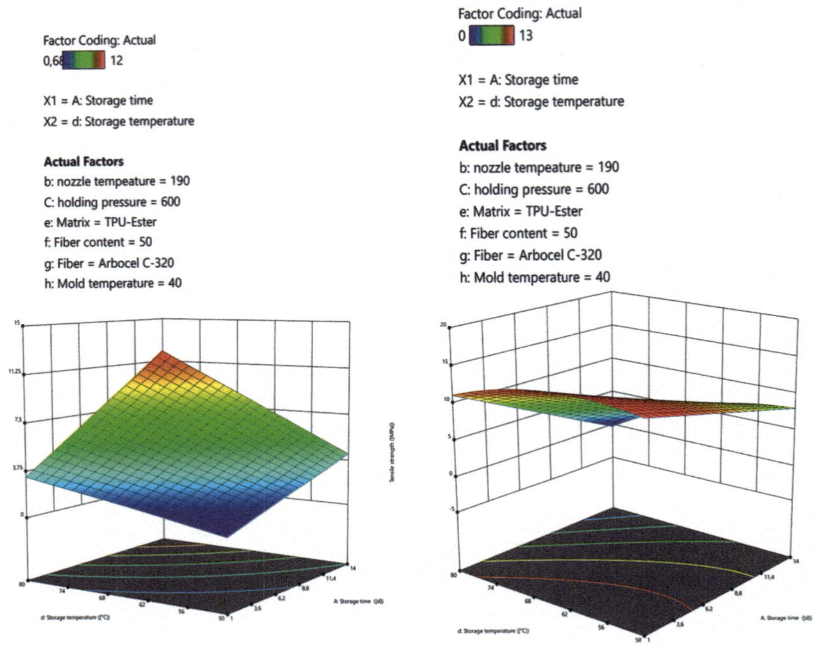


The investigations of the influence of the fibre content show that the decrease of the mechanical properties is stronger with higher filled TPU (Figure 24). It has also been shown that the decrease in tensile strength is lower for the ether-based TPU which is more stable against hydrolysis. Further approaches to investigate the aging behaviour are the dynamic mechanical behaviour, the influence of thermo-oxidative aging, and the influence of temperatures below the glass transition temperature (< -30 °C) on the mechanical properties.

Due to the thermoplastic processability of TPU, another starting point is the recycling of wood-filled TPU and the influence on the mechanical properties, fibre-length degradation, and fibre decomposition. For this purpose, test specimens are manufactured, then shredded and injection-moulded again. Over five cycles, the degradation of the properties can be detected, and, subsequently, a limit value for the maximum recycling cycle of wood-filled TPU can be defined. Furthermore, the flow behaviour is detected by means of MFR so that conclusions can be drawn about the thermally induced chain degradation. Another focus of the investigation is the use of discarded wood-based materials, such as particleboard, OSB, or MDF, for use as filler material. In particular, the influence of the binders on the compound or specimen quality regarding the increase in fibre-matrix adhesion or the influence on the strength is a starting point for the series of investigations. Finally, the influence of recycling on the life cycle assessment (LCA) regarding the $CO_2$ equivalent will be elaborated.

Based on the knowledge gained regarding processing, aging, and recycling behaviour, a technology carrier in form of a MDF-WPC structure is finally produced using injection moulding and bonding technology. For this purpose, suitable carrier material from the furniture industry is selected. Then the surface bonding between carrier material and wood-fibre-reinforced TPU is specifically influenced to create a multi-component structure. Finally, the mechanical behaviour is modelled, and approaches for the separation and recycling of the individual components are developed.

With wood-fibre reinforcement of TPU, new ways for the use of natural-fibre-reinforced plastics are available. Wood-fibre-reinforced TPUs have a distinct advantage over non-reinforced plastics in the reduction of the consumption of finite resources and micro-plastic emissions. As wood content increases, consumption and use of fossil-based plastics decrease. As a result, less micro-plastic pollutes the environment. Furthermore, the wood content captures $CO_2$ and leads to better mechanical properties, resulting in increased longevity compared to unfilled plastics. In contrast, however, the higher density of wood-filled TPU, as compared to unfilled TPU, increases $CO_2$ emissions during transport. (Friedrich, 2021) When recycling wood-filled TPU, which allows $CO_2$ to be isolated for a longer period, the $CO_2$ footprint is increased by the preparation process in terms of shredding, re-drying, compounding, and injection moulding. Due to the thermal load for the fibres, only components that are used for components subject to less mechanical stress can then be produced. In this context, thermal wood-fibre degradation can be minimised via additives or fibre-conserving process control during compounding and injection moulding.

So far, research has shown that wood-fibre-reinforced TPUs can be processed well in the injection moulding process and exhibit good mechanical properties even after recycling. Based on these findings and through the development of LCA and the multi-component wood-WPC composite structure, new market potentials have opened up for the industry. Thus, the society's acceptance of natural-fibre-reinforced plastics can be increased due to the pleasant tactile sensations and smells. However, society is also deceived by the wood-like appearance of the surface, which lowers the image for sustainable materials (Friedrich, 2021). Nevertheless, with this project and the right marketing of such materials, synergy effects can be developed among society, industry, and natural-fibre-reinforced plastics, in particular with respect to recycling. Recycling also becomes more important in other disciplines, such as metal processing.

## 3.3 Friction-induced recycling process for aluminium rejects

An approach to the energy-efficient and resource-efficient recycling of different aluminium scrap is the use of a friction-induced process principle. The process principle presented here uses friction occurring between the die and the material (the aluminium scrap) for heating besides generating the pressure required for extrusion of a semi-finished product. The basis of the recycling process is the Conform process principle, which was invented and patented in the 1970s to rework wire semi-finished products (Etherington, 1974). In this project, the process principle has been applied to the problem of energy-efficient recycling of aluminium scrap, and a test rig has been set up. Figure 25 shows the process principle of the tool system realised at the Paderborn University. A major advantage of this process principle compared to the conventional processes presented for the production of semi-finished aluminium products as well as other solid-state recycling processes is the fact that it is a continuous process principle. Therefore, the central component of the experimental setup is a wheel with a circumferential groove driven by a powerful geared motor. The materials to be recycled in the initial basic tests are dry-produced aluminium chips, which are filled into the groove of the wheel through a continuous filling system and carried along by it. In the further course of a quarter revolution, the cross-sectional area of the wheel groove is steadily reduced by the engagement of a tool insert, thus compacting the aluminium chips. Due to the continuous compression, the friction between the alu-

*Figure 25: Process principle of the friction-induced recycling process*

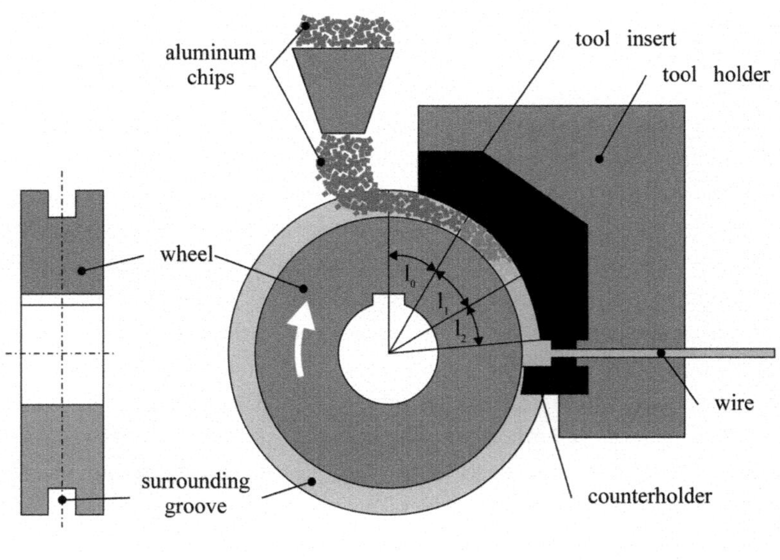

minium chips and the wheel or the tool increases and thus also the temperature in the system. After a quarter turn, the complete cross-sectional area of the wheel groove is filled by a counter holder. The now plasticised material is deflected and extruded through a shaping opening in the form of a die.

For complete recycling or complete bonding of the individual aluminium components, strong deformation must be ensured at a simultaneously high temperature. The deformation is implemented by the reducing tool insert as well as the counter holder. The friction-induced process approach ensures a steady increase in temperature from the start of the process as well as keeping it constant during the stationary process phase. The investigations carried out were started at room temperature with respect to the temperature in the tool system as well as in the chips. Depending on the rotation speed of the wheel, the aluminium alloy used, and the design of the tool system, the temperature measured on the outside of the tool system is increased to a final stationary temperature within a few minutes. This final steady-state temperature can and is kept constant over the course of the investigation. For the recycling process of the wrought alloy EN-AW-6060 at a rotation speed of 11 rounds per minute to a wire with a diameter of 5 mm, the final steady-state temperature is around 300 °C. Compared with the conventional and melt-metallurgical recycling process presented previously, with process temperatures of around 680 °C, a significant reduction in the processing temperature is possible.

The aim of the initial investigations of the friction-induced recycling process is to demonstrate the feasibility of the process and to describe the process in terms of influences of various parameters. Some examples of process parameters that can be specifically influenced before starting any investigation are the rotation speed of the wheel, the geometric design of the tool system, the material of the aluminium chips under investigation, and the filling rate of the wheel. Certain parameters, such as the filling rate of the wheel, have only a marginal or subordinate influence on the process as well as the mechanical properties of the semi-finished product produced. Other parameters, such as the rotation speed of the wheel, have an influence on the relative speed between the workpiece and the material, and thus also on friction. This, in turn, has an influence on the temperature or heating rate. In addition to parameters that can be specifically influenced, the friction-induced recycling process also has parameters that are set as a function of the previously mentioned parameters. These parameters cannot be changed directly by an action but are set indirectly based on a defined parameter combination. Examples of parameters are the temperature measured on the outside of the tool system, the torque to be applied to keep the rotary motion constant, and the discharge or production rate of the semi-finished product. A challenge in process control is the fact that the characteristic variables usually represent the target variables. For a defined process, the process temperature and the discharge rate usually has to be set specifically. For this purpose, various relationships between the process parameters and the characteristic quantities have been broken down in the course of the investigations. One example is the dependence of the hardness on the process temperature as well as the rotation speed of the wheel. During the start-up or heating phase of the process, the die temperatures have been recorded and assigned to the different sections of the wire produced. A correlation can be established between the hardness as well as the external temperature of the tool as a function of the rotation speed. This shows that the hardness decreases with increasing temperature. However, this is only true up to a temperature of around 280 °C, which corresponds almost to the final steady-state temperature. Above this temperature, constant mechanical properties are achieved. Compared with the low rotation speed of 6 rpm, the higher rotation speed of 10 rpm shows lower strength values in the start-up phase at the same temperatures. However, when a temperature of 280 °C is reached, constant mechanical properties considering the hardness are achieved regardless of the rotation speed.

Based on the findings of the mutual influences of the process parameters and the characteristic values, the validation of the processability of different aluminium alloys with the friction-induced recycling process is to be investigated. This represents the precondition for the diverse application of the friction-induced recycling process in the various manufacturing and production technology fields. Figure 26 shows the cross-sectional area as well as the mechanical hardness for four exemplary aluminium alloys. The alloy EN-AW-1350 is considered to be an example of an almost pure aluminium alloy, which is frequently used in the field of electrical engineering due to its high electrical conductivity. The age-hardenable wrought alloy EN-AW-6060 is primarily used for the investigation of the friction-induced recycling process. The reason for this is its frequent use in the field of civil engineering and to produce semi-finished products with arbitrary cross-sections. In the aerospace field, EN-AW-7075, which is also age-hardenable and a high-strength alloy, is used to ensure low weight in addition to high strength. AlSi10Mg is used as an example of a casting alloy in order to cover this area of application as well, with sometimes high quantities of swarf produced on a daily basis. For all four alloys considered, it is shown that good and complete mould-filling is achieved with respect to the surface. Both macroscopically and microscopically, individual chips can no longer be identified. For all alloys, it is true that the chips, which were previously a few millimetres in size, can be recycled into a full semi-finished product. The semi-finished product is extruded at a constant discharge rate in the steady state of the recycling process. With regard to the mechanical properties, which are considered in Figure 26 below as an example based on Vickers hardness, typical relationships can be determined for the different alloys. The aluminium EN-AW-1350, which is virtually pure without the addition of alloying elements, exhibits the lowest degree of hardness, and the high-strength alloy EN-AW-7075, as expected, is the highest. The hardness is evenly distributed over the surface and shows comparable variations compared to reference samples. In a direct comparison of the average hardness of alloy EN-AW-6060 to conventionally produced reference samples in the solution-annealed condition, comparable properties of the recycled semi-finished products are found. Future investigations should validate the possibility of selective heat treatment of the recycled semi-finished products to adjust the strength.

*Figure 26: Cross-section and strength of four alloys investigated as examples*

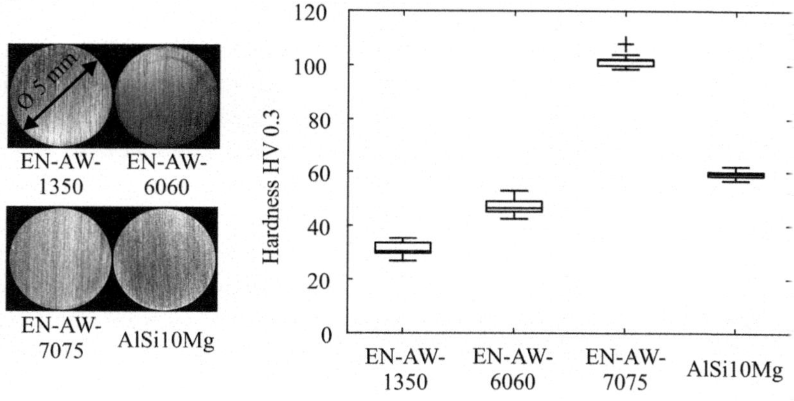


In addition to achieving comparable mechanical properties, the efficiency of material and energy input, which is important for a recycling process, is assessed. For this purpose, the friction-induced recycling process is compared with the conventional process chains for the production of semi-finished aluminium products described above. To produce one kilogramme of a round aluminium profile using the friction-induced recycling process, approximately 8.68 MJ of electrical energy is required for the low rotation speed of the wheel of 6 rpm. If the rotation speed is increased to 11 rpm and thus the discharge rate is also significantly increased, 9.86 MJ are required per kilogramme of aluminium. The amount of energy specified here is required by the gear motor and is determined by means of the electrical power consumption of the frequency converter. In addition to overcoming the idling torque, a large part of the energy is required to overcome the frictional resistance among the tools as well as the aluminium. Possibilities for reducing the energy input of the friction-induced recycling process are seen in a change of the friction surfaces on the outside of the grooved wheel. By reducing the friction surfaces, the frictional resistance and thus the amount of energy introduced should be reduced. However, a change in the friction surfaces also has an influence on process parameters, such as temperature, and should therefore be considered comprehensively in future investigations. The advantages of the friction-induced recycling process over both primary and secondary aluminium production are, on the one hand, a significant reduction in the amount of energy required. On the other hand, existing resources can be utilised. Scrap materials and other auxiliary materials are not required at all, at least not in the recycling process of dry-produced aluminium flakes. The salt slag produced in secondary aluminium production can be avoided by applying the friction-induced recycling process, thus protecting the environment. Another advantage is the direct production of semi-finished products. As described, the ingots produced by the primary or secondary production process have to be processed into semi-finished products in a second process step by extrusion. This step is omitted, since recycling and shaping are carried out directly in the friction-induced recycling process. The compact design of the overall plant and the low acquisition costs compared with the equipment used for conventional production mean that the process can also be used in small or medium-sized companies. By integrating recycling into the business environment, emissions and costs, which are caused by the decentralised collection and the transport of the scrap materials, can be avoided.

The investigations described above have in common that aluminium scrap used was produced in the form of chips in a controlled and dry machining process. If foreign materials in the form of iron powder or steel chips are added in a defined mass fraction of up to 30%, this has a positive influence on the strength and uniform elongation. Minor impurities, which cannot be avoided in the industrial environment during production, negatively influence the process or the mechanical properties of the semi-finished products produced. Contamination of the aluminium chips with a cooling lubricant commonly used in manufacturing technology, on the other hand, shows significant deterioration of the mechanical properties even with small amounts of the cooling lubricant. For the application of the process in all areas of manufacturing technology, it is necessary to develop possibilities and methods for the removal of contamination. One method for this is the formation of an interdisciplinary working group with the aim of (electro-) chemical pre-treatment of the rejects to be recycled. Based on the results of the ECUF project (Electrochemically Supported Joining of Sheet Metal Materials) from the DFG priority funding programme 1640, a possibility for the removal of cooling lubricants as well as other rejects is to be developed (Schmidt et al., 2014). In addition to the removal of foreign substances, to what extent the removal of the natural oxide layer of the aluminium chips can have a positive effect on the joint strength can and should also be investigated.

A future objective of investigation is to improve the production chain of user-specific products and finished products continuously. In this context, the spectrum of components produced from rejects or scrap is to be extended from semi-finished products to finished products. This is to be achieved by combining the friction-induced recycling process with the friction spinning process, which is also being investigated. Friction spinning has been developed within the framework of the TRR30 collaborative research centre with the aim of combining the two sub-processes of friction welding and spinning. Through synergetic effects, it is possible to extend process boundaries. Similarities to the friction-induced recycling process are found in the process principle due to the fact that the heat required for plasticising the material is generated in a friction-induced manner (Lossen, 2019). The exchange of process knowledge from the fields of both processes can and should help to gain a deeper understanding of the process and to develop a process combination. A first step in the direction of a direct manufacturing process of user-specific components from scrap is the production of semi-finished products, which are usually processed with the friction spinning process. One example is a tube with an outside diameter of 40 mm and a wall thickness of 5 mm. This must first be produced with the friction-induced recycling process and then formed with the friction spinning process. Another application-related field for recycled semi-finished products is joining with adaptive friction elements. The combination of the two processes into a resource-efficient and energy-efficient manufacturing process represents the final step of the investigations.

With the friction-induced recycling process, an alternative to the direct recycling of semi-finished aluminium products has been presented and described. The investigations carried out so far have demonstrated the processability of aluminium chips from a wide range of alloys and the possibility of producing user-specific semi-finished products with good mechanical properties. In further interdisciplinary research projects, the aim is to investigate in detail and improve the process with regard to chemical pretreatment of the different aluminium rejects as well as the combination with friction spinning.

### 3.4 Interfacial design for catalytic recycling of carbon-fibre-reinforced thermoset polymers

There is a desperate need for research of alternative methods and processes of CFRPs, as a valuable lightweight material with limited recycling treatment methods. With these prospects, chemical recycling was conducted in this project in order to reclaim carbon fibre from CFRPs made from Prepregs under mild conditions. This prepreg consists of 60% carbon fibre and 39% epoxy resin, plus 1% additives (unidirectional carbon-fibre-epoxy prepreg). After the curing process, the composite undergoes chemical recycling at 160 degrees Celsius by utilizing aluminium nitrate as catalyst and dimethylacetamide as solvent. This solvent has the ability to penetrate the dense structure of the cured epoxy matrix, as it has been shown in the Figure 27, and then the catalyst is able to do its task to cleave the chemical bond between carbon and nitrogen for around 5-7 hours. Separated carbon fibre will be washed with acetone and water and left to dry in the oven for one day. The results are the clean surface of fibres and also the solid form of the recovered epoxy matrix. After the degradation reaction, the matrix resin is almost completely removed from the carbon fibres. Recycled fibre has been analysed mechanically and chemically by TGA, Raman Spectroscopy, XRD, XPS, SEM, and EDX.

*Figure 27: Principle of catalytic degradation of cured epoxy resin (CEP)*

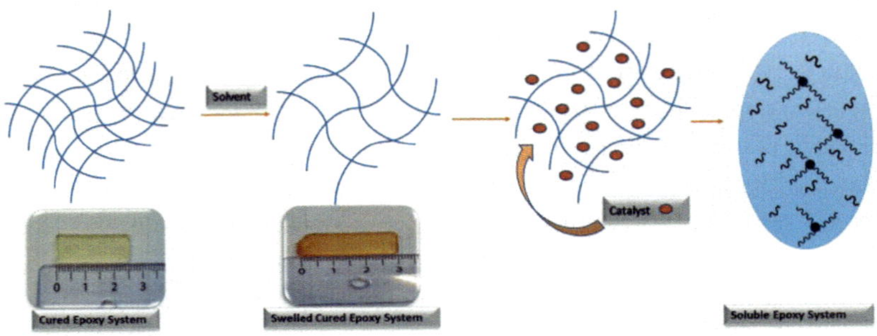


Raman spectroscopy is a non-destructive technique providing a quick and easy structural characterisation of carbon materials. The degree of graphitisation of recycled fibres was characterised by Raman spectra. By interpreting the Raman spectrum, we have the clues to confirm the crystallinity, carbon atoms hybridisation, disorders and defects, and the thickness of the layers of graphene. Graphitic structures display two prominent peaks at 1330 and 1580 cm−1, which correspond to the D band (the vibrations of the sp3-hybridised carbons) and G band (in-plane vibration of sp2 carbon atoms), respectively. Generally, the intensity ratio of the D and G bands (ID/IG) is a measure of the level of defects and the degree of functionalisation that is introduced into the graphene sheets. ID/IG value has been compared to distinguish SP2 and SP3 orbitals of carbon atoms. This ratio has been changed from 1.73 for virgin fibre to 1.85 for reclaimed fibre. The G peak is attributed to the SP2 hybrid orbital of the carbon atom, and the D peak is assigned to the $SP^3$ hybrid orbital of the carbon atom. The C-O and C=O bonds will strengthen the intensity of the D peak, so Raman spectra can confirm that the surface of fibres has not been oxidised considerably.

On the other hand, the thermostability of fibres was detected by TGA (Thermal Gravimetry Analysis). The thermal behaviour of virgin fibre and recycled fibre is comparable, and there is no weight loss in recycled fibre after the exact time and the result of 100% degradation ratio. The weight of reclaimed CF remained unchanged, just like virgin CF after treatment. They both follow the same pattern by changing the temperature, indicating a satisfactory degradation efficiency.

The degradation matrix, which is Bisphenol A of epoxy Di glycidyl ether, has been optimised by changing the temperature, amount of catalyst, and time to achieve the best and most efficient degradation ratio without damaging the surface of fibres and destroying the mechanical, physical and chemical properties of them. The optimised reaction is with a 15% (W) catalyst at 160×c in 7 hours and a 20% catalyst in 5 hours. Under these conditions, the $D_r$ (degradation ratio) is almost 100%. It means a total recovery of carbon fibre from CFRP.

The surface morphology of the recycled fibres was detected by SEM (Scanning Electron Microscopy). The SEM micrographs of the recovered CFs showed smooth surfaces after the exact time and catalyst concentration.

The steps of recycling to reach a smooth surface have been shown by SEM images (Figure 28, Figure 29):

*Figure 28: Raman spectroscopy and XRD*

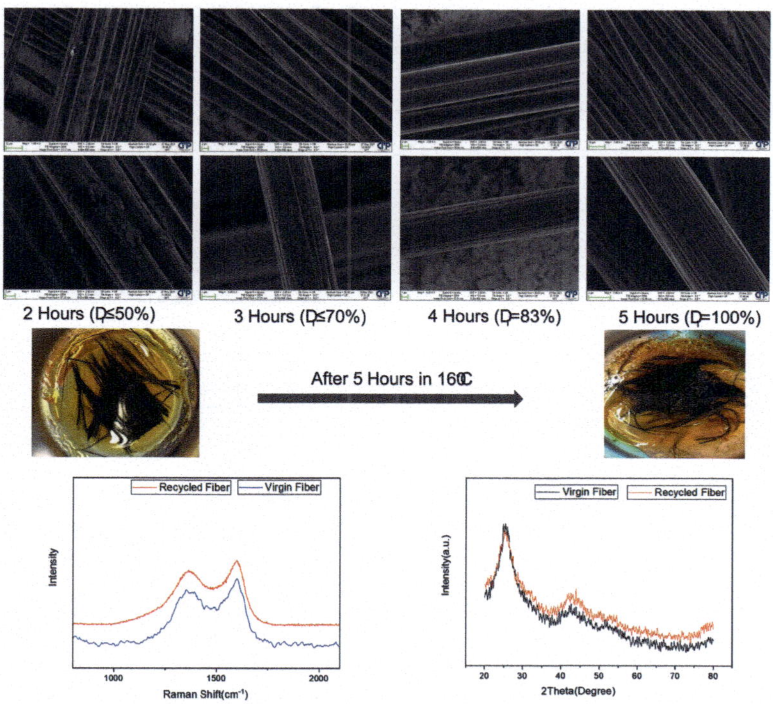

*Figure 29: XPS (X-ray photoelectron spectroscopy); left – virgin fibre, right – recycled fibre*

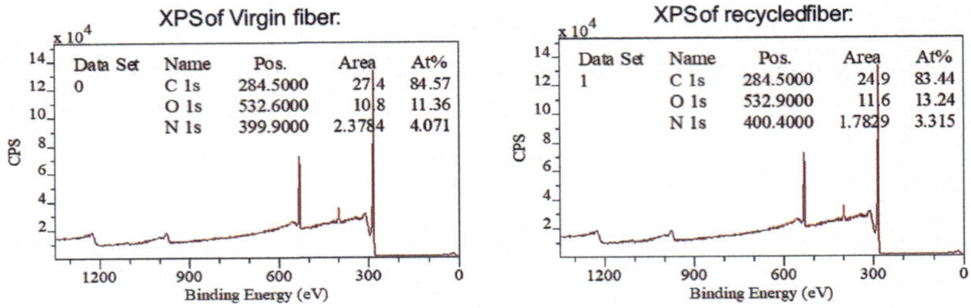


The tensile strength of the monofilament of recycled carbon fibre is an important indicator of the reusing ability of the fibre. By this test, the extent to which the fibre can be stretched without breaking is measured. Results show no significant differences in tensile strength between virgin carbon fibre and recycled ones. EDX (Energy Dispersive X-ray Analysis) has been carried out to detect the element present on each of the samples (Figure 30). As it is clear, the amount of oxygen in

*Figure 30: EDX (energy dispersive X-ray analysis)*

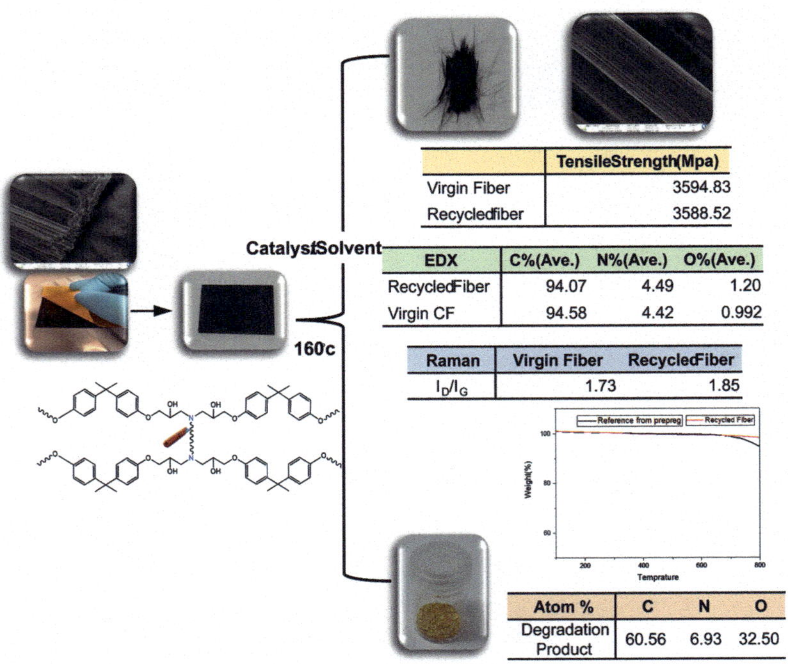

the recycled fibre is not considerably higher. Also, the functional groups on the surface of recycled CF were detected by XPS. In addition, it shows not very significant changes in the percentage of oxygen on the surface of the fibres. XRD also shows that the crystallinity structure of fibres has not been destroyed by utilising the catalyst in the solvent system.

On the other hand, some analytical measurements have been performed on degradation products to clarify the structure of the degraded epoxy matrix and the catalyst to examine the ability to re-use them in further processes. The existence of nitrogen in the chemical structure of the degradation product can confirm the cleavage of the bond between carbon and nitrogen in the cured composite.

The high efficiency of Al $(No_3)_3$/DMAc is attributed to the strong coordination effect of aluminium nitrate with the C-N bonds and the strong swelling ability of dimethylacetamide solvent, which worked together to break down the chemical bonds of the cross-linked polymer. Furthermore, mild degradation temperature (< 200°C) and low catalyst concentration imparted little damage to the recovered fibres in comparison with other recycling methods at high temperatures.

## 3.5 Green synthesis of graphene nano composites for automo3bile applications

Increased environmental awareness and current economic situations tempt people today to use nanomaterials with biodegradable polymers in developing new composite materials because of their exciting properties such as a high surface area

The growing trend to substitute conventional steel and cast iron in vehicles for lightweight purposes leads to the development of automotive components with lighter materials. Replacing cast iron and traditional steel components with lightweight materials, such as high-strength steel, magnesium (Mg) alloys, aluminium (Al) alloys, carbon fibre, and polymer composites can directly reduce the weight of a vehicle's body and chassis by up to 50 percent (Elmarakbi & Azoti, 2015). Lightweight materials are another essential technology that can improve passenger vehicle fuel efficiency by 6–8% for each 10% reduction in weight while also making electric and alternative vehicles more competitive (Joost, 2012). In search of new lightweight materials, graphene-based composite materials have attracted scholarly and industrial interest because of their attractive properties.

Graphene belongs to a new class of carbon nanomaterials-two-dimensional material made up of conjugated **Sp2** carbons arranged in a honeycomb structure (Novoselov et al., 2012). With enhanced electrical conductivity and a high degree of, mechanical strength, high thermal conductivity and, high optical transparency, graphene holds great promise as the next wonder super material. Such an ideal is, however, achievable only if large scale production of high-quality graphene is achieved on a large scale. Generally, graphene production is divided into two approaches: bottom-up and top-down. The bottom-up approach seeks to build graphene sheets from scratch; on the other hand, the top-down approach relies on the fundamental idea of extracting layers of graphene from graphite. Both methods provide graphene of contrasting quality and yield. However, in terms of high yield and low cost, the top-down approach via chemical oxidation and reduction is the most convenient method to date. Moreover, graphene obtained via such chemical treatment is important for many applications like coatings, paint/ink, transparent conductive layers, bio applications, composites, and energy storage.Green synthesis promotes the partial or total substitution of chemicals that are potentially harmful to the environment with more environmental friendly ones while decreasing energy consumption.

Recently, researchers have developed green production methods for synthesising green graphene using environmentally friendly biomass resources (e.g., sugar, chitosan, alfalfa plants, foodstuffs) (Zhu et al., 2010; Ruiz-Hitzky et al., 2011; Muramatsu et al., 2014; Singh et al., 2017). The main objective of the green production method is to utilise fewer toxic chemicals and natural precursors (Singh et al., 2017). Rice husk is the worldwide highest production of agriculture material which totals approximately 120 million tons per year globally (Tuck et al., 2012), and its effective utilisation is required.

Current work provides an overview of the green synthesis of graphene as polymer reinforcements within composite material for automotive applications. The synthesis process of graphene from rice husk was performed in accordance with the process described by Muramatsu (2014) with a few modifications to ease the process.100 g of raw rice husk was purchased from the local rice mill and washed several times with distilled water and dried in the open air for 24 hours. The dried rice husk was grounded and heated in a microwave oven (700 watts for ~ 4 minutes). The obtained solid residue was called rice husk ash (RHA). The RHA was chemically activated using KOH with an impregnation ratio of 1:4 of KOH powder. The mixture was then compacted in a graphite crucible. Next, the crucible was placed in the midpoint of a larger graphite crucible. The empty space around the graphite crucible was fully covered by sufficiently pressing and packing the sacrificial fine graphite powder. The sacrificial graphite powder is used to prevent oxidation on the mixture from air at high temperatures. The crucibles were heated at ~900°C for 2 hours. After the chemical activation process was performed, the post-treatment was carried out whereby chemically activated RHA was poured in 250 ml deionised water (DI water) and stirred for 30 minutes to remove potassium ion residue. The sample was centrifuged at 3000 rpm for 30 minutes. Then, the sample was sonicated in 250 ml of DI water for 5 minutes. After that, the sample was rinsed in 500 ml DI water using filtration. The sample was dried in the oven for 24 hours at 80 °C to remove moisture. The results concluded that it is possible to synthesise graphene using rice husk as a raw material by microwave processing. Characterisation has been done by various techniques like XRD, FTIR, FESEM, and Raman spectroscopy analysis. It has confirmed the presence of graphitic structure. In this research, graphene was successfully synthesised by activating rice husk ash (RHA) (using microwave method) and KOH with a 1:4 impregnation ratio. Raman spectroscopy analysis confirmed the presence of graphitic structure.

The study investigated the synthesis of green graphene by reusing biomass waste and was successfully done, and research continues to integrate graphene as polymer reinforcements within composite materials for automotive applications.

## 3.6 Artificial neural networks in material simulations

Modern engineering demands high precision simulations to further enhance the state of the art. An ideal supplement would be the digital twin, a computational copy of reality, which makes experiments and manipulations accessible and versatile. Using in silico experiments, a product could be designed and tested completely virtually, which limits the need for manufacturing prototypes and allows for more flexibility.

The complexity of the underlying physics, as well as the computational effort, counter such approaches. For complex structures, extended numerical computations must be carried out. A crash simulation can easily take days to weeks. In addition, the more involved material models get, the higher the computational costs will be. Consideration of micromechanical effects, which are dominant in modern heterogeneous materials, poses a double burden to the simulation, namely the micro-computation and the macro-computation. Furthermore, the development of material models is time-consuming and demands highly trained experts. These factors drive the costs for high-precision simulations.

Additional cost drivers are uncertainties which arise due to natural fluctuations in microstructures and material parameters on the one hand, as well as due to measurement, manufacturing, and model errors on the other hand. To capture these uncertainties in simulations, several hundreds or thousands of individual computations must be carried out, which is a huge cost multiplicator.

An alternative to traditional computational approaches, which are often tailored to a specific problem, is given by the current rise of artificial neural networks. These models can represent a broad class of functions, which means that they can be used to solve a broad class of problems.

An (artificial) neural network is a complex composition of simple functions called neurons. These neurons are stacked into layers, whereas the layers form a network. Although artificial neural networks were inspired by the human brain, the modern formulation merely consists of simple matrix multiplications to map an input to an output. But as a network can consist of a huge number of neurons, their collective representative power leads to astonishing results, which lead to improvements in fields like autonomous driving, speech recognition, and so forth.

Recently their potential was recognised in the scientific community, and hundreds of papers have been published in the past years.

A neural network encodes its behaviour in a large set of parameters, so-called weights. These weights can be adjusted, which influences the behaviour of the network. To solve a certain task, these weights are optimised with special algorithms. This process is called training. An untrained network produces just random noise, whereas a trained network can recognise faces or solve complex mathematical equations. Although the training process can be very demanding with respect to mathematical complexity and computational effort, it is only a one-time effort. After training, a neural network can process information very fast and can be reused again and again. It is not uncommon for a neural network to outperform numerical methods in forwarding problems by a factor of $10^4$ or more with respect to execution wall time.

Classical approaches to neural networks work in the so-called data-driven regime. One significant subclass is formed by supervised learning. Here, a neural network is trained with the aid of training data. Iteratively, the network is fed with inputs, and its outputs are compared with correct solutions obtained otherwise, perhaps by experimental data, which has similarities to regression problems. After each iteration, the weights are updated, and the error between predictions and correct solutions gets smaller and smaller, finally reaching the desired accuracy. While the training involved is theoretically typically less, the computational effort is very high. Often large training data sets demand terabytes of storage space and large networks, which consume many computational resources. Another problem is gathering data. Many different training samples need to be provided during training so that the network not only learns from the available data but also generalises to the unseen data. Typically, in the field of image processing, more than 10,000 pictures are required. In micromechanics, to obtain a single image from a CT-scanner, several hours pass. Tensile tests last several minutes to hours, and often far fewer than 100 samples can be practically obtained. One can circumvent this problem by adding artificial data, but this introduces errors and biases.

One possible way to overcome the problem of big data regimes is to introduce physical knowledge into the neural networks themselves. For hundreds of years, physicists, mathematicians, and mechanists invented sophisticated mathematical models, which can be used to guide the neural network during training to the correct behaviour with only one view of training samples or even zero views. This approach is called physics-informed neural networks.

In continuum mechanics, the response of a structure is described by partial differential equations. These can be seen as restrictions and requirements for a solving equation. Once the solving equation is found, the differential equations are fulfilled, and quantities of interest, like displacements and stresses, can be calculated easily. Every loading, structure, and material combination has a different solving equation.

Finding these equations is only possible for simple problems, and often traditional computer methods must be used to approximate them. With the help of physics-informed neural networks, these solving equations can be found for arbitrary complex settings. The drawback with respect to supervised learning approaches is that the physics-informed neural network does not generalise to different cases and is tailored to one specific combination of loading, structure, and material. The advantages lie in the absence of training data needed for training, as only the differential equations of the specific situation under investigation are required.

But the precise material laws are not known for all materials yet some extra experimental data may be given. In the case of recycled materials, a lack of specific mathematical formulations of the material behaviour after several recycling steps prevents the usage of pure physics-informed neural networks and traditional computational methods. In this case, a mixture of supervised learning and physics-informed neural networks becomes attractive. This approach can be seen in the middle of a regime of no data but high physical knowledge and a regime of big data with no physical knowledge. The main idea is to restrict the learning process to known physical laws which includes some data from experiments as well. The neural network then closes the gap between our current mathematical knowledge and the experimental data at hand.

Artificial neural networks open a new exciting field in material modelling. Their flexibility makes them attractive in a broad range of applications. Especially the multifield character can bring together the extensive knowledge gained in the long-standing field of continuum mechanics and extra experimental data, typical in engineering contexts.

To this end, the aim of the dissertation is to propose a full end-to-end multi-scale simulation environment utilising artificial neural networks in the context of continuum micromechanics. The main goals are:

- Microstructural characterisation and synthetic generation of artificial microstructures
- Parameter identification and inverse problems
- Microstructural analysis and computational homogenisation
- Multi-scale analysis

In Henkes (2021a), the author showed the power of artificial neural networks in the context of multi-scale uncertainty quantification of complex microstructures. Heterogeneous materials are subjected to uncertainties in their microstructure topology as well as their material parameters. These uncertainties stem from natural variability, manufacturing processes, and measurement accuracies, among other factors. A typical microstructure, consisting of a matrix material with spherical inclusions, is shown in Figure 31.

*Figure 31: Microstructure, consisting of a matrix material with spherical inclusions*

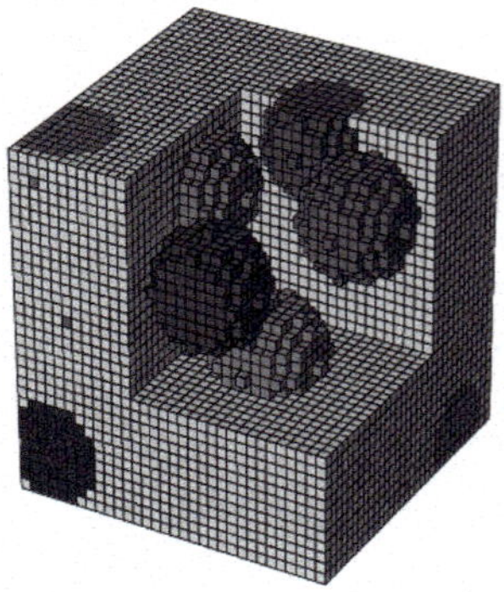

Suppose the uncertain material parameters of the single constituents, namely matrix and inclusion, are known, possibly due to extensive experimental investigations. In that case, it is possible to infer the macroscopically uncertain response of the macro material from this knowledge. This uncertain homogenisation process is computationally very demanding. The usage of artificial neural networks accelerates this process, turning a calculation that would take an hour or possibly even days into mere minutes. This is achieved by learning the homogenisation process and then applying stochastic methods, such as the Monte-Carlo simulation or polynomial chaos expansion. The degree of accuracy of this approach is high, while leading to huge computation speed-ups.

Another project (Henkes at al., 2021b) deals with the governing equations of linear elasticity without applying standard numerical methods like FEM or FFT but instead using artificial neural networks directly. The microstructure below, a matrix with irregular inclusions (WPC), is subjected to unidirectional loading. Then, a physics-informed neural network is used to find a global solution to the boundary-value problem. To enhance the accuracy of the solution, a domain decomposition approach was used.

The residual energy and stress (in the axial direction from left to right) fields can be seen in Figure 32. The artificial neural network can resolve complex fields and capture the underlying microstructure without the use of any data.

With these findings in mind, confidence about the "black box" neural networks is gained. As neural networks can capture the underlying physics accurately, many possible fields in engineering sciences can profit from this new technology.

*Figure 32: Residual energy and stress fields (in the axial direction from left to right)*

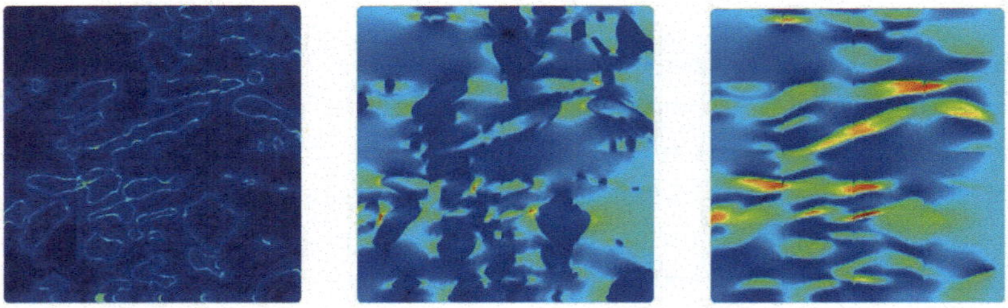

If neural networks help engineers to understand better and predict the, possibly uncertain, material response of heterogeneous materials, they will be able to use them in products more often. In the case of WPC, due to its complex fibre topology, which stems from the natural process of growth and the following industrial manufacturing process, the underlying physics is not fully understood yet. Artificial neural networks, amplified by physical knowledge already known and real-world experimental data, can bridge the unknown to be used in state-of-the-art simulation environments.

This can lead to optimal usage of such materials in structures, reducing the overall number of resources needed.

## References


Abdelbasir, S. M., Hassan, S. S. M., Kamel, A. H., & El-Nasr, R. S. (2018). Status of electronic waste recycling techniques: a review. *Enviromental Science and Pollution Reseach,* Vol. 25, 16533–16547. https://doi.org/10.1007/s11356-018-2136-6

Alireza, A., (2008). Wood-plastic composites as promising green-composites for automotive industries. *Bioresource Technology,* Vol. 99, Issue 11, 4661-4667 https://doi.org/10.1016/j.biortech.2007.09.043

Altenbach, H., Altenbach, J., & Kissing, W. (2004). *Mechanics of Composite Structural Elements.* 2. Ed. Springer Publisher. https://doi.org/10.1007/978-981-10-8935-0

Arnette, A. N., Brewer, B. L., & Choal, T. (2014). Design for sustainability (DFS): the intersection of supply chain and environment. *Journal of Cleaner Production,* Vol. 83, 374–390. https://doi.org/10.1016/j.jclepro.2014.07.021

Bauer, S. (2003). Design for X. Ansätze zur Definition und Strukturierung. Proceedings of the 14th Symposium on Design for X, 1-8. https://www.designsociety.org/publication/27590/Design+for+X+%E2%80%93+Ans%C3%A4tze+zur+Definition+und+Strukturierung

Baker, A., Dutton, S., & Kelly, D. (Eds.) (2004). *Composite Materials for Aerospace Structures.* 2. Ed., ISBN 1-56347-540-5

Bender, B., & Gericke, K. (2021). *Pahl/Beitz Konstruktionslehre. Methoden und Anwendung erfolgreicher Produktentwicklung.* 9. Ed., Springer. https://doi.org/10.1007/978-3-662-57303-7

Kirchner, E., & Neudörfer, A. (2020) Grundregeln der Gestaltung. In B. Bender, & K. Gericke (2021). *Pahl/Beitz Konstruktionslehre. Methoden und Anwendung erfolgreicher Produktentwicklung (467-523).* 9. Ed., Springer. https://doi.org/10.1007/978-3-662-57303-7_14

Boehm, B. W. (1988): A spiral model of software development and enhancement. *Computer,* Vol. 21, Issue 5, 61–72. https://doi.org/10.1109/2.59

Boin, U. M., Linsmeyer, T., Neubacher, F., & Winter, B. (2000). *Stand der Technik in der Sekundäraluminiumerzeugung im Hinblick auf die IPPC-Richtlinie.* Federal

Enviroment Agency – Austria, M-120. https://www.umweltbundesamt.at/fileadmin/site/publikationen/M120.pdf

Boothroyd, G., Dewhurst, P., & Knight, W. A. (Eds.) (2010). *Product Design for Manufacture and Assembly*. CRC Press. ISBN 9781420089271

Breiing, A. & Knosala, R. (1997). *Bewerten technischer Systeme. Theoretische und methodische Grundlagen bewertungstechnischer Entscheidungshilfen*. Springer Berlin. https://doi.org/10.1007/978-3-642-59229-4

Breuer, U. P. (1997). *Beitrag zur Umformtechnik gewebeverstärkter Thermoplaste*. Dissertation, Technische Universität Kaiserslautern. https://kluedo.ub.uni-kl.de/frontdoor/index/index/docId/4716

Brüggemann, S., Brüssel, C., & Härthe, D. (2018). *Nachhaltigkeit in der Unternehmenspraxis. Impulse für Wirtschaft und Politik*. Springer Gabler Wiesbaden. https://doi.org/10.1007/978-3-658-23065-4

Campbell, F. C. (2010). Structural Composite Materials. ASM International. ISBN: 978-1-61503-037-8

Cappelli, F., Delogu, M., Pierini, M., & Schiavone, F. (2007). Design for disassembly: a methodology for identifying the optimal disassembly sequence. *Journal of Engineering Design*, Vol. 18, Issue 6, 563–575. https://doi.org/10.1080/09544820601013019

Caulfield, D. F., Jacobson, R. E., Sears, K. D., & Underwood, J. H. (2001). Fiber reinforced engineering plastics, *Proceedings of the 2nd International Conference on Advanced Engineered*. https://www.srs.fs.usda.gov/pubs/9097

Chiu, M. C., & Kremer, G. E. (2011). Investigation of the Applicability of Design for X Tools during Design Concept Evolution: A Literature Review. *International Journal of Product Development*, Vol. 13, Issue 2, 132-167. https://doi.org/10.1504/IJPD.2011.038869

Cooper, D. R., & Allwood, J. M. (2012). Reusing steel and aluminum components at end of product life. *Environmental Science & Technology*, Vol. 46, Issue 18, 10334–10340. https://doi.org/10.1021/es301093a

Corbière-Nicollier, T., Gfeller Laban, B., Lundquist, L., Leterrier, Y., Månson, J.-A. E., & Jolliet, O. (2001). Life cycle assessment of biofibres replacing glass fibres as reinforcement in plastics. *Resources, Conservation and Recycling*, Vol. 33, Issue 4, 267-287, https://doi.org/10.1016/S0921-3449(01)00089-1

Council for the Environment and Infrastructure (Rli) (2015). *Circular Economy. From Wish to Practice*. ISBN 978-90-77323-25-0

Cross, N. (2000. *Engineering Design Methods: Strategies for Product Design*. 4. Ed. New York: Wiley & Sons Inc. ISBN: 978-0-470-51926-4

Cruz Sanchez, F. A., Boudaoud, H., Camargo, M., & Pearce, J. M. (2020). Plastic recycling in additive manufacturing: A systematic literature review and opportunities for the circular economy. *Journal of Cleaner Production*, Vol. 264, 121602. https://doi.org/10.1016/j.jclepro.2020.121602

Dowlatshahi, S. (1996): The role of logistics in concurrent engineering. *International Journal of Production Economics*, Vol. 44, Issue 3, 189–199. https://doi.org/10.1016/0925-5273(96)00173-9

Dyckhoff, H. (2000). *Umweltmanagement. Zehn Lektionen in umweltorientierter Unternehmensführung*. Springer Berlin, Heidelberg. ISBN 978-3-540-66966-1

Ehrlenspiel, K., & Meerkamm, H. (2013). *Integrierte Produktentwicklung. Denkabläufe, Methodeneinsatz, Zusammenarbeit*. 5. Ed. Carl Hanser Publisher. ISBN 978-3-446-43548-3

Eigner, M., Dickopf, T., Apostolov, H., Schaefer, P., Faißt, K.-G., & Keßler, A. (2014). System Lifecycle Management. Initial Approach for a Sustainable Product Development Process Based on Methods of Model Based Systems Engineering. In S. Fukuda, A. Bernard, B. Gurumoorthy, & A. Bouras (Eds.). *Product Lifecycle Management for a Global Market*. PLM 2014. IFIP Advances in Information and Communication Technology, Vol 442, Springer Berlin, Heidelberg. https://doi.org/10.1007/978-3-662-45937-9_29

Ellen MacArthur Foundation (2013). Towards The Circular Economy Vol. 1: an economic and business rationale for an accelerated transition. https://ellenmacarthurfoundation.org/towards-the-circular-economy-vol-1-an-economic-and-business-rationale-for-an

Elmarakbi, A., & Azoti, W. L. (2015). Novel composite materials for automotive applications: concepts and challenges for energy-efficient and safe vehicles, *10th International Conference on Composite Science and Technology ICCST/10.*

Etherington, C. (1974). Conform - A New Concept for the Continuous Extrusion Forming of Metals. *Journal of Engineering for Industry*, Vol. 96, Issue 3, 893–900. https://doi.org/10.1115/1.3438458

Europäisches Parlament (2008). 2008/98/EG: Directive 2008/98/EC of the European Parliament and of the Council of 19 November 2008 on waste and repealing certain Directives. *Official Journal of the European Union*, 312, p. 3-30.

Evens, T., Bex G. J., Yigit, M., de Keyzer, J., Desplentere, F., & van Bael, A. (2019). The Influence of Mechanical Recycling on Properties in Injection Molding of Fiber-Reinforced Polypropylene. *International Polymer Processing*, Vol. 34, Issue 4, 398–407. https://doi.org/10.3139/217.3770

Faerber, M., Jochaud, F.,Stöber, C., Jablonski, S., Meerkamm, H., Knowledge Oriented Process Management For DfX. International Design Conference 2008, 777-784, https://www.designsociety.org/publication/26721/KNOWLEDGE+ORIENTED+PROCESS+MANAGEMENT+FOR+DFX

Ford, D., & Ryan, C. (1981). Taking technology to market. Harvard Business Review, Vol. 59, Issue 2, 117–126. https://www.osti.gov/biblio/6132739

Fiksel, J., & Wapman, K. (1994). How to design for environment and minimize life cycle cost. *Proceedings of 1994 IEEE International Symposium on Electronics and The Environment*, 75-80, https://doi.org/10.1109/ISEE.1994.337290

Freund, T. (2018). *Konstruktionshinweise zur Beherrschung von Unsicherheit in technischen Systemen*. Dissertation. Technische Universität Darmstadt. https://tuprints.ulb.tu-darmstadt.de/id/eprint/7231

Freund, T., Würtenberger, J., Lotz, J., Rommel, C., & Kirchner, E. (2017). Design for Robustness. Systematic Application of Design Guidelines to Control Uncertainty. *Proceedings of the 21st International Conference on Engineering Design* (ICED 17) Canada, 277–286. ISBN: 978-1-904670-92-6

Friedrich, H. E. (Eds.) (2017). *Leichtbau in der Fahrzeugtechnik*. Springer Vieweg Wiesbaden. https://doi.org/10.1007/978-3-658-12295-9

Friedrich, D. (2021). *Angewandte Bauphysik und Werkstoffkunde naturfaserverstärkter Kunststoffe. Eine Anleitung für Studium und Praxis*. Springer Fachmedien Wiesbaden. https://doi.org/10.1007/978-3-658-30938-1

Gajski, D. D., & Kuhn, R. H. (1983). Guest Editors' Introduction: New VLSI Tools. *Computer*, Vol. 16, Issue 12, 11–14. https://doi.org/10.1109/MC.1983.1654264

Gangil, B., Ranakoti, L., Verma, S., Singh, T., & Kumar, S. (2020). Natural and Synthetic Fibers for Hybrid Composites. In Khan, A., Rangappa, S. M., Jawaid, M., Siengchin, S. & Asiri, A. M. *Hybrid Fiber Composites: Materials, Manufacturing, Process Engineering* (1-15). Wiley-VCH Publisher. https://doi.org/10.1002/9783527824571.ch1

Geyer, E. (1976). Produktplanung. Ideenfindung, Ideenbewertung, Ideenverfolgung. In Rationalisierungs-Kuratorium der Deutschen Wirtschaft, & H. H. Moll (Eds.). *RKW-Handbuch Forschung, Entwicklung, Konstruktion (F+E): ergänzbares Handbuch für Wissenschaft, Technik, Wirtschaft und Verwaltung. Grundwerk*. Schmidt. ISBN: 978-3-5030-1197-1

Gräßler, I. (2004). *Kundenindividuelle Massenproduktion. Entwicklung, Vorbereitung der Herstellung, Veränderungsmanagement*. Springer Berlin, Heidelberg. ISBN: 978-3-5402-0554-8

Gräßler, I., & Yang, X. (2016). Interdisciplinary development of production systems using Systems Engineering. *Procedia CIRP*, Vol. 50, 653-658. https://doi.org/10.1016/j.procir.2016.05.008

Gräßler, I., Hentze, J., & Yang, X. (2016). Eleven Potentials for Mechatronic V-Model. International Conference Production Engineering. *Production Engineering and Management*, 6th International Conference, Vol. 1, 257-268.

Gräßler, I., Scholle, P., & Pottebaum, J. (2017b). Integrated Process and Data Model for Agile Strategic Planning. In: Vajna, Sandor (eds.) : 11th International Workshop on Integrated Design Engineering, 207

Gräßler, I., Pöhler, A., & Hentze, J. (2017a). Decoupling of Product and Production Development in Flexible Production Environments. *Procedia CIRP*, Vol. 67, 548-553. https://doi.org/10.1016/j.procir.2017.01.040

Gräßler, I., & Pöhler, A. (2018). Intelligent devices in a decentralized production system concept. *Procedia CIRP*, Vol. 67, 116-121. https://doi.org/10.1016/j.procir.2017.12.186

Gräßler, I., Dattner, M., & Bothen, M. (2018). Main feature list as core success criteria of organizing requirements elicitation. *R&D Management Conference*, 1-16. https://doi.org/10.17619/UNIPB/1-679

Gräßler, I., & Pöhler, A. (2019). Human-centric design of cyber-physical production systems. *Procedia CIRP*, Vol. 84, 251-256. https://doi.org/10.1016/j.procir.2019.04.199

Gräßler, I., Oleff, C., & Scholle, P. (2020). Method for Systematic Assessment of Requirement Change Risk in Industrial Practice. *Applied Sciences*, Vol. 10, Issue 23, 8697. https://doi.org/10.3390/app10238697

Gräßler, I., & Hesse, P. (2021). Digitaler Zwilling zur Gestaltung der Prozesse im End-of-Life. Produktdaten für das Recycling einer Produktinstanz. In H. Biedermann, W. Posch, & S. Vorbach (Eds.). *Digitalisierung im Kontext von Nachhaltigkeit und Klimawandel (135–148)*. Vol. 9. Nomos Verlagsgesellschaft. https://doi.org/10.5771/9783957102966-135

Gräßler, I., & Pottebaum, J. (2021). Generic Product Lifecycle Model: A Holistic and Adaptable Approach for Multi-Disciplinary Product–Service Systems. *Applied Sciences*, Vol. 11, Issue 10, 4516. https://doi.org/10.3390/app11104516

Gross, D., Hauger, W., Schröder, J., & Wall, W. A. (2009). *Technische Mechanik 1*. Springer Berlin Heidelberg. https://doi.org/10.1007/978-3-540-68397-1

Güley, V. (2014). *Recycling of aluminum chips by hot extrusion*. Dissertation, Technische Universität Dortmund. ISBN: 978-3-8440-2476-0

Habenicht, G. (2016). *Kleben - erfolgreich und fehlerfrei*. Springer Fachmedien Wiesbaden. https://doi.org/10.1007/978-3-8348-8316-2

Hansen, F. (1968). *Konstruktionssystematik*. 3. Ed. VEB Verlag Technik Berlin.

Henkes, A., Caylak, I., & Mahnken, R. (2021a). A deep learning driven pseudospectral PCE based FFT homogenization algorithm for complex microstructures. *Computer Methods in Applied Mechanics and Engineering*, Vol. 385, 114070. https://doi.org/10.1016/j.cma.2021.114070

Henkes, A., Wessels, H., & Mahnken, R. (2021b). Physics Informed Neural Networks for direct solution of continuum mechanical governing equations in complex microstructures. *Computer Methods in Applied Mechanics and Engineering*, Vol. 393, 114790. https://doi.org/10.1016/j.cma.2022.114790

Herrmann, C. (2010). *Ganzheitliches Life Cycle Management. Nachhaltigkeit und Lebenszyklusorientierung in Unternehmen*. Springer Publisher. https://doi.org/10.1007/978-3-642-01421-5

Heshmati, A. (2018) A review of the circular economy and its implementation. International Journal of Green Economics, Vol. 11, Issue 3-4, 251-284. https://doi.org/10.1504/IJGE.2017.089856

Horwath, I., Dohmeier-Fischer, S., Weiß-Borkowski, N., & Tröster, T. (2018). From Empowerment to Innovation: Inter- and Transdisciplinary Research Methods in Lightweight Engineering. *INTED2018 Proceedings*, 7060-7068. https://doi.org/10.21125/inted.2018.1651

Hubka, V. (1992). Design for Quality and Design Methodology. *Journal of Engineering Design*, Vol. 3, 5–15. https://doi.org/10.1080/09544829208914744

Isaksson, O., & Eckert, C. (2020). Product Development 2040: Technologies are just as good as the designer's ability to integrate them. *Design Society Report* DS107, https://doi.org/10.35199/report.pd2040

Ishii, K., Eubanks, C. F., & Di Marco, P. (1994). Design for product retirement and material life-cycle. Material & Design, Vol. 5, Issue 4, 225-233. https://doi.org/10.1016/0261-3069(94)90007-8

Jacobson, R., Caulfield, D., Sears, K., & Underwood, J. (2002). Low temperature processing (LTP) of ultra-pure cellulose fibers into nylon 6 and other thermoplastics, *Proceedings of the Sixth International Conference on Woodfiber - Plastic Composites* (127-133). ISBN: 0892529181

Jahn, T., Bergmann, M., & Keil, F. (2012). Transdisciplinarity: Between mainstreaming and marginalization. *Ecological Economics*, Vol. 79, 1-10. https://doi.org/10.1016/j.ecolecon.2012.04.017

Jawaihr, I. S., Wanigarathne, P. C., & Wang, X. (2005). Product Design and Manufacturing Processes for Sustainability. In M. Kutz (Eds.). *Mechanical Engineers' Handbook. Manufacturing and Management (414–443)*. 3. Ed., John Wiley & Sons. https://doi.org/10.1002/0471777463.ch12

Joost, W.J. (2012). Reducing Vehicle Weight and Improving U.S. Energy Efficiency Using Integrated Computational Materials Engineering. *The Journal of The Minerals, Metals & Materials Society*, Vol. 64, 1032–1038. https://doi.org/10.1007/s11837-012-0424-z

Kipp, T., & Krause, D. (2008). Design for Variety. Efficient Support for Design Engineers. *Proceedings DESIGN 2008, the 10th International Design Conference*, 425–432.

Klein, B. (2013). *Leichtbau-Konstruktion. Berechnungsgrundlagen und Gestaltung*. Springer Fachmedien Wiesbaden. https://doi.org/10.1007/978-3-658-02272-3

Klenk, F., Häfner, B., Lanza, G., & Wagner, M. (2019). Kreislaufwirtschaft in globalen Wertschöpfungsnetzwerken. *Industrie 4.0 Management*, Vol.35, 29–32. https://doi.org/10.30844/I40M_19-6_S25-28

Krause, D., & Gebhardt, N. (2018). *Methodische Entwicklung modularer Produktfamilien. Hohe Produktvielfalt beherrschbar entwickeln*. Springer Vieweg Berlin Heidelberg. https://doi.org/10.1007/978-3-662-53040-5

Kriwet, A., Zussman, E., & Seliger, G. (1995). Systematic Integration of Design-for-Recycling into Product Design. *International Journal of Production Economics*, Vol. 38, Issue 1, 15–22. https://doi.org/10.1016/0925-5273(95)99062-A

Kuo, T.-C., Huang, S. H., & Zhang, H.-C. (2001). Design for manufacture and design for 'X': concepts, applications, and perspectives. *Computers & Industrial Engineering*, Vol. 41, Issue 3, 241–260. https://doi.org/10.1016/S0360-8352(01)00045-6

Kuo, P.-Y., Wang, S.-Y., Chen, J.-H., Hsueh, H.-C., & Tsai, M.-J. (2009). Effects of material compositions on the mechanical properties of wood–plastic composites manufactured by injection molding. *Materials & Design*, Vol. 30, Issue 9, 3489–3496. https://doi.org/10.1016/j.matdes.2009.03.012

Lachmayer, R., Rettschlag, K., & Kaierle, S. (Eds.) (2020). *Konstruktion für die Additive Fertigung 2019*. Springer Vieweg Berlin Heidelberg. https://doi.org/10.1007/978-3-662-61149-4

La Mantia, F.P., & Morreale, M. (2011). Green composites: A brief review. *Composites Part A: Applied Science and Manufacturing*, Vol. 42, Issue 6, 579-588. https://doi.org/10.1016/j.compositesa.2011.01.017

Lienig, J. (2006): *Layoutsynthese elektrischer Schaltungen. Grundlegende Algorithmen für die Entwurfsautomatisierung*. 1. Ed. Springer Berlin Heidelberg. https://doi.org/10.1007/3-540-29942-4

Lossen, B. (2019). *Ein Beitrag zur Herstellung von hybriden Bauteilen mittels Reibdrücken*. Dissertation. Shaker Publisher. ISBN: 978-3-8440-6729-3

Machi, L. A., & McEvoy, B. T. (2016). *The Literature Review: Six Steps to Success*. 2. Ed. Corwin Press. ISBN: 978-1-4522-4088-6

Mahnken, R. (2011). *Lehrbuch der technischen Mechanik-Band 3: Dynamik: eine anschauliche Einführung*. Springer Vieweg Berlin Heidelberg. ISBN: 978-3642198373

Mahnken, R. (2016). *Lehrbuch der Technischen Mechanik-Band 1: Starrkörperstatik: Grundlagen und Anwendungen*. Springer Vieweg Berlin Heidelberg. https://doi.org/10.1007/978-3-662-52785-6

Mahnken, R. (2019). *Lehrbuch der Technischen Mechanik-Band 2: Elastostatik: Mit einer Einführung in Hybridstrukturen*. Springer Vieweg Berlin Heidelberg. https://doi.org/10.1007/978-3-662-58166-7

Mapleston, P. (2001). Additive suppliers turn their eyes to wood/plastic composites. *Modern Plastics*, Vol. 78, Issue 8, 52.

McConnell, V. P. (2010). Launching the carbon fiber recycling industry. *Reinforced Plastics* Vol. 54, Issue 2, 33–37. https://doi.org/10.1016/S0034-3617(10)70063-1

McDonough, W., & Braungart, M. (2002). *Cradle to Cradle. Remaking the Way We Make Things*. 7. Ed. North Point Press. ISBN: 978-0-8654-7587-8

Meng, F., McKechnie, J., Turner, T. A., & Pickering, S. J. (2017). Energy and environmental assessment and reuse of fluidised bed recycled carbon fibers. *Composites Part A: Applied Science and Manufacturing*, Vol. 100, 206–214. https://doi.org/10.1016/j.compositesa.2017.05.008

Meng, F., Olivetti, E. A., Zhao, Y., Chang, J. C., Pickering, S. J., & McKechnie, J. (2018). Comparing life cycle energy and global warming potential of carbon fiber composite recycling technologies and waste management options. *ACS Sustainable Chem. Eng.*, Vol. 6, Issue 8, 9854-9865. https://doi.org/10.1021/acssuschemeng.8b01026

Mishnaevsky, L., Branner, K., Petersen, H. N., Beauson. J., McGugan, M., & Sørensen, B. F. (2017). Materials for wind turbine blades: an overview. *Materials*, Vol. 10, Issue 11, 1285. https://doi.org/10.3390/ma10111285

Moritzer, E., & Bürenhaus, F. I. (2021). Influence of processing parameters on fiber length degradation during injection molding. *SPE (Society of Plastics Engineers) Antec 2021 Proceedings*: The Annual Technical Conference for Plastic Professionals. ISBN: 978-1-7138-3075-7

Moritzer, E., & Richters, M. (2021). Characterization of wood-filled thermoplastic polyurethane for the injection molding process. *Journal of Applied Polymer Science*, Vol. 138, Issue 38. https://doi.org/10.1002/app.50968

Mörtl, M., & Schmied, C. (2015). Design for Cost. A Review of Methods, Tools and Research Directions. *Journal of the Indian Institute of Science*, Vol. 95, 379–404.

Mulder, W., Blok, J., Hoekstra, S., & Kokkeler, F. (2012). *Design for maintenance. guidelines to enhance maintainability, reliability and supportability of industrial products*. University of Twente. ISBN: 978-94-6190-993-0

Muramatsu, H., Kim, Y. A., Yang, K. S., Cruz-Silva, R., Toda, I., Yamada, T., Terrones, M., Endo, M., Hayashi, T., & Saitoh, H. (2014). Rice husk-derived graphene with nano-sized domains and clean edges. *Small*, Vol. 10, Issue 14, 2766-2770. https://doi.org/10.1002/smll.201400017

Nair, A. B., & Joseph, R. (2014). 9 - Eco-friendly bio-composites using natural rubber (NR) matrices and natural fiber reinforcements. Chemistry, Manufacture and Applications of Natural Rubber, 249-283. https://doi.org/10.1533/9780857096913.2.249

Novoselov, K. S., Falko, V. I., Colombo, L., Gellert, P. R., Schwab, M. G., & Kim, K. (2012). A Roadmap for Graphene. *Nature*, Vol. 490, 192-200. https://doi.org/10.1038/nature11458

Okorie, O., Salonitis, K., Charnley, F., Moreno, M., Turner, C., & Tiwari, A. (2018). Digitisation and the Circular Economy. A Review of Current Research and Future Trends. *Energies*, Vol. 11, 3009. https://doi.org/10.3390/en11113009

Pahl, G., & Beitz, W. (1977). *Konstruktionslehre. Handbuch für Studium und Praxis*. 1. Ed., Springer Berlin, Heidelberg. https://doi.org/10.1007/978-3-662-02288-7

Pahl, G., Beitz, W., Feldhusen, J., & Grote, K.-H. (2007). *Engineering Design. A systematic approach*. 3. Ed., Springer London. https://doi.org/10.1007/978-1-84628-319-2

Pan, Y., & Li, H. (2016). Sustainability evaluation of end-of-life vehicle recycling based on emergy analysis: a case study of an end-of-life vehicle recycling enterprise in China. In *Journal of Cleaner Production*, Vol. 131, 219–227. https://doi.org/10.1016/j.jclepro.2016.05.045

Pickering, S. J., & Turner, T. A. (2014). Research and development in support of carbon fiber recycling. Composites and Advanced Materials Expo: Combined Strength. Unsurpassed Innovation., CAMX 2014, Orlando.

Pohl, C., Krütli, P., & Stauffacher, M. (2017). Ten Reflective Steps for Rendering Research Societally Relevant, *GAIA - Ecological Perspectives for Science and Society*, Vol. 26, Issue 1, 43–51. https://doi.org/10.14512/gaia.26.1.10

Ponn, J., & Lindemann, U. (2011). *Konzeptentwicklung und Gestaltung technischer Produkte. Systematisch von Anforderungen zu Konzepten und Gestaltlösungen*. Springer Berlin, Heidelberg. https://doi.org/10.1007/978-3-642-20580-4

Potting, J., Hekkert, M., Worrell, E., & Hanemaaijer, A. (2017). *Circular Economy. Measuring innovation in the product chain*. PBL Publisher, No.: 2544

Prakash, M., & Laxminarayana, H. P. (2019). A Review on Micro Drilling of Glass Fiber Reinforced Polymer Composites. International Journal for Research in Applied Science & Engineering Technology (IJRASET), Vol. 7, Issue 5, 3612-3615. https://doi.org/10.22214/ijraset.2019.5592

Pulkkinen, A., Martikainen, A., & Kuusela, J. (2012). A framework of Design for Procurement. *Proceedings of 18th International Conference on Engineering* (ICE). https://doi.org/10.1109/ICE.2012.6297662

Raabe, D., Tasan, C. C., & Olivetti, E. A. (2019). Strategies for improving the sustainability of structural metals. *Nature*, Vol. 575, 64–74. https://doi.org/10.1038/s41586-019-1702-5

Radovanovic, I. (2007). *Verarbeitung und Optimierung der Rezeptur von Wood-Plastic Composites*. Dissertation, Universität Osnabrück. https://osnadocs.ub.uni-osnabrueck.de/handle/urn:nbn:de:gbv:700-2007041315

Redtenbacher, F. (1863). *Der Maschinenbau*. 2. Ed. Karlsruhe: Verlagsbuchhandlung von Friedrich Bassermann (Friedrich Bassermann Publishing Bookshop).

Regenfelder, M., & Ebelt, S. (2012). Strategies of Waste Prevention - A New Prevention Hierarchy. *Proceedings of Management of Technologies - Step to Sustainable Production (MOTSP)*, 397–404.

Rogers, D. S., & Tibben-Lembke, R. (2001). An Examination of Reverse Logistics Practices. *Journal of Business Logistics*, Vol. 22, Issue 2, 129–148. https://doi.org/10.1002/j.2158-1592.2001.tb00007.x

Roth, K. (2000). *Konstruieren mit Konstruktionskatalogen. Band 1: Konstruktionslehre*. 3. Ed. Springer Berlin, Heidelberg. https://doi.org/10.1007/978-3-642-17466-7

Rowell, R. M. (Ed.) (2013). *Handbook of Wood Chemistry and Wood Composites*. 2. Ed. Boca Raton: CRC Press Taylor & Francis Group. ISBN: 978-1-4398-5381-8

Ruiz-Hitzky, E., Darder, M., Fernandes, F.M., Zatile, E., Palomares, F. J., & Aranda, P. (2011). Supported graphene from natural resources: Easy preparation and applications. *Advanced Materials*, Vol. 23, Issue 44, 5250-5255. https://doi.org/10.1002/adma.201101988

Sathishkumar, T. P., Naveen, J., & Satheeshkumar, S. (2014). Hybrid fiber reinforced polymer composites – a review. Journal of Reinforced Plastics and Composites, Vol. 33, Issue 5, 454–471. https://doi.org/10.1177/0731684413516393

Schmidt, H.C., Rodman, D., Grydin, O., Ebbert, C., Homberg, W., Maier, H.J., & Grundmeier, G. (2014). Joining with Electrochemical Support: Cold Pressure Welding of Copper – Weld Formation and Characterization. *Advanced Materials Research*, Vols. 966-967, 453–460. https://doi.org/10.4028/www.scientific.net/AMR.966-967.453

Schröder, C. (2013). *Verfahrenstechnische Entwicklung zum Hinterspritzen von Echtholzfurnieren mit Wood-Plastic-Composites* (WPC). Dissertation, Paderborn University. Shaker-Publisher. ISBN: 978-3-8440-2186-8

Schuh, G., & Klappert, S. (2011). *Technologiemanagement*. 2. Ed., Springer Berlin Heidelberg. https://doi.org/10.1007/978-3-642-12530-0

Schwarz, H.-G. (2004). Aluminum Production and Energy. *Encyclopedia of Energy*, 81–95. https://doi.org/10.1016/B0-12-176480-X/00372-7

Sears, K., Jacobson, R., Caulfield, D., & Underwood, J. (2001). *Composites containing cellulosic pulp fibers and methods of making and using same*. U.S. Patent WO 00/21743.

Singh, P., Bahadur, J., & Pal, K. (2017). One-step one chemical synthesis process of graphene from rice husk for energy storage applications. *Graphene*, Vol. 6, Issue 3, 61-71. https://doi.org/10.4236/graphene.2017.63005

Soo, V. K., Peeters, J., Paraskevas, D., Compston, P., Doolan, M., & Duflou, J. R. (2018). Sustainable aluminium recycling of end-of-life products: A joining techniques perspective. *Journal of Cleaner Production*, Vol. 178, 119–132. https://doi.org/10.1016/j.jclepro.2017.12.235

Soo, V. K., Compston, P., & Doolan, M. (2018). The Impact of Joining Choices on Vehicle Recycling Systems. *Procedia CIRP*, Vol. 69, 843–848. https://doi.org/10.1016/j.procir.2017.11.009

Srinivas, H. (2022). *Moving towards a Circular Economy: More than Just 3Rs!* GDRC Research Output - Concept Note Series E-097. Kobe, Japan: Global Development Research Center. https://www.gdrc.org/uem/waste/more-3r.html

Stark, R., Anderl, R., Thoben, K.-D., & Wartzack, S. (2020). WiGeP-Positionspapier: „Digitaler Zwilling". *Zeitschrift für wirtschaftlichen Fabrikbetrieb*, Vol. 115, 47-50. https://doi.org/10.3139/104.112311

Steidl, E., Sobczak, L., & Pretschuh, C. (2018). Monitoring of Injection Molding Tool Corrosion and Effects of Wood Plastic Compound's Moisture on Material Properties. *International Polymer Processing*, Vol. 33, Issue 1, 66–75. https://doi.org/10.3139/217.3382

Steinhilper, R., & Rieg, F. (2012). *Handbuch Konstruktion*. Carl Hanser Publisher. ISBN: 978-3-446-43000-6

Stewart, R. (2011). Rebounding automotive industry welcome news for FRP. *Reinforced Plastics,* Vol. 55, Issue 1, 38-44. https://doi.org/10.1016/S0034-3617(11)70036-4

Strange, T., & Bayley A. (2008). *Sustainable Development: Linking Economy, Society, Environment.* OECD Publishing. https://doi.org/10.1787/9789264055742-en

Sy, M., & Mascle, C. (2011). Product design analysis based on life cycle features. *Journal of Engineering Design,* Vol. 22, Issue 6, 387–406. https://doi.org/10.1080/09544820903409899

Synnes, E. L., & Welo, T. (2015). Design for Automated Assembly of Large and Complex Products: Experiences from a Marine Company Operating in Norway. *Procedia Computer Science,* Vol. 44, 254–265. https://doi.org/10.1016/j.procs.2015.03.052

Tchana Toffe, G., Oluwarotimi Ismail, S., Montalvão, D., Knight, J., & Ren, G. (2019). A Scale-up of Energy-Cycle Analysis on Processing Non-Woven Flax/PLA Tape and Triaxial Glass Fibre Fabric for Composites. *Journal of Manufacturing and Materials Processing.* Vol. 3, Issue 4, 92. https://doi.org/10.3390/jmmp3040092

Tekkaya, A. E., Güley, V., Haase, M., & Jäger, A. (2012). Hot Extrusion of Aluminum Chips. *ICAA13 Pittsburgh,* 1559–1573. https://doi.org/10.1007/978-3-319-48761-8_235

Teschner, R. (2013). *Glasfasern.* Springer Vieweg Berlin, Heidelberg. https://doi.org/10.1007/978-3-642-38329-8

Tiefel, T. (Ed.) (2008). *Gewerbliche Schutzrechte im Innovationsprozess.* Deutscher Universitätsverlag Wiesbaden. https://doi.org/10.1007/978-3-8350-5496-7

Tiefel, T. (2007). Technologielebenszyklus-Modelle - Eine kritische Analyse. In T. Tiefel (Hg.). *Gewerbliche Schutzrechte im Innovationsprozess (pp. 25–49),* Deutscher Universitätsverlag Wiesbaden. https://doi.org/10.1007/978-3-8350-5496-7_2

Tseng, M. M., Wang, Y., & Jiao, R. J. (2017). Mass Customization. In The International Academy for Production Engineering, L. Laperrière & G. Reinhart (Eds.) (2017). *CIRP Encyclopedia of Production Engineering,* Springer Berlin, Heidelberg. https://doi.org/10.1007/978-3-642-35950-7_16701-3

Tuck, C. O., Perez, E., Horvath, I. T., Sheldon, R. A., & Poliakoff, M. (2012). Valorization of biomass: Deriving more value from waste. *Science,* Vol. 337, Issue 6095, 695-699. https://doi.org/10.1126/science.1218930

Unterweger C., Brüggemann O., & Fürst C. (2013). Synthetic fibers and thermoplastics short-fiber-reinforced polymers: Properties and characterization. *Polymer Composites,* Vol. 35, Issue 2, 227-236. https://doi.org/10.1002/pc.22654

Vajna, S., Weber, C., Zeman, K., Hehenberger, P., Gerhard, D., & Wartzack, S. (2018). *CAx für Ingenieure.* Springer Vieweg Berlin, Heidelberg. https://doi.org/10.1007/978-3-662-54624-6

Vanderreydt, I., Rommens, T., Tenhunen, A., Mortensen, L. F., & Tange, I. (2021). *Greenhouse gas emissions and natural capital implications of plastics (including biobased plastics).* Eionet Report – ETC/WMGE 2021/3

van Kleef, E., van Trijp, H. C. M., & Luning, P. (2005). Consumer research in the early stages of new product development: a critical review of methods and techniques. *Food Quality and Preference,* Vol. 16, Issue 3, 181–201. https://doi.org/10.1016/j.foodqual.2004.05.012

Vita, A., Castorani, V., Germani, M., & Marconi, M. (2019). Comparative life cycle assessment of low-pressure RTM, compression RTM and high-pressure RTM manufacturing processes to produce CFRP car hoods. *Procedia CIRP,* Vol. 80, 352–357. https://doi.org/10.1016/j.procir.2019.01.109

Wang, S., Xing, X., Zhang, X., Wang, X., & Jing, X. (2018). Room-temperature fully recyclable carbon fiber reinforced phenolic composites through dynamic covalent boronic ester bonds. *Journal of Materials Chemistry A,* Vol. 6, Issue 23, 10868–10878. https://doi.org/10.1039/C8TA01801D

Widerøe, F., & Welo, T. (2013). Using contrast material techniques to determine metal flow in screw extrusion of aluminium. *Journal of Materials Processing Technology,* Vol. 213, Issue 7, 1007–1018. https://doi.org/10.1016/j.jmatprotec.2012.11.013

World Commission on Environment and Development (1987). *Report of the World Commission on Environment and Development: Our Common Future* (Brundtland Report). https://digitallibrary.un.org/record/139811

Wögerbauer, H. (1943). *Die Technik des Konstruierens.* 2. Ed., Verlag von R. Oldenbourg.

Yuan, Q., Wu, D., Gotama, J., & Bateman, S. (2008). Wood Fiber Reinforced Polyethylene and Polypropylene Composites with High Modulus and Impact Strength, *Journal of Thermoplastic Composite Materials,* Vol. 21, Issue 3, 195-208. https://doi.org/10.1177/0892705708089472

Zhu, C., Guo, S., Fang, Y., & Dong, S. (2010). Reducing sugar: New functional molecules for the green synthesis of graphene nanosheets. *ACS Nano,* Vol. 4, Issue 4, 2429-2437. https://doi.org/10.1021/nn1002387

# Case Study III: Challenges of lightweight design, vehicles, and rescuers

*Emine Fulya Akbulut Irmak, Hendrik Hanses, Ilona Horwath, Thomas Tröster*

Planet Earth reflects the energy received from the sun back into space as infrared radiation. The way these radiation fluxes are absorbed by the atmosphere is related to the chemical composition of the atmosphere of our planet. Certain gases, called greenhouse gases, have the property of being less transparent to infrared radiation than to incoming solar energy. It means that the atmosphere becomes less transparent to infrared radiation, causing the significant warming of the Earth's surface as a greenhouse. There is already some greenhouse effect in our atmosphere because otherwise the global temperature of the Earth's surface would be much cooler than its current temperature. Therefore the problem the whole world is dealing with is not the present greenhouse effect but the greenhouse gas effect caused by human activities and negatively affecting the planet's habitability (Bartiaux & van Ypersele, 1993).

A global emission reduction must be pursued to enable a sustainable climate. The only way to achieve this is to balance the concentration of greenhouse gases in the atmosphere. One of several ways to reach this goal is to adopt the principles of different responsibilities among countries, such as population, consumption, and technology (United Nations, 1992). However, one such parameter which affects climate change that many other parameters are directly or indirectly related to is the size of the human population. Thus, a larger population means more emissions and correspondingly needs to take more action to meet a specific climate target. However, this explanation cannot be related directly to the unarguably lower carbon emissions in less populated countries. In countries with a high standard of living, the environmental impact of population growth and distribution, along with unsustainably high consumption rates, must be considered and interpreted through appropriate parameters (Wolfgang, 2009).

The world has arrived at a broad consensus that greenhouse gas emissions from human activities have significantly influenced global warming ever since the first Industrial Revolution. A significant level of this carbon emission stems from industrial activities. Moreover, iron and steel, cement, chemicals and petrochemicals, pulp and paper, and aluminium productions are responsible for a noteworthy percent of the most carbon-intensive energy-related emissions, which are associated with the combustion of fossil fuels (IEA, 2009; Naudé, 2011; Tol, 2009). Most of the energy-intensive industries are generally located in developing countries. Although many plants in these countries (for the aluminium, cement, and fertilizer industries) have the latest technology with the lowest specific energy utilisation, old and inefficient facilities continue to serve in industrialized countries. Nevertheless, the industrial sector has achieved reductions in energy and emission intensity by adopting energy efficiency, sustainability criteria, and certain reduction technologies throughout history, especially in energy-intensive industries. It should not be ignored that the innovations in technology and in practical use also meet several other criteria, such as cost competitiveness, safety, and legal requirements, and are gaining customer acceptance (Metz et al., 2007).

Economic growth has increased the demand for transportation in technologically advanced and developing countries. As the transportation network facilitates trade and accelerates development, it has been on the agenda as an increasing need day by day.

The increasing industrialization has created the need for large shipments of goods and materials over significant distances. Thus systems that will transport people and goods cheaply and efficiently come to the forefront as the main facilitators of economic development. It is precisely in these matters that public transportation plays a critical role in urban areas. However, neither could buses maintain their popularity against private vehicles, nor did rail mass transit systems gain ground outside the busiest cities in the industrialized world. Therefore motorisation has spread day by day, causing some concerns. The gradual growth in the size, weight, and power of passenger cars exacerbate the energy and environmental concerns about motorisation. Although the efficiency of vehicle technology has improved steadily over time, many of the benefits of these improvements have evolved towards increased power and size at the expense of enhanced fuel efficiency (Metz et al., 2007).

With the effect of producing more efficient engines, increasing the body aerodynamics, and decreasing the rolling resistance of the tyres, a stable improvement is observed in the performance of automobiles. In addition, lowering the weight of a car also reduces the load on the suspension parts, which provides a longer lifespan. Furthermore, the use of these materials can lead to significant fuel savings and a lower carbon footprint during transportation. Lightweight structures are the focal points of the automotive and aerospace industries, significantly, as they reduce weight while maintaining structural strength. Although they are light and durable, these materials are generally more costly (Hovorun et al., 2017).

Modern cars are made up of cast iron and steel parts, followed by aluminium alloys, plastics, rubber, glass, and non-ferrous materials. Although the usage rates differ from vehicle to vehicle, steel still has a high percentage in vehicle structure today. Due to its properties, such as increased strength, stiffness, fatigue, crashworthiness, and formability, it has been used in the manufacturing of car bodies for a long time (Hovorun et al., 2017). In addition to high-performance material properties, requirements such as lower emissions to protect the environment must also be met. Satisfactory mechanical properties can sometimes be a contradictory parameter in achieving low emissions. However, reducing the full vehicle weight, starting with the regional parts, can be a general solution. When the amount of load that various vehicle components are exposed to and must withstand is blended and analysed with years of experience, it can be noted that the weight savings can reach approximately 50% in body-in-white (BIW) applications (Tisza & Czinege, 2018).

Metallic materials that are often referenced in the application of lightweight construction principles in automobile manufacturing are high-strength steels and high-strength aluminium alloys (Tisza & Lukács, 2018). However, applying the multi-material concept may be the most appropriate solution. Thus, the performance of the parts, where necessary in the vehicle, can be improved locally. The multi-material concept is widespread in today's automobile body manufacturing.

For instance, the A8 model vehicle, developed by Audi in 1994, has an almost entirely aluminium white body and sheds light on the vehicle technology that was in use in the past. Careful examination shows that only steel is used for the B-pillars, and approximately less than 10% of the body structure consists of steel material. In the same model vehicle, launched in 2018, a multi-material body structure consisting of more than about 40% steel draws attention. The material variety ranges from ultra-high-strength steel materials to carbon fibre reinforced plastic materials. It is proven that the effect of the production methods developed by technology over time for this increase is undeniable (GCC, 2017).

According to the historical evolution of conventional vehicles, an increase in weight is associated with the high safety standards that are more critical day by day. Likewise, the high safety standards found in conventional vehicles are significant in fully electric cars as well. These vehicles already have a sturdy battery, and therefore they are more sensitive to the weight of body structure components.

All vehicles, regardless of the power source, must focus on the safety of their passengers in the event of an accident because when a vehicle preserves its structural integrity as much as possible despite the dynamic load it is exposed to; that means that it puts the passengers trapped in the vehicle at lower risk. Unfortunately, on the contrary, the high-protection vehicle structure obtained by using high-strength materials can become a problem for rescue teams when it comes to rescuing passengers. Therefore, in addition to the rescue teams' skills and experience, the rescue equipment sector, which constantly needs to improve its performance parallel to vehicle technology, emerges. These tools must be high-pressure and able to quickly cut through parts made of aluminium, high-strength steel, and even fibre material in the event of an accident.

Any rescue operation is a specialised team effort that requires following a previously standardised rescue procedure with sufficient equipment by a trained team to rescue survivors trapped inside the vehicle after an accident. People trapped inside the vehicle are often seriously injured, which means that rescue teams must react quickly.

The first actions to be taken in the event of an accident do not differ much from those required for conventional vehicles with gasoline or diesel engines. However, the lack of knowledge about electric vehicles can mean increasing operational time for rescuers. In an accident involving electric vehicles, the high-voltage system must be turned off by the rescue teams and secured against being switched on again. The team must be aware of the fact that high-voltage cables are never cut, and insulating gloves must always be worn to prevent electric shock in rescue operations (Wöhrl et al., 2021).

Since each electric car design is different from conventional ones, the cable harnesses are also designed differently for each vehicle. When it comes to the constantly developing technology and mass production speed, such a situation turns into a highly complex problem for rescue teams. To prevent this, vehicle manufacturers publish rescue manuals for each model. This manual contains all the necessary information for rescue teams, from high voltage cables to battery design (Volkswagen AG, 2020a). However, it is not always realistic to use this in the field since it is a highly extensive guide. The rescue data guide is used, provided that the fire brigade has the technology for this. Rescue manuals also explain the meaning of each symbol used in the manual in a chart (Volkswagen AG, 2020b). In the event of an accident involving a vehicle, rescue teams should carry out their rescue activities based on the manual that belongs to the vehicle in question.

The method used by the fire brigade when rescuing persons in conventional vehicles, typical rescue points of a car, and the techniques used for the necessary equipment were discussed in detail by expert firefighters in the workshop carried out by Weber Rescue in Meiningen. However, it should be noted that firefighters present only technical rescue examples according to specific, accident scenarios during the training. These techniques must be adapted to the specific situation. In a rescue operation, some procedures must be followed sequentially after the accident site has been secured. The first step is to check the material of the car body with a magnet before initiating rescue operations. In this way it can be determined whether the material used in the relevant parts of the vehicle is aluminium or steel. The next step is to break the glass window of the car with equipment that looks like a metal pen with a spring on it. The equipment is positioned at the corner of the window to be broken, pressure is put on the spring, and sudden force is applied to the glass. This procedure is applied to other windows.

This process is continued with the spreading process on the doors. The hydraulic spreader is placed effectively with the help of the gaps created in the door area.

If the gap is not wide enough for the hydraulic spreader, the spreader applies the compression process. This continues until a utilisable gap is obtained. Then the spreader is placed in this gap, and the spreading process continues until the door lock points are damaged. After the door is released from the lock points, the same method is applied to the door junction points, where the expansion process continues until the doors are removed entirely. The doors are separated first from the lock points and then from the junction points, Figure 1.

*Figure 1: A car door is opened in the lock and junction area by hydraulic spreader*

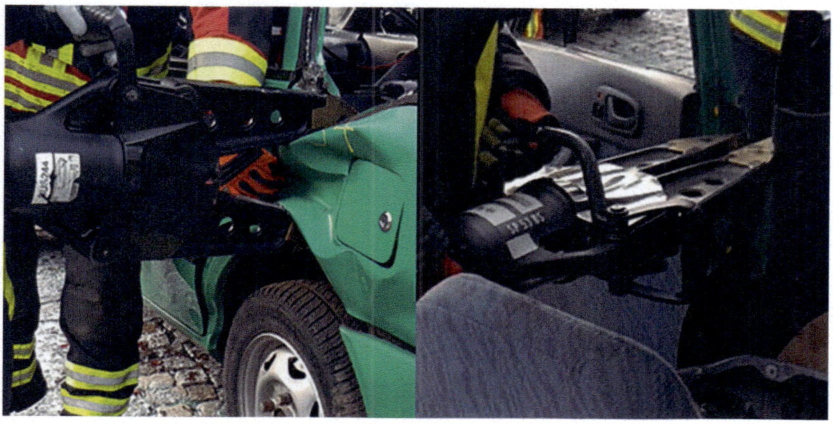

The next step is to cut the B-pillar of the vehicle so that firefighters can reach the people trapped inside the car more easily. This cutting process is completed in two stages, using hydraulic scissors from the top and bottom of the vehicle's B-pillar, Figure 2.

*Figure 2: Large footwell opening by hydraulic scissors*

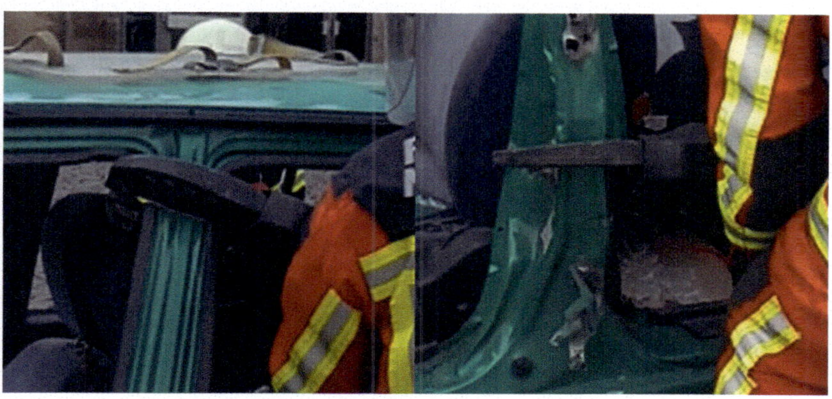

If necessary, the tailgate of the car should also be removed. In this case, the connexion points between the tailgate and the vehicle are cut with the help of the hydraulic scissors. If the vehicle's tailgate is locked, this lock point is first opened by the hydraulic spreader. After having opened the lock all the way, firefighters should cut the connexion points of the tailgate. Finally, after making sure that all connexions of the vehicle's roof with the body and pillars are cut, the vehicle roof is fully opened using a hydraulic rescue ram, Figure 3.

*Figure 3: Removing the tailgate and opening the roof*

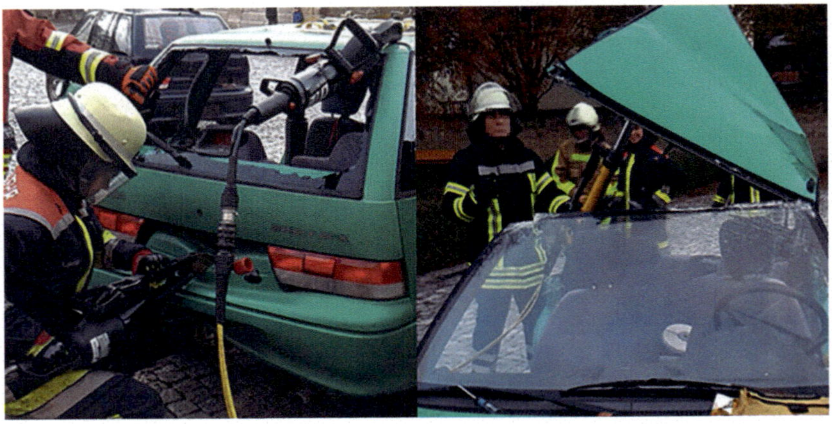

On the basis of this information, on the training day organised for female firefighters, the hydraulic rescue cutter RSU 180 Plus was used to cut vehicle parts. According to the standards, these scissors perform best at a weight of approximately 16.7 kg. The SP 50 BS hydraulic rescue spreader used in spreading processes has a weight of roughly 17 kg. During training, the rescue operation was carried out on two conventional cars. Since the training area has a flat and open ground, rescue equipment with a hydraulic pipe was used. If the space is not a flat and open ground, a battery-powered version of rescue tools should be used instead. However, the fact that rescue operations can be carried out with the battery-powered version means that firefighters must carry approximately 3.9 kg extra weight throughout the process. This is a lot of weight that has the potential to impede the firefighters' performance in a rescue operation regardless of their gender. As stated before, the body material of the vehicle was checked with a magnet before starting the rescue operation. The old model Suzuki Swift GLX car used in this training has an aluminium body, as does the 1994 Audi A8 mentioned before. To clarify, hydraulic rescue equipment with medium performance standards was sufficient for these vehicles. The presence of steel material in the vehicle body may require hydraulic rescue equipment, preferably from the highest performance class. The higher the performance of equipment, the heavier its weight. This causes the weight to increase to the range of approximately 20 - 25 kg, not counting the battery, in the existing hydraulic scissors and spreader rescue tools of different companies (Holmatro, 2022; Lukas Hydraulik GmbH, 2019; Weber-Hydraulik GmbH, 2019). Weights at this level are increasingly difficult for a firefighter to manage in a controlled manner during a rescue operation.

It is worth bearing in mind that a successful operation depends not only on the performance of the rescue equipment used, but also on the health of the firefighters involved in the process. One reason behind this is the possibility that the firefighter may have back issues since that is one of the most common health issues in Western Societies (Bundesärztekammer 2018, Damm et al 2016). Under these circumstances, the equipment, which is already quite heavy, is even more challenging for firefighters in a relatively poor physical condition. Some rescue team members who had back surgery shared their experiences in training, stating that they had difficulty lifting the equipment and placing the equipment on the vehicle correctly while using this gear during the procedure. It is undisputed that the impeccable success of rescue operations is vital. However, it is also unacceptable that the factors are not removed that make healthy fire department personnel, who actively participate in the processes as firefighters hesitate to apply the skills and technical knowledge they have due to the unfavourable health conditions they will later suffer.

The health of the rescue workers is just as important as that of everyone else. Therefore the equipment developers must do their utmost to ensure that the equipment is user-friendly and not harmful to its operators' health. This can be achieved, among other things, by reducing the weight of the equipment. Consequently, in the current project, studies were carried out to reduce the weight of and to redesign a product, which is already on the market as a hydraulic rescue spreader, based on the aforementioned reasons.

## The lightweight design of a hydraulic rescue spreader under engineering aspects

Engineering design is defined as the use of scientific principles, technical knowledge, and imagination to describe how a mechanical system performs predetermined functions (Fielden, 1963). Based on this definition, the current project focused on the lightweight design of a product commercially available as a hydraulic rescue spreader so as to achieve the aforementioned functions. In addition, it was decided not to share the critical data of the tool in this study due to the confidentiality agreement signed with the company.

The investigations started with the study of the working principle and performance of the mechanism of the equipment in question. It was shown in the initial observations that the nominal pressure under which this equipment operates is the same as that of the seven other pieces of equipment classified by performance under the title of hydraulic rescue spreader. This sheds light on how the mechanism design affects the performance of powerful equipment operating under heavy loads. In addition, Table 1 containing a few of the main features has been submitted for examination to illuminate the general properties of the equipment. The hydraulic rescue spreaders in this table were classified according to different technical characteristics, such as dimensions, weight, spreading distance, and spreading force in the operating range (Weber-Hydraulik GmbH, 2019).

*Table 1: Technical data of hydraulic rescue spreaders (Weber-Hydraulik GmbH, 2019)*

| Name | Dimensions (LxWxH) **(mm)** | **Weight (kg)** | **Spreading distance (mm)** | **Spreading force in working range (kN)** | **Nominal Pressure (bar)** |
|---|---|---|---|---|---|
| SP 40 C | 708 x 269 x 188 | 9,8 | 515 | 40 | 700 |
| SP 44 AS | 708 x 250 x 190 | 13,3 | 610 | 44 | 700 |
| SP 49 | 791 x 248 x 199 | 19,9 | 710 | 49 | 700 |
| SP 53 BS | 836 x 299 x 216 | 20,3 | 800 | 53 | 700 |
| SP 54 AS | 821 x 282 x 200 | 16,9 | 735 | 55 | 700 |
| SP 50 BS | 854 x 282 x 200 | 17,1 | 805 | 50 | 700 |
| SP 64 BS | 879 x 307 x 210 | 20,1 | 820 | 64 | 700 |
| SP 84 CS | 790 x 307 x 210 | 19,8 | 660 | 82 | 700 |

The mechanism of the hydraulic rescue spreader consists of an assembly of rigid bodies connected by joints to transfer and transform a force and motion. As a result of the choice of the tool to be handled in the project, its structural features were examined, and the basic mechanism was roughly defined. The force transmitted to the arms at different opening positions by the piston in the hydraulic cylinder under the hydraulic spreader body was calculated analytically. These calculations were first examined in three different positions. The first position was the force transmitted to spreader tips when the equipment was closed entirely. The second position was the force level when the tool reached the midpoint of the maximum opening distance. The third and final position was the force distribution of the equipment when it was fully open. Data from these points was compared with data acquired from experiments and simulations in the further work packages of the project. The main parts of a hydraulic rescue spreader are shown in Figure 4 for clarity.

The pressure available in the hydraulic cylinder is the same in all hydraulic rescue spreaders and is 700 bar. It is known that, regardless of the source of the force, the force acting perpendicular to the unit surface is called pressure (P), and the force acting perpendicular to the whole surface is called the pressure force (F). In this study, the forces extending through the piston towards the joint points on the spreader and the tips of the spreader arms were calculated using simple engineering calculations based on the piston surface measurements inside the cylinder. In the following equation, it is shown that the pressure, which is given by (P), is the perpendicular force, represented by (F), acting on the unit surface area, symbolized by (A).

The design of the hydraulic rescue spreaders available on the market is generally identical. The design diversity that seems to be negligible in these tools, apart from minor design differences, may cause structural results that significantly affect performance, contrary to what is believed. The properties of the spreader used in the current project were investigated experimentally and numerically.

*Figure 4: Hydraulic rescue spreader parts (Weber-Hydraulik GmbH, 2019)*

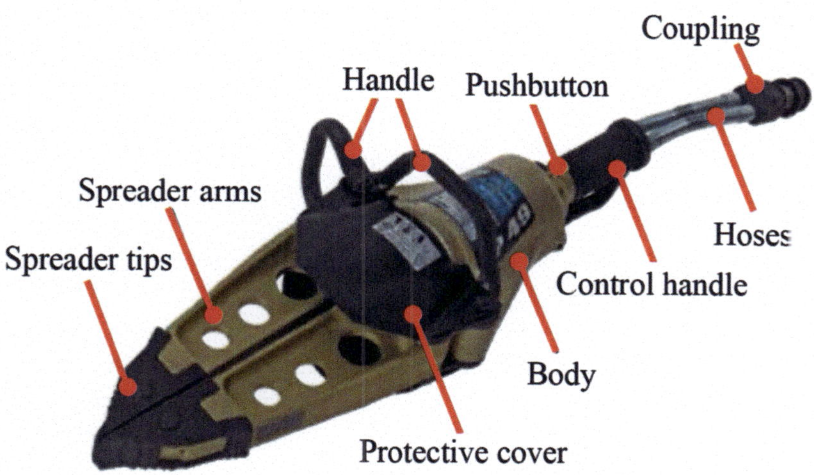


The main mechanical properties refer to maintaining the current performance level of the spreader. These features are a hydraulic system triggering the tool, the total opening distance between the spreader tips, and the force transmitted by the spreader arms not falling below the current level.

Although the features observed under the title of kinematics sound more detailed, they leave the design area more accessible than mechanical properties. The data here is as follows: the structure, consisting of a series of rigid bodies and connexions, must be planar with one degree of freedom (DOF) and must only open and close in a planar fashion without rotational movements. The structure is triggered linearly by force from the hydraulic system. Except for the joints connected to the linear trigger system, the other joints must be revolute only. The spreader tips must start from the fully closed position with the movement of the linear trigger system and complete its activity until it reaches a certain opening distance. The last-but-not-least, significant feature of double-acting equipment is its symmetrical structure, Figure 5.

It is known that a reduction in the number of bars in a mechanism contributes to reducing the overall mass. To consider the kinematic requirements, Grübler's equation for planar mechanism, stated below, has been studied.

M, L, and J represent the number of DOF, the number of links, and the number of joints in the mechanism, respectively. Since the spreader system has one DOF and has revolute and prismatic connexions, L corresponds to an even number (Norton, 1999). In addition, the degree of freedom of the mechanisms depends on the number of parts, the number of joints, and the degree of freedom of the joint, not the size of the parts.

As a result of the investigations, it was concluded that a two or four-bar connexion is not possible. Because if a link has no symmetry on the other side of the y-centreline, it must be on the centreline and can only translate along the y-centreline. In addition, if the number of joints is double, the prismatic joint must be on the centreline and one of the revolute joints. Most hydraulic rescue spreaders available on the market have a six-bar linkage system. It has also been determined that linkage consisting of eight bars is not possible. As a result, it is neither attainable to design the connexions symmetrically nor easy to position the necessary joints appropriately. In this study, the different design results of the six-bar connexion system were analysed.

The second stage in the project was determined as the force measurement at the tips of the tool by positioning the hydraulic rescue spreader on a flat surface at different opening positions. The surface of the test area preferred at this stage has a grid structure. This floor is ideal for thick metal blocks connected to load cells to limit the spreader at different opening distances. One of the two points to be considered is that the spreader tip is located in the centre of the load cells. Thus, an excessive difference in the force on the load cells during loading time is avoided. This prevents the occurrence of bending moments in the system. The bending moment damages the system and prevents reliable data from being obtained. Another point to be considered is that the jagged spreader tip is made of hardened steel and can damage the surface of the metal block connected to the load cells. A thin metal sheet is placed between the spreader and the metal block in the load cells so as not to damage the surface of this structure. During the spreader performance test phase, ten experiments consisting of five different opening distances with two repetitions for each were carried out. In addition, the GOM Aramis digital image correlation system was applied to obtain detailed calculations regarding displacement on the tool, Figure 6. This system facilitates the acquisition of precise strain measurements of the part. This measurement requires that the surface of the tool first be painted entirely with a special white paint and then sprayed black to form small uniform dots. While measuring, the initial position of black dots on the white paint is considered as a reference, and two cameras record their movements throughout the test.

*Figure 5: Mechanism of the spreader*

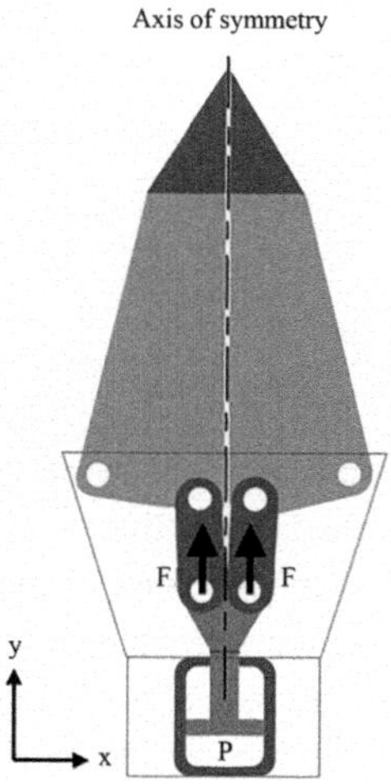


| Links | Joints | Revolute Joints |
|---|---|---|
| 6 | 7 | 6 |

M=3(L-1)-2J

M=1 degree-of-freedom

The trend of force-time performance tests is presented in Figure 6. As seen clearly, the curvature of the force-time curve appears steeper at the beginning of the test. This variation of the curvature refers to the contact of the spreader tip and the moment of penetration. Then the joint point connecting the spreader tip and the arm point is fixed, and the parts move together. With the fixation of the connexion, the curvature of the curve changed, and the force value reached the maximum after a while. In addition, the simultaneous achievement of the same maximum force values of the experiments belonging to each test group is proof that the tests confirm each other.

*Figure 6: Preparation of the test field of the spreader*

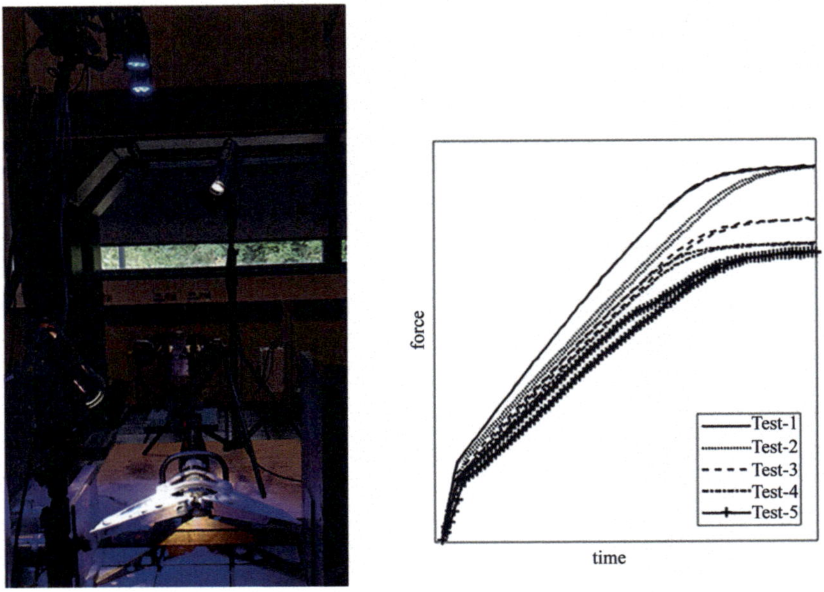


The force values corresponding to the specific opening distance measures were obtained from the test and first compared with the analytical calculations. These force values are used as input for structural analysis simulations. It is known that the more consistent the calculations are with the experiments, the more reliable the analytical and numerical model results will be. In such studies, numerical modelling and validation of simulations are highly significant. Validated numerical models make it possible to collect data in details that cannot be obtained in experiments, as well as to obtain information about possible results by changing the practical, experimental conditions. This means saving both time and costs of setting up the experiments. For this reason, in the present project, the numerical model of each experimental group was prepared and verified by considering the force, time and displacement parameters obtained from the experiment. Data collected from simulations are the fracture parameters investigated to determine the stress distribution on the arm and the load-carrying capacity of the arm under different conditions. The goal of using that information is to design a lighter spreader arm.

Numerical models can be roughly grouped under two main headings, explicit and implicit. With an explicit algorithm, the new state is used to directly calculate the current data of a particular system at a different time than the present time. By contrast, an implicit analysis cannot be calculated directly from the former case; it finds a solution by solving a combined system of equations containing both the current and subsequent states of the given scenario. That is, it requires nonlinear solution algorithms. This method may be more challenging to implement. In the current project, the implicit numerical model method was preferred in order to model the experiments numerically. Therefore, the next step after the analytical comparison is to compare and validate the results of the implicit numerical model with respect to the respective experiments.

After the tests were proven to be consistent with each other, the first preparations for the simulation studies were planned. These preparations are about understanding the properties of the material used in the spreader arm in detail. Thus, the examination stages involve determining the structure, hardness and mechanical properties of the material. The data obtained from these stages were used as input for simulation studies. Within the scope of this project, Ls Dyna commercial software was used for simulation studies, and HyperMesh programme was preferred for the preparation of the numerical model.

One of the many applications of X-ray computed tomography scanning (CT-scan) in industry is the detection of porosity and other defects in metal parts. Defects include unintended porosity, rough surfaces, and design deviations that can vary significantly among samples. Unintended porosity in the structure will affects the mechanical properties of the structure adversely. Due to the operating conditions of the spreader arm, there should be no undesirable features in the material structure. For this purpose, within the scope of the project, first, the arm material of the spreader was examined, and then its structure was inspected via CT-scan. The material, which is produced with production methods that require a highly promising material structure, has been proven to consist of a homogeneous structure that does not contain any pores, precisely as it should be.

The studies were continued with the uni-axial tensile test, for which the specimens were produced by wire erosion method from the metal block, under quasi-static loading. The tests, uni-axial tensile, shear tensile and notched tensile, required to obtain all the necessary parameters within the scope of the project, were carried out in sets of five repetitions each. In addition, the experiments that were carried out to understand whether the material exhibits anisotropic behaviour were repeated with samples cut at 0 degrees, 45 degrees and 90 degrees. Altogether, forty-five tests were performed for material characterisation studies. According to the information obtained from the test results, it was determined that the mechanical material properties, such as elastic modulus, yield stress, ultimate stress, and fracture strain, are related to each other. One of the uni-axial tensile experimental results was chosen as a reference for material characterisation studies. It is required that the curve selected as a reference must contain neither the lowest nor the highest values. Therefore, a stress-strain curve with average mechanical properties was selected as a reference. Since there is no plastic deformation or fracture on the equipment, many parameters can seem unnecessary. However, the project aims to estimate the most unstable area and possible fracture mechanism in a particular scenario numerically. Plastic material properties were used for this purpose in the numerical material model card in the simulation.

Material characterisation studies begin with the conversion of the obtained engineering strain-stress curves into true strain-stress curves. In engineering strain-stress calculations, the cross-sectional area of the specimen is considered constant. However, in reality, the situation is entirely different. As the tensile test continues, the cross-sectional area of the sample becomes narrow. In the simulation, a material card is created to introduce the material information. In addition to the main material properties, the hardening curve is often added to the material card. Therefore, true stress and true plastic strain curves are used to fit the hardening curve. Figure 7 explains the sequence of the material characterisation process. Using the true stress-strain curve in the plastic region, the fit of the hardening curve was calculated by MATLAB in the form of Hockett-Sherby hardening law and implemented in the material card. All calculations, including the fracture properties of the material, were validated, and a good correlation between tests and numerical results was obtained.

*Figure 7: Material characterisation process*

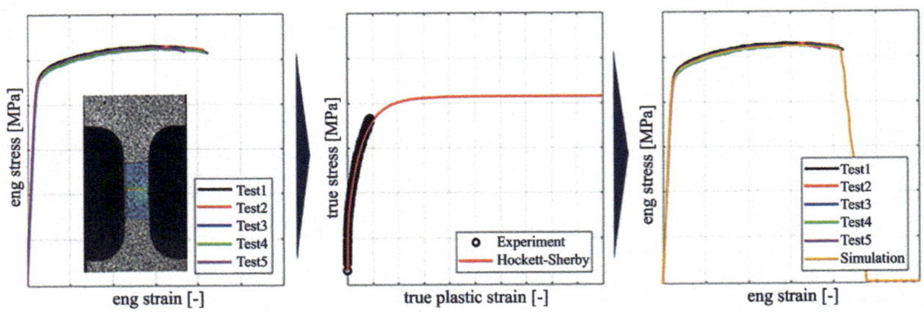


Another stage of the simulation studies are the surface analysis studies of the hydraulic rescue spreader. These studies do not yet include the fracture properties, since the priority belongs to the design. Structural analysis studies, which were carried out using non-linear implicit analysis methods, first started with the fully closed position. Here, the boundary conditions for the joint points and the opening distances were applied as in the experiments. The closer the methods applied in the simulation to the real ones, the closer the analysis results are to the real ones. It is challenging to use all the loads on the equipment in the simulation the same way as in the experiment. For this reason, realistic applications are implemented, and the differences in the results are accepted up to a certain level. Numerical models were prepared based on the displacement data measured at the same point and the time data as in the experiments. The simulation results of the respective experiments were compared to the experiments in the form of a force-time curve, and a good correlation was observed, Figure 8. The validated results of the numerical model were considered as a guide for the creation of the new design of the tool.

*Figure 8: Comparison of experiment and numerical study*

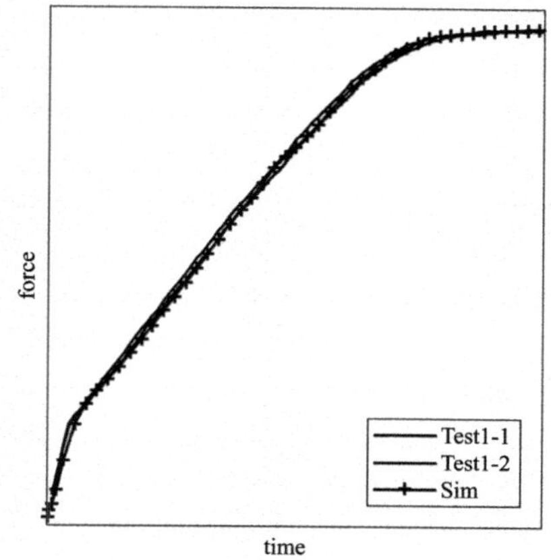


After the structural analysis studies were completed, the topology optimisation studies started. The OptiStruct programme was preferred for this work package. Topology optimisation aims to remove the material from the body that has no load distribution under any circumstances at the existing design in the recalculated analysis. Another way is to expand the design volume to get a unique design different from the current one. The next step from the problem analysis stage in the design sequence is to propose and evaluate possible solutions and select the most promising one. This process is usually successfully concluded by taking the economical and feasible production methods and the ergonomics of the offered solution into account. Considering the models that were previously validated in Ls Dyna, the spreader arm was analysed this time in OptiStruct under different loading conditions, and the topology optimisation results were examined. A standard model was determined by considering all loading conditions. Significant findings have been obtained that shed light on weight reduction in the arm of the spreader, which has the title of being the lightest in its class. In accordance with the confidentiality agreement, detailed images and results are going to be published in future publications.

## Development of operational and demand-oriented firefighting equipment

German fire brigades undertook more than 4.5 million operations in 2019. If the ambulance service operations are excluded (ambulance service conducted 2,663,910 emergency rescues and 508,105 ambulance transport), there were still 1.3 million operations in 2019. These operations are broken down by category and frequency: 17% fires and explosions, 0.01% catastrophe alarms, 48% technical assistance, 3% animals/insects, 15% other, and 17% false alarms. (Deutscher Feuerwehrverband e. V., 2021)

These operations can be very different from each other, and the fire brigades are regularly confronted with new challenges. Rescue operations must be carried out optimally, often in the shortest possible time. In the course of this contribution, the focus will be on technical assistance operations. Here, a constantly changing situation is the state of the art of modern vehicles. The automotive industry is committed to reducing fuel consumption for environmental reasons. Reducing the weight of vehicles is an essential contribution to lowering fuel consumption (Taub et al., 2019). At the same time, the safety properties must be retained or improved. Common materials for vehicle construction, low-carbon steel, and cast iron, are being replaced by materials with higher specific strength and stiffness (Taub et al., 2019). These materials with higher specific strength and stiffness are high-strength steels, aluminium, magnesium, and polymer composites (Taub et al., 2019). Figure 9 shows the change in the material composition of vehicles from 1970 to 2020 related to the mass (Todor & Kiss, 2016). This underlines the constantly changing situation for the emergency services in this field.

*Figure 9: Change in material compositions in vehicles from 1970 to 2020 according to (Miller et al., 2014).*

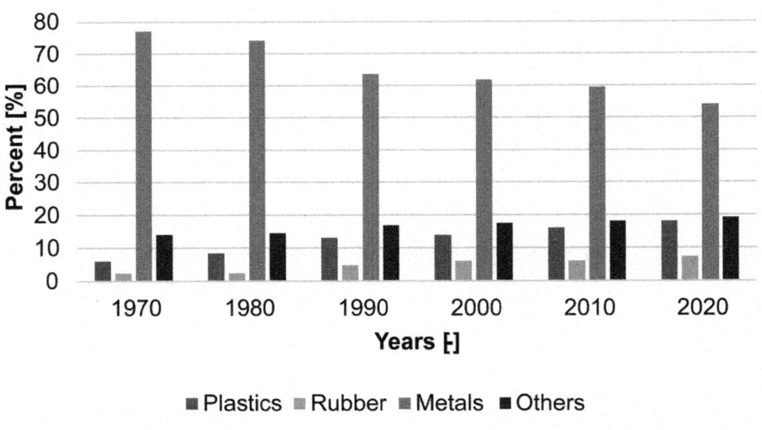


Replacing parts made of conventional materials, such as metals, with parts made of, for example, composite or composite materials contributes to weight reduction of the vehicle. This leads to higher fuel efficiency and improved vehicle power-to-weight ratio, resulting in higher vehicle performance. (Todor & Kiss, 2016)

This poses new challenges for rescue services, which will be further illustrated using the example of rescue scissors. Fibre composite materials generally do not pose a problem for rescue scissors with respect to their cutting force. But their brittle behaviour during cutting can cause parts to be scattered and endanger people during the rescue operation. In addition, toxic dust is produced during the destruction of the structure. (Spanner, 2018, p. 66)

Rescue scissors can reach the limits of their cutting force in the case of reinforced pillars in vehicles. The following diagramme (Fig. 10) shows the working pressures of hydraulic rescue scissors when cutting a B-pillar (Dürr et al., 2014). A comparison between vehicle models from 1994 and 2006 has shown that the required cutting force has more than doubled in some cases. From today's perspective, the vehicles that have been compared are outdated, but it can be assumed that this trend continues. This statement is justified, among other things, by the constantly increasing safety requirements for the vehicles. Moreover, current figures are not publicly available.

In conclusion, it can be said that vehicles are getting safer, but modern vehicle technology makes it more difficult to rescue people from them after an accident. Alternative power sources for vehicles also create new challenges and pose novel risks. These are just two examples of vehicles, but new challenges are not limited to this area.

*Figure 10: Working pressure depending on vehicle model year and cutting position according to (Dürr et al., 2014).*

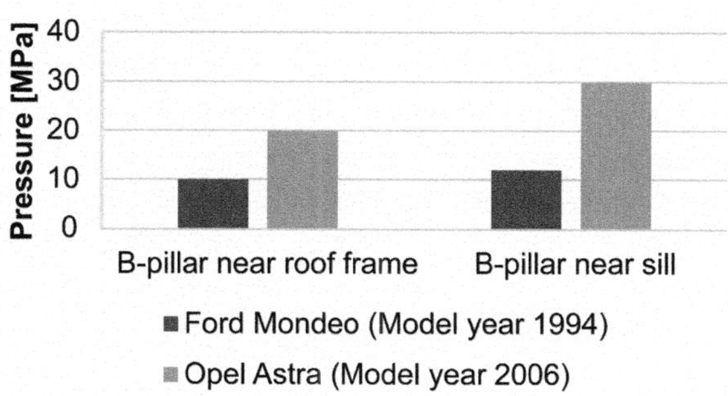


## From the perspective of the general public

In order to imagine what relevance traffic accidents have for the general public, selected statistics and studies are discussed below. In Europe, traffic accidents are the leading cause of death among young people between the ages of 5 to 29 (Jackisch et al., 2016). In 2020, there were over 2.2 million road accidents in Germany; 11.2% of these accidents caused personal injuries (Statistisches Bundesamt, 2021). A survey in the area of Hanover from 1985 to 2003, which analysed the accidents resulting in personal injuries, showed that a person was trapped in 9.5% of these accidents (Westhoff et al., 2007, p. 248).

## From the perspective of the fire brigade

From the fire brigade's point of view, according to the statistics at the beginning of this article, 14% of all operations are technical assistance operations. Time management plays a significant role in pre-hospital trauma care, from the accident to arrival at an appropriate trauma centre. The rule of the "golden hour of shock" is widely used in pertinent literature: it explains that the recovery of trauma patients is better if they receive the necessary care within one hour. Although this rule is controversial, the care of severely injured patients always remains time-critical (Weigeldt et al., 2018). The ADAC (German Automobile Club) has stated that the number of vehicle accidents in which people can be rescued within 50 minutes has fallen: 40 % of people were rescued in less than 50 minutes between 1990 and 1992; 20 % were rescued in less than 50 minutes between 2005 and 2007 (ADAC, 2019). The reason for the longer rescue times results, among other things, from higher standards of materials, which make it more difficult to reform the structure. Another point is the new technologies, such as new power drives, airbags, or restraint systems, which have to be taken into account during the rescue.

## Rescue equipment

In the previous sections, the relevance of technical assistance operations for the fire brigade, but also for the general public, was shown. The importance of an optimal rescue process after a traffic accident is undeniable. The conditions, such as time pressure or the complex position of the vehicle, train, lorry, or debris, constitute barriers that are not easy to overcome. Therefore, a well-functioning and high-performance rescue system is essential to support the rescue teams during their work. These rescue devices should also be lightweight and user-friendly. Furthermore, these steps will help to protect the health of emergency services.

*Figure 11: Example illustration of various rescue systems (Weber Rescue, 2020).*

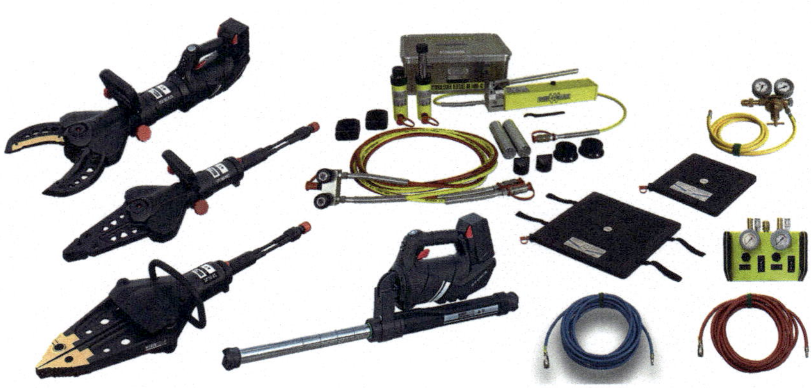

It is vital to have good cooperation among the participants of technical rescue to minimize the rescue time and improve the patient's chances of survival. The effort required for a technical rescue depends significantly on the materials used in the vehicle, the dynamics of the accident, and the patient's state of health (Faul et al., 2021).

The use of equipment in the field of technical rescue requires the users to have the necessary practical and theoretical training. Structural solutions, which help to perform a technical rescue, are needed. (Jasiuk et al., 2019, p. 63) In order to get an idea of the equipment, Figure 11 shows examples of rescue tools. These are (from left to right) the rescue scissors, the combi tool, the spreader, the hydraulic lifting kit, the rescue ram, and the lifting bag system.

This research aims to provide a basis for developing firefighting equipment that suits the use and needs optimally. The basis will be used for the optimisation focusing on a selected rescue tool to achieve these goals. This tool should be optimised for operational and demand orientation after using the developed basis of this research. To develop rescue tools that meet the various technological and practical challenges of first responders, an interdisciplinary and transdisciplinary approach is required, which will be outlined later.

## Optimal equipment – not only important in the field of rescue services

Prior to that, the importance of operational and demand-oriented equipment should be discussed. The term equipment is not to be reduced to physical devices but also includes the support provided by technical and software solutions. In general, it is important that the equipment people use in their daily work is suitable and adapted to their needs. Only by using optimal equipment can it be ensured that the equipment contributes to the reduction of the user's workload. This reduction in workload pertains not only to the physical workload but also to the mental workload because the mental workload is made up of the totality of external influences acting on a person (Bengel et al., 1997, p. 40).

It is important to have the necessary tools available, especially if they are required to rescue people's lives. This concerns the tools of the emergency and rescue services. For example, firefighting equipment should be optimally designed for its use and developed according to the requirements. On the one hand, this helps to reduce the physical workload during rescue operations and training; on the other hand, the tools are also decisive for the success of the rescue operations. Furthermore, optimisation according to the user's requirements can make it possible for the tools to be used by a larger number of users.

At this point, there is a certain gap. On the one hand, not all fire departments are equipped with the latest technology. One reason for this is that the communes are responsible for the maintenance of the fire departments in Germany. On the other hand, in some cases there is a knowledge gap between the development and the users, depending on the rescue tool. For example, rescue equipment is sometimes used in ways that are different from what it has originally been intended for, or there are problems in the field that were not known at the development stage. Another issue is the standardisation. According to European standard, rescue scissors, for example, which are used to cut vehicles after an accident to rescue a trapped person, do not have to be tested on vehicles. However, it should be made clear that the producers of rescue equipment do carry out such tests.

## Development methodology

The research project can be divided into two objectives to assist in the development of operational and demand-oriented firefighting equipment. On the one hand, the project shows which steps help to better consider the aspect of operational and demand orientation in the development of new rescue equipment. Furthermore, a direct application of these steps on a selected rescue device is carried out within the project, where this part of the project is to be seen as a validation at the same time. This research is also carried out in cooperation with the Weber Hydraulic company, which, in addition to its expertise that has been garnered over many years, also provides material and rescue equipment for tests. On the following pages, special attention will be paid to the survey and the interdisciplinary and transdisciplinary cooperation within the framework of the research project.

To return to the point of the importance of the interdisciplinary and transdisciplinary approach, the factors influencing the success of a rescue operation must be considered first. Handling strategy, ergonomics, and handling are closely correlated with each other during the use of rescue tools and emergency equipment. Several factors affecting this situation can be mentioned. Examples are the weight, the tool functions (special features), and the user's skills.

The weight of the rescue equipment creates a high hurdle for the members of the rescue team. The weight of rescue scissors, for example, ranges from under 4 kilogrammes (pedal cutting scissors) up to more than 25 kilogrammes (opening width and cutting force of the rescue scissors are highly dependent on the weight of the rescue scissors). For other rescue tools, it could be even more. Optimisation using lightweight construction methods should help to reduce the weight. Different loading conditions should be investigated experimentally and numerically to optimise the chosen rescue tool during this research.

On the operating side, the success in using rescue systems also depends largely on the skills of the user (Hessische Landesfeuerwehrschule, 2020). This insight should also be used for research. The knowledge of experts from practice, procurement, leadership, and much more are to be included via different survey studies. This allows taking into account essential information from the field, which otherwise would not have been considered.

The focus of the research is on the German rescue organisations. This is mainly because, in Germany, the municipalities are responsible for providing an adequate fire brigade, which, in some cases, is a special situation as contrasted with other countries.

## Study design

To close the gaps in expertise that have already been mentioned and to enable the development of the selected rescue tool in a way that is suitable for use and needs, the first part of the research project involves a survey conducted via an online questionnaire. Figure 12 shows the structure of the questionnaire. After the questions concerning the individual, a differentiation is made between the different organisations, whereby similar but organisation-specific points are asked in several sections. The individuals are asked questions about their experience in the organisation, their location, available rescue equipment, operations and training or personal experience with rescue equipment. In the last section that pertains to the selected rescue tool, the same questions are again asked in all parts.

*Figure 12: Paths in the questionnaire according to the organisation of the participants.*

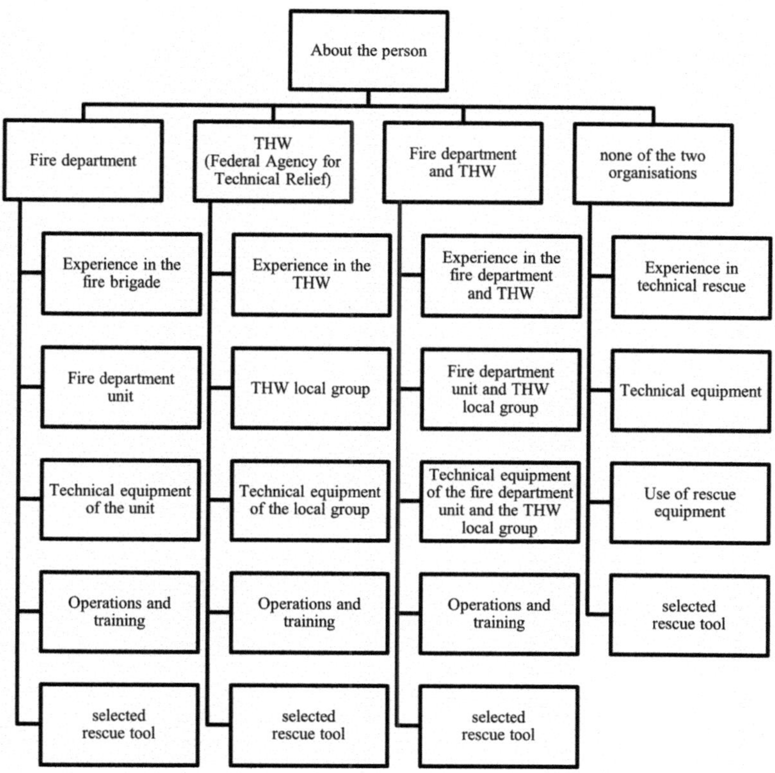

The questions regarding the selected rescue tool are classified according to the individual research questions. These questions are particularly relevant for optimising the selected rescue equipment. The analysis is to be taken into account directly in optimisation. In this way, this part forms one of the interfaces between development and the user field. The part on the selected rescue equipment can be summarised in the following groups of questions:

- How useful is a reduction in the weight from the user's point of view?
- How important is a compact and robust design for the users?
- How useful is a modification of the drive from the user's point of view?
- Which further optimisations make sense from the user's point of view?
- In which application scenarios is the tool used and how is it used?

The questionnaire is shared with various groups on social media, thus reaching a large cross-section of society with an interest in firefighting, technical rescue or rescue equipment manufacturing. In addition, it was sent specifically to fire departments as well as to certain groups of people in the fire departments and local groups of the Federal Agency for Technical Relief (THW) in Germany.

## Analysis of the survey: first results

The survey made it possible to answer various research questions directly from the users' points of view. In addition to the survey on technical rescue, the research also included various participatory observations, for example at the technical rescue XXL workshop for female firefighters. Altogether, 392 experts and practitioners took part in the survey, mainly from the fire brigade and the technical aid organisation (THW) in Germany. More specifically, 50% of the participants are from the fire brigade, 47.2% from the THW, 2.6% are in the fire brigade and THW, and 0.3% are in neither organisation. Most of the participants regularly use rescue tools, which will be shown later.

Participants included 96.7% male, 3.1% female and 0.3% diverse. For comparison, on 31 December 2018, the proportion of women in the volunteer fire brigade was 9.9% and 1.7% in the professional fire brigade (Deutscher Feuerwehrverband e. V., 2020). In the voluntary sector of the THW, the proportion of women in 2020 was 6.4% (Bundesanstalt Technisches Hilfswerk [THW], 2020). Compared to the number of women in the volunteer fire brigade and the THW, the percentage of women in the survey sample is less than the percentage in the organisation. This distortion is counteracted by a separate analysis according to gender.

Most of the participants are between 30 and 39 years old. The proportion of respondents under 20 or over 60 was, as expected, the lowest. It is also remarkable that the proportion of those aged 50 to 59, at 13.3%, is significantly lower than the ranges from age 40 to 49 (23.7%) or 20 to 29 (20.9%). At this point, an analysis is made according to age groups as well. This makes it possible to determine whether certain problems and concerns are particularly prevalent in certain age groups.

## Personal use of rescue equipment

The personal questions also included how often the participants use rescue equipment themselves. The majority of the participants in the survey (41%) use rescue equipment once a quarter during their training. 35% train with rescue equipment once a month. During operations, the majority use rescue equipment once a year (36%), followed by 34% of participants who use rescue equipment once a quarter during operations.

Rescue equipment is used weekly in operations and exercises by only one percent of the participants. In contrast, 13% do not use rescue equipment at all in operations, and one percent of the participants does not even use it during training. Figure 13 illustrates the distribution in detail. The distribution shows that almost all participants regularly use rescue equipment, although the frequency varies significantly. This highlights the relevance of a simple mode of operation that is also successful with less regular use.

*Figure 13: Frequency of use of rescue equipment — operation vs. training.*

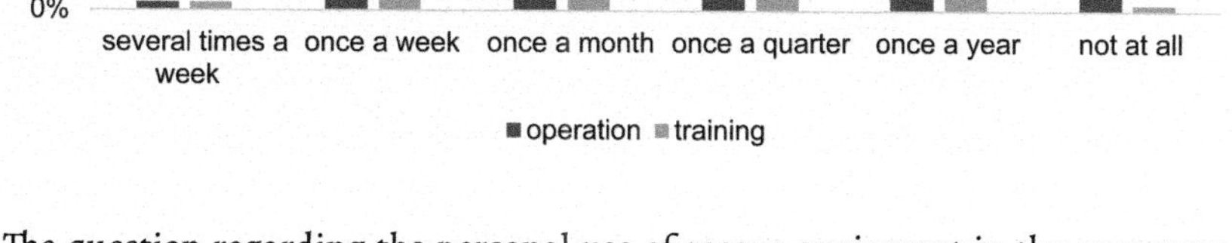


The question regarding the personal use of rescue equipment in the survey was also broken down by specific rescue equipment. The rescue tools selected are the rescue scissors, spreader, combi tool, rescue cylinder, hydraulic winch, lifting bag system and hydraulic lifting kit. Figure 14 shows a detailed breakdown according to the types of rescue equipment; distinctive points are evaluated below. Several times a week, all of the rescue tools are used by less than 0.3% of the participants. Once a week, the selected rescue tools are used by 0.5% to 4.6% of the participants – depending on the rescue tool. Spreader (4.6%), rescue scissors (4.3%), and rescue cylinder (3.8%) are ahead of the other rescue tools in weekly use. Also, in monthly use, most participants use spreaders (23.0%), rescue scissors (22.2%), and rescue cylinders (18.1%). The most frequently unused rescue tool is the combination tool, which is not used at all by 63.0% of the participants. Most participants use the lifting bag system (44.6%), the spreader (42.9%), the rescue shears (42.6%), the hydraulic lifting kit (34.2%), and the rescue cylinder (30.1%) once a quarter. The hydraulic winch is used most frequently – by 39.0% of the participants – once a year. On the one hand, the frequency of use can be used to give an estimate of how heavy the burden is on the emergency teams. On the other hand, the knowledge can be determined in relation to other questions in the survey.

*Figure14: Frequency of use of certain rescue equipment in comparison.*

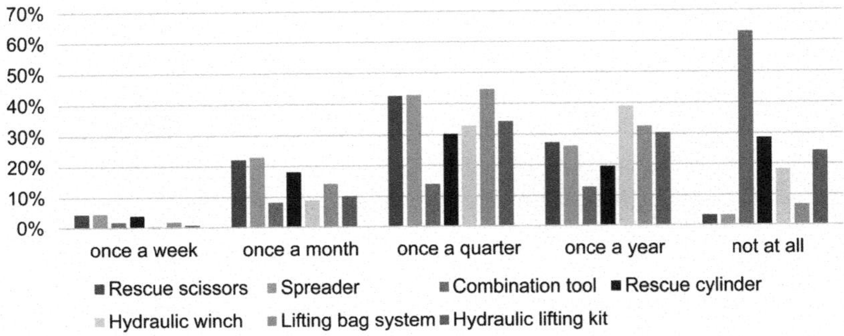


The survey also explored the views of the respondents and their units on the issue of battery-powered rescue equipment. 43% of the participants are neutral regarding the topic of battery-powered rescue equipment since they currently do not use battery-powered rescue equipment and are not positive or negative about it. For 6% of the participants, none of the given answer options apply. 20% of the participants would like to purchase battery-powered rescue equipment in the future. 23% of the participants already use battery-powered rescue equipment and are very satisfied (14%) or satisfied (8%) with it. Only 1% are dissatisfied. 8% of the participants do not want to purchase battery-powered rescue equipment in the future. This distribution suggests that there are more supporters of battery-powered rescue equipment than participants who are against battery-powered rescue equipment.

## Experience in the fire brigade or THW

To determine the quality of the knowledge of the participants, various questions were asked regarding active work in the organisation. The question of how long the participants have been active in the fire brigade also shows that most of them (57.8%) have been active for more than 20 years and have thus been able to gain a great deal of experience. Overall, 90.8% of the participants from the fire brigade have been active in the fire brigade for at least 10 years. Also, in THW, 44.1% of the participants from this area have been active for more than 20 years. Another 35.4% have been active in THW for more than 10 years. Thus, there is also a wealth of experience regarding participation in this survey.

The response to the question, which training courses have already been attended by the participants from the fire brigade sector, clearly shows that the participants from the fire brigade are for the most part highly skilled. Especially the technical assistance training course, which is relevant for answering these questions, was completed by 83.5% of the participants. Many of the participants also have leadership qualifications. Overall, the participants of the fire brigade are well-qualified to take part in this survey.

The THW participants also have a large proportion of leaders who took part in the survey. Thus, 24.1% of the participants from the THW are group leaders, 15.9% are platoon leaders and 4.6% are platoon squad leaders. Training officers (5.1%) and technical advisors (3.1%) are also represented. This also shows the high qualifications of the THW participants.

## Experience regarding the selected rescue tool

The survey also identifies the competence specifically related to the selected rescue tool. The majority of the participants assess their level of knowledge as good (52.6%) to very good (35.7%) regarding the selected rescue tool. Only 10.5% of the participants have little or no knowledge. 0.3% do not give any information.

## Next steps

A further analysis of the survey will link the participants' backgrounds to their experience in particular rescue scenarios and tools. These insights have the advantage for the optimisation that, first of all, it is known exactly what the rescue equipment is used for. This makes it possible to adapt the rescue equipment exactly to the needs and, if appropriate, to skip functions that are not necessary. Rescue equipment that is better adapted to the needs of the emergency services will, in turn, result in a more efficient rescue operation in the field. The selected rescue equipment is to be optimised in the direction of lightweight construction considering the specific results from the survey. For this purpose, various lightweight construction methods are to be applied. The next step is a simulation using the Finite Element Method. On this basis, a prototype will be developed. The text "Hydraulic Rescue Spreaders: Challenges of lightweight design, vehicles, and rescuers," in this book, outlines potential further steps.

## References

ADAC (2019). Kostenlos Karte kann Ihr Leben Retten. https://www.adac.de/info-testrat/adac-im-einsatz/motorwelt/Rettungskarte.aspx

Bartiaux, F., & van Ypersele, J. P. (Eds.) (1993). The role of population growth in global warming. *International Union for the Scientific Study of Population* (IUSSP), Vol. 4, 33-54. ISBN: 2-87108-030-5.

Bengel, J., Singer, S., & Kuntz, V. (1997). Psychische Belastungen des Rettungspersonals. In J. Bengel (Ed.), *Psychologie in Notfallmedizin und Rettungsdienst* (pp. 39–56). Springer. https://doi.org/10.1007/978-3-642-97961-3_3

Bundesanstalt Technisches Hilfswerk (2020). *Jahresbericht 2020*. https://www.thw.de/SharedDocs/Downloads/DE/Hintergrund/Jahresberichte/jahresbericht_2020.pdf?__blob=publicationFile

Deutscher Feuerwehrverband e. V. (Ed.) (2020). *Feuerwehr-Jahrbuch des Deutschen Feuerwehrverbandes 2020: Herausforderung Corona-Pandemie*. DFV.

Deutscher Feuerwehrverband e. V. (Ed.) (2021). *Feuerwehr-Jahrbuch des Deutschen Feuerwehrverbandes 2021: Flutkatastrophe 2021 - Feuerwehr unverzichtbar*. DFV. https://www.feuerwehrverband.de/presse/statistik/

Dürr, C., Unger, T., Müller, U. (2014). Tertiäre Sicherheit – Rettung aus modernen Fahrzeugen nach einem Unfall. In: Siebenpfeiffer, W. (eds) Leichtbau-Technologien im Automobilbau. ATZ/MTZ-Fachbuch. Springer Vieweg, Wiesbaden. https://doi.org/10.1007/978-3-658-04025-3_26

Faul, P., Albert, J., & Schweigkofler, U. (2021). Technische Rettung und Kooperation mit der Feuerwehr. *Notfallmedizin up2date*, Vol. 16, Issue 01, 43–62. https://doi.org/10.1055/a-1196-2669

Fielden, G.B.R. (1963). *Engineering Design: Report of Royal Commission*. London: HMSO.

GCC (2017, May 12). *Audi puts steel back in the new A8*. Green Car Congress. Energy, technologies, issues and policies for sustainable mobility. https://www.greencarcongress.com/2017/05/20170512-audia8.html

Hessische Landesfeuerwehrschule (2020). *TH-VU-Ausbildung: Lehrunterlage zur technisch-medizinischen Rettung nach Verkehrsunfällen mit Personenkraftwagen*. hlfs.hessen.de.

Holmatro (2022). *Rescue tools*. Booklet. https://www.holmatro.com/sites/default/files/downloads/en/brochure-rescue-tools-en-4715.pdf

Hovorun, T. P., Berladir, K. V., Pererva, V. I., Rudenko, S. G., & Martynov, A. I. (2017). Modern materials for automotive industry. *Journal of Engineering Sciences*, Vol. 4, Issue 2, F8-F18. https://doi.org/10.21272/jes.2017.4(2).f8

IEA (2009). *Global gaps in clean energy research, development, and demonstration*. International Energy Agency. Paris. https://www.iea.org/reports/global-gaps-in-clean-energy-research-development-and-demonstration

Jackisch, J., Sethi, D., Mitis, F., Szymański, T., & Arra, I. (2016). European facts and the global status report on road safety 2015. *Injury Prevention*, Vol. 22 (Suppl 2), A29. https://doi.org/10.1136/injuryprev-2016-042156.76

Jasiuk, E., Szarpak, A., Zielinski, R., & Madziala, M. (2019). Organisation of technical rescue operations in the national rescue system. *Disaster and Emergency Medicine Journal*, Vol. 4, Issue 2, 63–67. https://doi.org/10.5603/DEMJ.2019.0013

Lukas Hydraulik GmbH (2019). *Instruction manual for rescue equipment: Spreaders*. https://lukas.com/manuals/public/downloads/1600416392.pdf

Metz, B., Davidson, O., Bosch, P., Dave, R., & Meyer, L. (Eds.) (2007). *Climate change 2007: Mitigation of climate change*. Cambridge University Press. ISBN: 978 0521 88011-4

Miller, L., Soulliere, K., Sawyer-Beaulieu, S., Tseng, S., & Tam, E. (2014). Challenges and Alternatives to Plastics Recycling in the Automotive Sector. *Materials*, Vol. 7, Issue 8, 5883–5902. https://doi.org/10.3390/ma7085883

Naudé, W. (2011). Climate change and industrial policy. *Sustainability*, Vol. 3, Issue 7, 1003–1021. https://doi.org/10.3390/su3071003

Norton, R. L. (1999). *Design of machinery: An introduction to the synthesis and analysis of mechanisms and machines* (2nd ed.). McGraw-Hill series in mechanical engineering. McGraw-Hill. ISBN: 0-07-048395-7

Spanner, H. (2018). *Einsätze mit Faserverbundwerkstoffen*. Kohlhammer. ISBN: 978-3-17-031103-9

Statistisches Bundesamt. (2021). Straßenverkehrsunfälle nach Unfallkategorie, Ortslage. https://www.destatis.de/DE/Themen/Gesellschaft-Umwelt/Verkehrsunfaelle/Tabellen/polizeilich-erfasste-unfaelle.html;jsessionid=839D33E-5F2A4B17ED138D9499E00E674.live741

Taub, A., Moor, E. de, Luo, A., Matlock, D. K., Speer, J. G., & Vaidya, U. (2019). Materials for Automotive Lightweighting. *Annual Review of Materials Research*, Vol. 49, Issue 1, 327–359. https://doi.org/10.1146/annurev-matsci-070218-010134

Tisza, M., & Lukács, Z. (2018). High strength aluminium alloys in car manufacturing. IOP Conference Series: Materials Science and Engineering, Vol. 418, 12033. https://doi.org/10.1088/1757-899X/418/1/012033

Tisza, M., & Czinege, I. (2018). Comparative study of the application of steels and aluminium in lightweight production of automotive parts. *International Journal of Lightweight Materials and Manufacture*, Vol. 1, Issue 4, 229–238. https://doi.org/10.1016/j.ijlmm.2018.09.001

Todor, M.-P., & Kiss, I. (2016). Systematic approach on materials selection in the automotive industry for making vehicles lighter, safer and more fuel–efficient. *Applied Engineering Letters*, Vol. 1, Issue 4, 91–97.

Tol, R. S. J. (2009). The economic effects of climate change. *Journal of Economic Perspectives*, Vol. 23, Issue 2, 29–51. https://doi.org/10.1257/jep.23.2.29

United Nations (1992). *Report of the united nations conference on environment and development.* Rio de Janeiro. ISBN: 92-1-100498-5

Volkswagen AG (03/2020a). *Guide for rescue workers.*

Volkswagen AG (08/2020b). *Rescue Manual Volkswagen ID.4.* https://www.volkswagen.de/idhub/content/dam/onehub_pkw/importers/de/besitzer-und-nutzer/wichtige-kundeninformationen/rechtliches/rettungsdaten/downloads-en/rescue-datasheets/Volkswagen_ID-4_SUV_2020-08_5d_Electric_EN.pdf

Weber Rescue (2020). *Rettungsgeräte: Hydraulische und pneumatische Rettungssysteme mit Zubehör.*

Weber-Hydraulik GmbH (2019). *Operating instructions hydraulic rescue equipment: Spreader.*

Weigeldt, M., Erbe, R., & Gondert, M. (2018). Technisch-medizinische Rettung beim Verkehrsunfall. *Notfall + Rettungsmedizin,* Vol. 21, Issue 8, 707–722. https://doi.org/10.1007/s10049-018-0536-2

Westhoff, J., Haasper, C., Otte, D., Probst, C., Krettek, C., & Richter, M. (2007). „Einklemmungstrauma" im Strassenverkehr. Unfallanalyse, Verletzungsschwere und -verteilung eingeklemmter PKW- und LKW-Insassen der Jahre 1983-2003 [Motor vehicle accidents with entrapment. A medical and technical investigation of crash mechanism, injury pattern and severity of entrapment of motor vehicle occupants between 1983 and 2003]. *Chirurg,* Vol. 78, Issue 3, 246–253. https://doi.org/10.1007/s00104-006-1260-x

Wöhrl, K., Geisbauer, C., Nebl, C., Lott, S., & Schweiger, H.-G. (2021). Crashed electric vehicle handling and recommendations—State of the art in Germany. *Energies,* Vol. 14, Issue 4, 1040. https://doi.org/10.3390/en14041040

Wolfgang, L. (2009). *What can demographers contribute to understanding the link between population and climate change.* Population Network Newsletter, 41.

# Case Study IV: Individualized Medical Technology using Additive Manufacturing

*Dennis Menge, Dennis Milaege, Kay-Peter Hoyer, Hans-Joachim Schmid, Mirko Schaper*

The high demand for individual products with the lowest possible price poses challenges for many manufacturing companies in today's globalised markets. The emerging technology of additive manufacturing, currently present in the media, is mentioned as a possible answer to the question of how customised products can be manufactured cost-efficiently and performance-efficiently (Lachmayer & Lippert, 2017).

The individualisation of medical devices through additive manufacturing is addressed in this publication. First, basic principles regarding individualisation of products and additive manufacturing concerning medical technology are highlighted. Based on this information, the main section of this publication focuses on possible challenges to interdisciplinary collaboration for engineers, possible intervention measures, and the accessibility of additive manufacturing to society. The potential of additive manufacturing for the production of medical devices is demonstrated utilising a Case Study from the Medicine Cluster of the NRW research college "Leicht – Effizient – Mobil" (FK-LEM). Finally, fundamental key statements and results are summarised.

In essence, this publication will answer the following key questions:

- What does interdisciplinary collaboration mean for engineers?
- Which access to institutions providing 3D solutions does society have with respect to additive manufacturing technology?
- Which challenges are currently still limiting the meaningful benefits of additive manufacturing for the use of medical devices in society?

# 1 Fundamentals

## 1.1 Individualisation through economic and social change

The individualisation of products is no longer a short-term trend but is recognised as a successive development triggered by various factors. The role of individual stakeholders and the importance of individual products for economic and social change are discussed in more detail below.

### Economic change

The market transformation from a seller's to a buyer's market is essentially determined by the demand for products and is a typical phenomenon of the 20th century in the Western world. At the same time, market conditions have significantly changed over time through technological progress in production systems. Thus, industrial mass production became society's primary objective at the beginning of the 20th century. The markets were characterised by rapidly growing demand and limited supply. The introduction of the division of labour and the design of more effective and standardised production systems, such as the use of assembly lines, resulted in an enormous increase in productivity. Despite the measures taken, the one-sided sales orientation meant that the growing demand could only be partially satisfied, as the company was confronted with a scarce supply of product variants and could not choose between different product alternatives (Paul, 2007; Mattmüller, 2012; Heina, 1999).

*Figure 1: Evolution of manufacturing paradigms in the 20th century according to Koren, 2010.*

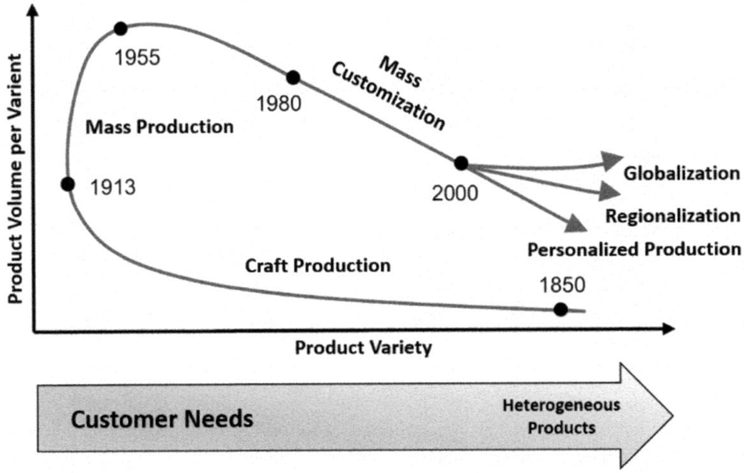

The economic growth in the 1970s resulted in a shift to a buyer's market in which the market supply exceeded the existing demand. The customer had the option of choosing from a wide range of products. To remain competitive, manufacturing companies had to adapt to the changing needs and demands of customers. The analysis of these individual customer needs plays an increasingly important role in satisfying actual emerging customer demand and ultimately positioning the company more successfully in the market. For the first time, product variety is increasing with decreasing product volume per individual variant (Schurawitzki, 1995). How the market changes and the needs of society are driving the paradigm shift is qualitatively shown in Figure 1. Currently, market globalisation is driving regionalisation and personalised production. Increasing daily market fluctuations are forcing manufacturing companies to produce even smaller quantities per product variant (Koren, 2010).

## Societal change

From a sociological point of view, the concept of individualisation has been significantly shaped by the sociologist Beck. Already in 1986, Beck described individualisation as a long-term process of society as a whole, in which each individual strives for self-determination and self-realisation (Beck, 1986). For a single individual, the "ascent of the ego" is increasingly at the forefront, and externally determined instances and social norms lose importance. In the course of development, however, the individual never has the possibility to free himself or herself from all social conditions. According to Beck, these merely change over time, since the process of individualisation is also dependent on social preconditions. In an individualised society, it is assumed that each person is granted individual freedom of opinion and decision, according to which he or she lives and acts. At the same time, however, responsibility and consequence must be assumed for one's actions. (Ewinger et al., 2016)

In literature, three social developments are frequently cited as drivers of individualisation. According to (Pillar, 2006), these include, above all, the continuing increase in prosperity across almost all population groups. In addition, shortening working hours leads to an increasing commitment to leisure time in all consumer classes. More specific hobbies and interests can be realised more intensively, leading to a transfer of social individualism to the material needs of society. In addition, the growing level of education is of decisive importance as people develop a stronger perception of their self-awareness and, as a result, tend to have a stronger urge to withdraw from social ideals. Hedonistic values, such as spontaneity, enjoyment, and self-development, replace existing life values, such as discipline and self-control. Hedonistic behaviour ultimately leads to heterogeneity in product demand at the aggregate level. Consequently, this leads to the growing importance of individualised products that are targeted to the new needs of individual consumers (Ewinger et al., 2016; Blecker & Friedrich, 2006).

In the 1990s, the process of social individualisation experienced a further essential push in addition to the points already listed. This is characterised in particular by globalisation and technological change. In addition to the rise of various information and communication technologies, the introduction of the World Wide Web and especially the global spread of the Internet are considered to be the driving force behind the process of social individualisation in many areas of life. Since the introduction of the Internet, around 80% of the German population has been using the Internet in Germany as of 2021. The Internet enables the international networking of society, resulting in increased communication and globalisation. Furthermore, the unrestricted exchange of information with others also has an impact on the decision-making and consumption behaviour of society. Consumption is no longer dependent on time and place. Around the clock, consumers have access to an individual, international variety of products that satisfy their needs. Moreover, they can use various comparison portals and their research to compare prices and select the most cost-effective provider. This leads to decreasing customer loyalty and increasing market transparency, which in turn leads to the establishment of the customer's position of power vis-à-vis the provider. Existing customer needs can also be recorded, analysed, and responded to more quickly via the internet and social media (Ternès et al., 2015; Ullrich, 2011; Ewinger et al., 2016).

## Mass customization

At this point, the question arises: How can manufacturing companies offer individual products economically in the course of economic market change and the social changes described above? The purchase price increases with the degree of individualisation of the product. The term "mass customisation" is often mentioned as a possible answer to this question. The term forms an oxymoron, combining the opposing concepts of mass production × the manufacture of large quantities of products of the same type × and customisation × to or by the customer. The primary goal of individual mass production is the manufacture of customised products with the efficiency of comparable mass production with defined standards. In line with the strategic goals, the cost and differentiation advantages of the respective paradigms are combined. The prices for customised products largely correspond to those of standard products, while the product characteristics are adapted to the individual requirements of the customers. Through appropriately designed organisational structures and production systems, customised products can be offered in the same price range as mass products, and the customer does not necessarily have to pay a corresponding surcharge for the customisation of a product (Pillar, 2006).

An important part of customised mass production is customer integration and interaction. First and foremost, this requires the creation of a suitable interaction platform between supplier and customer, where the customer's requirements and wishes regarding the product are communicated. In this context, we also speak about the creation of an interactive value chain. In addition, a suitable scope for design must be defined. This can vary from the selection of individual modules and parts to the customer's own ideas. The customer is thus actively involved in the production process as a "co-designer" and directly participates in product individualisation. This interaction often takes place via computer-based configurations. In this way, the customer gets in touch with the product virtually for the first time and is able to apply predefined changes to the product based on his or her experience (Ternès et al., 2015; Deutscher Dialogmarketing Verband, 2019).

The principle of customised mass production seems promising for manufacturing companies. In reality, individualised products are typically more expensive to manufacture than standard products due to the more complex production processes. However, if the customer has to pay for additional costs, these can be compensated by the personal design and the additional emotional benefits. Moreover, technological developments can positively change the possibilities and manufacturing prices of customised mass production. Additive manufacturing is an already established and promising manufacturing technology due to its high degree of design freedom and tool-free manufacturing. Also known as 3D printing, this technology is finding its way into private and industrial environments. The added value of additive manufacturing is not exclusively limited to the manufacture of individual products, but also serves the optimisation of companies in the economic sense (BMWi, 2015; **Rätsch, 2022**; Stember, 2020).

## 1.2 Additive manufacturing

Over the last two decades, additive manufacturing has grown into a cutting-edge manufacturing technology for products from a variety of industries. Current statistics forecast an increase in global market volume in billions of Euros by more than 100% for the year 2030 compared to 2020 for selected industries, such as aerospace, automotive, and medical technology, supporting the future importance of additive manufacturing across industries (Gebhardt & Schwarz, 2019).

Today, various additive manufacturing processes differ in terms of the material to be processed. Mainly polymers, metals, and ceramics in different aggregate states are used in industry and research. On the polymer side, the process of stereolithography (SLA) with liquid resins that cure a solid polymer under the influence of UV radiation has already become industrially established. Additive manufacturing with powdered polymers and metals is also of great industrial importance. Here, the two processes around selective laser sintering (SLS) for polymers and laser powder bed fusion (LPBF) for metals are worth mentioning. The basic principle of both processes is the local melting of the powder material by a laser to form a solidified component. In addition to the processing of liquid and powder materials, additive manufacturing also includes processes that work with solid or gaseous materials (Grund, 2015).

Despite a large number of additive manufacturing processes established, a common process route can be defined from the 3D CAD data set to the final component. In the first step, the generated CAD data set is converted into the standard triangulate language format (STL), which can be used by additive manufacturing technologies like LPBF (Figure 2). Then, as in all these processes, the component is

*Figure 2: General process route of LPBF*

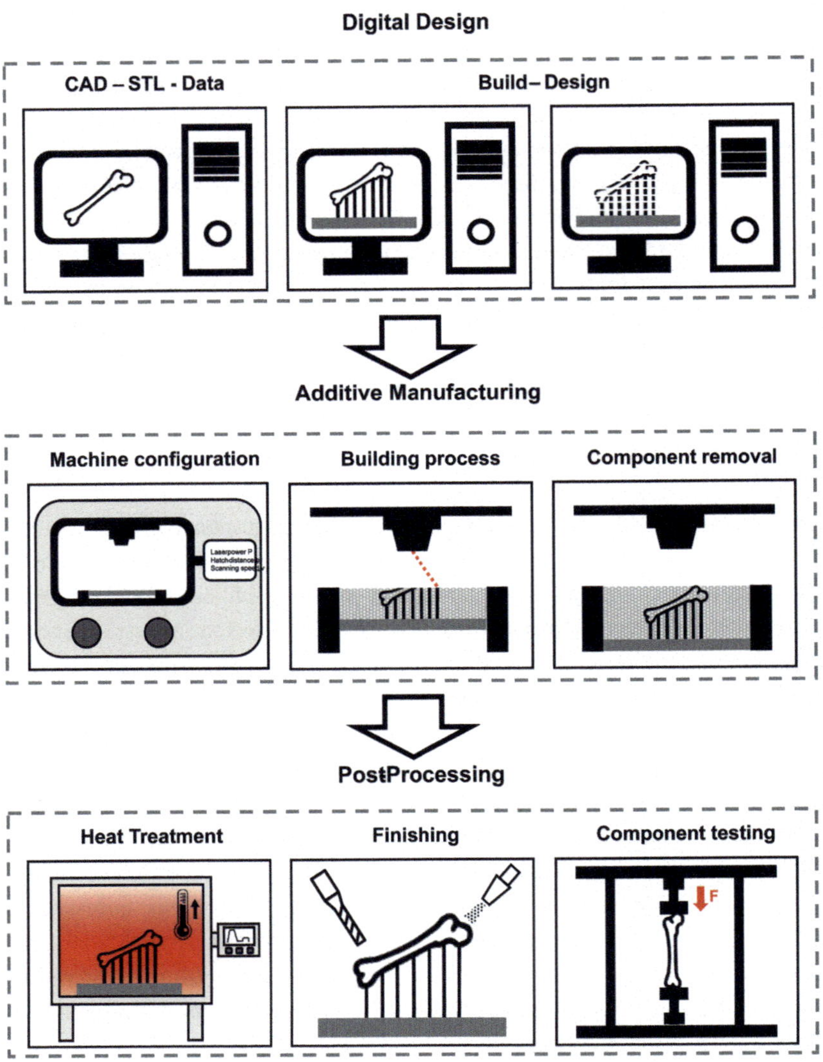

manufactured and provided by building up material layer by layer. Depending on the requirements of the component, a final post-processing of the printed component is necessary (Kumar et al., 2021; Kumke, 2018).

The principle of layer-by-layer component manufacturing allows structures to be produced from a two-dimensional geometry with any degree of complexity in the third dimension. This enables almost unlimited design freedom in the shape of additively manufactured components. Another advantage is the tool-free production, which eliminates the need for product-specific and moulding tools. Development costs for tools are eliminated, shortening the entire product development process. This implies that the unit costs are independent of the batch size. In industries such as medical technology, this fact offers the advantages of economical production and rapid availability of products compared to conventional manufacturing processes, in particular for patient-specific, individual aids with a quantity of one (Haleem & Javaid, 2020).

## 1.3 Additive manufacturing in medical technology

Medical technology generally describes the interdisciplinary cooperation between medicine and engineering, natural sciences or information sciences, developing medical applications.

### Potentials

In biomechanical terms, each person represents an individual with respect to their musculoskeletal system. For this reason, additive manufacturing is predestined for the development of patient-specific and stress-appropriate medical aids (Richard et al., 2017). Compared to the process route of additive manufacturing, which has already been explained above, the generation of radiological data of a patient is the starting point of further development. From clinical data, such as computed tomography (CT) or magnetic resonance imaging (MRI), visual 2D slice images can be converted into three-dimensional files. Likewise, a 3D scan of the affected organs or extremities is possible.

This allows the creation of an individual, customised design based on the anatomical structure of the patient (Huotilainen et al., 2014; Stelzer & Krzyzwinski, 2019). For the optimisation and individualisation of the generated 3D datasets, a large number of motion and loading studies, experiences as well as technical literature, can be used (Bogataj et al., 2015; Weigel & Nerlich, 2011; De Gruyter, 1953). They allow medical assistance to be tailored precisely to the person in question and in accordance with the load. The geometric shape of the medical device to be adapted can be designed almost indefinitely using additive manufacturing, which means, for example, that conventionally unfeasible details, such as lattice structures inside the component, can be manufactured. The medical device can thus be adapted to the patient's needs, resulting in an improvement in the quality of life through better fit and tolerability as well as an accelerated healing process with fewer complications. In addition, patient-adapted instruments can assist the surgeon, resulting in a reduction in surgical time (Richard et al., 2017).

### Material requirements for use in medical technology

In medical technology, the use of materials focuses on supporting or replacing cell or tissue functions in the human body. The material choice depends on the type and function of the tissue to be supported or replaced. For this reason, the requirements for the material in terms of properties and structure can vary widely. First and foremost, the mechanical properties are of the utmost importance. Depending on the functionality, the material must meet strength and fatigue requirements as well as minimum hardness and component stiffness. In addition to the mechanical properties, chemical and biological properties are important. A material implanted in the human body is exposed to a combination of mechanical stress and biological influences during its functional phase. To avoid damage to the recipient tissue, a certain biocompatibility must be ensured (Wintermantel & Ha, 2009; Hanawa, 2021). A so-called biomaterial has to be classified according to different property areas and resulting evaluation criteria as follows (Epple, 2003):

- Biological compatibility: e.g. immune reaction, osseointegration, cytotoxicity, etc.;
- Mechanical compatibility: e.g. strength, stiffness, etc.;
- Chemical compatibility: e.g. corrosion, degradation products, etc.

As can be seen, the property profiles cannot be divided strictly; hence a holistic development approach is required for biomaterials. The main objective is to ensure biocompatibility. In general, "biocompatibility" refers to the compatibility between a technical and a biological system, whereby the employed material causes a corresponding physical reaction after or during its use. Following a basic classification, a distinction can be made between structural and surface compatibility. Structural compatibility describes the adaptation of the biomaterial to the recipient tissue in terms of mechanical behaviour and refers to the shape as well as the internal structure. Surface compatibility refers to the adaptation of the chemical, physical, biological, and morphological surface properties. The purpose is to establish an interaction between the bioactivity of the biomaterial and the tissue. Whether and to what extent a biomaterial can be classified as biocompatible depends on the material, the preparation, and the application (Baldauf, 2016; Norrie, 2010; Abke, 2003). Biocompatibility can be divided as follows (Epple, 2003; Baldauf, 2016):

- **incompatible** materials are materials such as nickel or iron that produce substances in toxic concentrations or in form of antigens due to their lack of compatibility with the human organism and cause foreign body or inflammatory reactions;
- **biotolerant** materials, such as PMMA, Co-Cr alloys, only release a small number of substances in non-toxic concentrations; however, the release of toxic substances cannot be ruled out. Such materials are only partially used for long-term applications;
- **bioinert** materials, such as hydrocarbons or some titanium alloys, which lack participation in metabolism in general; accordingly, no toxic substances are released and are therefore not identified by the body as foreign bodies;
- **bioactive** materials, such as Ca-phosphate ceramics or magnesium, are characterised by a positive reaction with the recipient tissue, like promoted tissue formation by an adhesive bond between the material and the tissue.

Before a material can be successfully utilised in medical technology, it needs to have a certain degree of biocompatibility in addition to sufficient mechanical properties. For most applications, the material is required to withstand long and heavy loads and to be highly compatible with the recipient tissue. Currently, biocompatible metals, polymers, and ceramics are predominantly used in the manufacture of medical devices (Frank & Zitter, 1971; Schmidt et al., 2013).

## Applications of additively manufactured medical devices

The various additive manufacturing processes are establishing themselves in medical technology, particularly in the fields of dental technology and hearing acoustics. A denture or ear model can be generated by taking a 3D scan of the inside of the mouth or ear, which can then be used to manufacture, for instance, dentures or hearing aid capsules with 3D printers. In the field of dental technology, approximately 450 dental crowns per day are already produced in one building job cost-effectively using LPBF in Germany. In implant technology and prosthetics, surgical models, such as acetabular cup models with bone substitutes, and joints made of plastic or metal can be manufactured. In the field of bone replacement, additively manufactured implants, orthoses or prostheses are deployed in the reconstruction of skull or jawbones after fractures caused by accidents or tumour diseases. An additively manufactured skull cap made of plastic was transplanted for the first time in 2014, making it possible to completely replace the human skull. Additional examples of applications of additively manufactured medical products include finger, arm, and leg prostheses (Ehrenberg-Silies et al., 2015; Richard et al., 2019; Lachmayer & Lippert, 2017)

## 2 Interdisciplinarity in medical technology

The development of additively manufactured medical products involves interdisciplinary collaboration among natural sciences, engineering, and medicine. For example, at the beginning of the collaboration, medical literature and technical terms need to be translated to ensure a uniform language. As can be seen in the following section, there are challenges as well as potential in the case of interdisciplinary collaboration. Moreover, interdisciplinary collaboration transforms into transdisciplinary collaboration by involving society – in this context by involving medical staff and patients – which is illustrated by various examples and opportunities in chapter 3.4 and 4. Regarding the definition of transdisciplinarity, reference is made here to the Introduction and Case Study I.

### 2.1 Definition of terms, potentials, and challenges of interdisciplinary collaboration

Interdisciplinarity describes the involvement of two or more disciplines that have built a knowledge base of common research. In this context, disciplines are understood to be areas of expertise or research or specific collaborations of characters working on a scientific problem, who join together to conduct the necessary investigations and share the results obtained (Aboelela et al., 2007). The meaningfulness of any interdisciplinary collaboration is supported by the inclusion of different professional perspectives with respect to an existing problem in order to better obtain an answer or holistic view of a research topic (Choi & Pak, 2007). This can prevent an overly one-sided view of problems and stimulate advancement in generating ideas that go beyond the expertise and knowledge of individual disciplines. The integration of different ways of thinking, world views, and problem perspectives makes it more likely to find solutions to challenging problems (Bruner, 1991; Garland et al., 2006).

However, interdisciplinary collaboration can also affect team performance. Mello and Rentsch describe a low degree of information distribution, a lack of openness, and a great effort to build relationships as critical points for heterogeneous collaboration (Mello & Rentsch, 2015). Some publications also report frequent conflicts and lack of organisation, resulting in dissatisfying approaches to solutions. Often, the results will then fall short of the defined goals and have a psychological impact on people's health in the form of increased stress and dissatisfaction. As a result, there is reduced team performance and poorer group dynamics (Butler, 1998; Jehn, 1995; Jehn et al., 1999). According to Brandstädter (2019), the individuals involved pose a challenge to successful interdisciplinary collaboration due to their specifics, such as technical language, ways of thinking, goal orientation, etc. The challenges can be divided into five categories (Defila et al., 2000):

- **Communication:** The language basis represents the most important issue in communication among the disciplines involved. Technical terminological deficits in the meaning, translation or explanation of technical terms impede general comprehension. In addition to non-understanding, there is also the problem of misunderstanding, as the terms might have different meanings in each discipline and everyday language.
- **Subject description:** Disciplines differ in their worldview and ways of thinking, which leads to various perspectives regarding the object of investigation. This complicates the common description of the research goal due to different conflicts of interest, ways of thinking, and convictions.
- **Methodology:** Diverse perspectives with respect to a project complicate the choice of research and working methods. According to the discipline-specific view, disciplines differ in their understanding of which scientifically correct methods or working procedures should be applied. Therefore, the formulation of uniform common questions as well as the agreement with respect to the approach to be chosen might be complex.
- **Group dynamics:** Long-lasting interdisciplinary project collaboration is usually unfamiliar to all disciplines involved. Specific issues, such as lack of knowledge or competence in effectively managing interdisciplinary groups and work processes, can lead to negative team dynamics, ingroup-outgroup phenomena, and further conflicts.
- **Prejudice:** Each discipline's perspective of the world is unique. However, if these assumptions are interpreted as the "right" ones by the individual discipline representatives, this will lead to a major obstacle to successful collaboration. In addition, overestimation of the importance of one's own discipline's contribution often leads to prejudice. Moreover, prejudices are reinforced by an overestimation of one's own discipline's contribution to the research project.

Interdisciplinary cooperation is not automatically associated with a promising concept. Rather, the aforementioned challenges inhibit the development of potential. At this point, the question arises as to how the procedure for successful and, above all, effective interdisciplinary collaboration must be designed and what significant support measures for interdisciplinary collaboration are available. Medical technology in particular is dependent on the successful collaboration among different disciplines.

## 2.2 Support measures for interdisciplinary collaboration in medical technology

Corresponding intervention measures relating to the individual problem areas were derived from the identified challenges and can be used for interdisciplinary projects in the field of medical technology. Based on our experience with interdisciplinary collaboration, we only report communication problems (Table 1). This includes, in particular, the clarification of medical facts. In this case, for instance, reading up on and clarifying discussions with medical experts helped a great deal and were sufficient for a successful processing of the projects.

*Table 1: Support measures for better interdisciplinary collaboration in projects processed in Medicine Cluster of FK-LEM*

| Main problem | Support measures |
|---|---|
| Communication | Reading in professional literature<br>Professional discussions with medical staff<br>Attendance at basic medical lectures and workshops |

# 3 Potential of and accessibility to individual medical devices for society

The previous chapters highlight the benefits of additive manufacturing with respect to individualised medical technology and show the potential and challenges of interdisciplinary collaboration. Contact with additive manufacturing technology is often limited to engineers from industry or science. How can this technology be made accessible to society? The potential applications are manifold, and the technology could bring enormous benefits in quickly available, individually designed or patient-specific medical technology. However, some challenges, such as data protection, approval procedures, legal regulations, (Thompson, 2021) as well as the possible coverage of costs by health insurance have to be considered. To start with, the terms *medical device* and *aid* must be defined and differentiated from one another before the approval procedure and cost coverage are discussed. These aspects are essential for the applicability of additively manufactured, individual products and are not the subject of engineering education. In this way, a common language level with the medical sector is developed. Subsequently, the approval of additively manufactured medical devices is examined in particular, and the possibilities are considered as to how patients can gain access to individualised, additively manufactured medical devices or aids.

## 3.1 Definition of terms – Medical Device vs. Aids

To create the basis for understanding approval procedures that are necessary for the applicability of additively manufactured, individual medical devices, the two terms *medical technology* and *medical devices* are first defined and differentiated from one another.

The term *medical technology* is defined in the *Medical Device Regulation* (MDR[1]) or European Medical Device Regulation, which regulates placing on the market, availability on the market, and service of medical devices and their accessories for human use. According to the MDR, the term *medical device* is defined as follows:

***Medical device*** *means any instrument, apparatus, appliance, software, implant, reagent, material or other article intended by the manufacturer to be used, alone or in combination, for human beings for one or more of the following specific medical purposes:*

- diagnosis, prevention, monitoring, prediction, prognosis, treatment or alleviation of disease,
- diagnosis, monitoring, treatment, alleviation of, or compensation for, an injury or disability,
- investigation, replacement or modification of the anatomy or a physiological or pathological process or state,
- providing information employing in vitro examination of specimens derived from the human body, including organ, blood and tissue donations, and which does not achieve its principal intended action by pharmacological, immunological or metabolic means, in or on the human body, but which may be assisted in its function by such means.

*The following products are also considered medical devices:*

- devices for the control or support of conception;
- products specifically intended for the cleaning, disinfection or sterilisation of devices as referred to in Article 1(4) and of those referred to in the first paragraph of this point (according to the MDR).

However, medical devices according to the MDR are to be differentiated in some points from (medical) aids according to the *Aids Directive* ("Hilfsmittel-Richtlinie") according to Section 92 (1), Clause 2, No. 6, of the Fifth Book of the German Social Code ("Fünftes Buch Sozialgesetzbuch", SGB V). The *Aids Directive* has the aim of ensuring an adequate, expedient and economic supply to insured persons with

1 Medical Device Regulation – VERORDNUNG (EU) 2017/745

aids following the rules of medical practice and taking into account the generally accepted state of medical knowledge (Gemeinsamer Bundesausschuss, 2022). Aids according to this guideline are defined as follows:

**Aids** are material resources or technical products which are individually manufactured or supplied by the service provider as series-produced goods in an unmodified state or as a basic product with appropriate manual preparation, supplementation or modification. This may also include material resources or technical products which serve to bring medicines or other therapeutics intended for internal use into the body (e.g. certain syringes or inhalation devices). According to the legal regulations, aids include visual aids, hearing aids, body substitutes, orthopaedic and other aids. Aids also include accessories without which the basic products either cannot be used at all or cannot be used for the intended purpose. The designation also comprises the necessary modification, repair and replacement of aids, training in their use and, insofar as necessary to protect the insured person from unacceptable health risks, the maintenance and technical checks required according to the state of the art to maintain functionality and technical safety. (Gemeinsamer Bundesausschuss, 2022)

According to Wettlaufer (2021), ***aids*** are objects whose usage replaces, simplifies, supplements or enables an impaired bodily function. In addition to those mentioned in the definition, examples of assistive devices include prostheses, orthoses, wheelchairs, and inhalation devices. (Becker, 2021)

## 3.2 Approval procedure and cost coverage by the health insurance companies

In the following, the approval of aids and the coverage of costs by health insurance companies are discussed. After that, the approval of medical devices and subsequently the approval of additively manufactured medical devices are considered.

### Aids - Approval and cost coverage

By definition, the groups of medical devices and aids overlap. The intersection of both groups includes, for example, products that are used for the treatment or alleviation of diseases, disabilities and injuries. Medical devices that are not aids are products that are used by medical experts, such as clinical measuring devices, surgical drapes and many more. Aids are not medical devices if the manufacturer does not specify a purpose from which a qualification as a medical device results. Examples are toilet seats or guide dogs for the blind. (Wettlaufer, 2021)

For medical device manufacturers, it may be of economic interest whether their product can be declared as an aid. Because as an aid, the costs for the patient can be covered by the health insurance companies and offer the manufacturer increased sales potential and additional income. For this, it should, among other things, fall into a category of the *list of aids*, not be explicitly excluded as an aid according to §34 SGB V, and not fall under "general objects of daily use". (Wettlaufer, 2021) Moreover, the benefits for the manufacturer also mean benefits for patients, for whom more reimbursable medical devices are available.

In general, health insurance companies (here: statutory health insurance companies) cover the costs of aids if they are necessary in the respective case for a positive treatment result, the prevention of worsening of an illness, the counteracting of negative health development of a child or the prevention or counteracting of a disability.

The same also applies to the prevention of a possible need for long-term care (Bundesministerium für Gesundheit (2022a); Gemeinsamer Bundesausschuss, 2022). Furthermore, the qualification for care also includes the follow-up costs associated with the assistive device, such as maintenance, modification or replacement, as well as costs for instruction in the use of the device (Bundesministerium für Gesundheit (2022a)). However, the health insurer must approve the supply in advance even if a prescription has been issued by the attending doctor (Bundesministerium für Gesundheit (2022a)), or if the aid is listed in the *list of aids* (GKV Spitzenverband). The prescription with cost coverage by the health insurance company must therefore be covered by the health insurance company's service catalogue. However, due to the large number of medical devices as aids and the constantly new and further developments, it is also clear that not all products can be covered by the service catalogue of the health insurance funds. Due to the pressure to cut costs, the health insurance funds have only limited funds available for stable health insurance contributions, so the majority of products available on the market are not covered by the service catalogue of the health insurance funds. Therefore, a selection of products must be carried out for the service catalogue (Wabnitz, 2009). For example, aids that are to be classified as general objects of daily use or are excluded by the legal regulations according to § 34 paragraph 4 SGB V (various medicines and aids disputed by the Federal Ministry of Health with the approval of the Bundesrat from the therapeutic benefit), do not fall under the service obligation of the health insurance funds (Gemeinsamer Bundesausschuss, 2022). Furthermore, products are excluded in the absence of necessity and economic viability (Wabnitz, 2009). According to §33 SGB V, an aid is necessary if its use is indispensable and unavoidable in the individual case for the fulfilment of the intended purpose (Schulin, 1994). The provision of aid must also comply with the principle of economic efficiency according to §§ 2, 12 SGB V (Ihle, 2007), in that the provision must be sufficient, appropriate, economical and must not exceed a necessary level (Wagner & Knittel, 2022). It is also relevant that innovative medical devices are usually associated with innovative examination and treatment methods, which must first be reviewed by the "Gemeinsamer

Bundesausschuss" before the product can be covered by the health insurance fund (Schäfer, 2018). Thus, there are barriers and exclusions to the reimbursement of assistive devices.

The prescription for aids is made by contract physicians and must be formulated clearly. The decision for a prescription is made according to dutiful discretion within the framework determined by the law and this guideline to provide the insured with an adequate, appropriate and economical supply of aids according to the rules of medical art and the generally recognised state of medical knowledge (Gemeinsamer Bundesausschuss, 2022). In the context of this article, it should be noted that customised products are only permitted if the same purpose cannot be served by standard products, including ready-made and customised convection. Furthermore, it is prohibited for health insurance companies to cover the costs of new development including testing. When dispensing or handing over the aid to the patient, the authorised doctors should check whether the requirements specified in the prescription have been met and whether the aid is appropriate, particularly for individualised products (Gemeinsamer Bundesausschuss, 2022).

The previously mentioned *list of aids* is compiled and updated by the GKV-Spitzenverband (GKV: Gesetzliche Krankenkasse /statutory health insurance company) following Section 139 of the SGB V and lists the aids that are covered by the obligation of the health insurance funds to provide benefits. The *list of aids* thus provides comprehensive information about the obligation of the health insurance funds to provide benefits as well as about product type and quality, creates market transparency, and serves as an interpretation and orientation guide for the health insurance funds and other parties involved in the provision of health care. The inclusion of a product in the *list of aids* can be applied for by the manufacturer with proof of defined characteristics and quality features. The classification of aids in the directory is based on their function and area of application in various product groups, in which the quality and service requirements to be met by the manufacturer are defined by § 139 of the SGB V. The directory is freely accessible online with all information (GKV Spitzenverband).

For aids to be listed in the *list of aids*, they must fulfil certain requirements according to §139 SGB V, which must be proven by the manufacturer. These include functional suitability, safety, medical benefit (if required), information on safe and appropriate use, indication-related or use-related quality requirements, and requirements for service life and re-use. Indication-related or use-related quality requirements include, for example, functionality, usability, cleaning, compatibility and combination, size, weight and customisation options. For aids that are also medical devices, proof of functionality and safety is already given by the necessary "Communauté Européene" (CE) marking, which is discussed in the following section (Wettlaufer, 2021).

## Approval of medical devices

In the following, the approval and market access requirements for medical devices according to the MDR (EU-wide directive) are discussed. On a national level, the MDR is supplemented by the Medizinprodukterecht-Durchführungsgesetz (in short: MPDG) (Johner, 2019). The MDR regulates placing the device on the market, making it available on the market and putting medical devices into service for use on humans. Clinical trials conducted for these products also belong to their scope. According to the "Bundesgesundheitsministerium", the purpose of the EU regulations is to provide an efficient and robust legal framework to promote innovation and rapid accessibility while maintaining high safety standards and high benefits for patients (Bundesgesundheitsministerium).

Medical devices must be CE certified to be placed on the European market and put into service. For this purpose, the product must meet the essential safety and performance requirements. Medical device manufacturers are required to establish a specific quality management system to ensure the implementation of risk management for risk minimisation and clinical evaluation for each product. The requirements for the quality management system are listed in DIN EN ISO 13485 (Medical devices×Quality management systems×Requirements for regulatory purposes). During the development and manufacture of medical devices, the requirements defined in the MDR, which ensure the performance of the devices and the safety of patients, users and third parties, must be met. Fulfilment of and compliance with the requirements must be proven in the so-called conformity assessment procedure. Medical devices are classified into Risk Classes I, IIa, IIb and III. The classification is conducted by the manufacturer. Depending on the risk class of the medical device, the conformity assessment procedure must be carried out by an independent testing and certification agency, referred to in the MDR as a *notified body*. These institutions are designated in a state procedure organised at the European level and are constantly monitored by the relevant authority (Bundesministerium für Gesundheit (2022b)). *Notified bodies* in Germany are, for example, TÜV and DEKRA (Zentralstelle der Länder für Gesundheitsschutz, 25.01.22). The *notified bodies* examine the quality management system and not the product itself. Only for Class I products, can the manufacturers themselves assess the conformity. The characteristics and examples of the four risk classes are listed in Table 2. In general, the higher the risk and the longer the duration of use, the higher the risk class. Through a clinical evaluation, the manufacturer must continue to demonstrate medical performance and demonstrate an acceptable benefit to risk ratio. The requirements for clinical trials of medical devices are comprehensively regulated by the EU regulatiolemns and the MPDG and also include post-market clinical follow-up (according to the MDR; Zentralstelle der Länder für Gesundheitsschutz, 25.01.22). The product's compliance with all requirements and its technical safety are finally documented by the CE marking and the declaration of conformity. This means that the products can be marketed in the EU, but they are subject to constant monitoring to identify and record any risks that may subsequently arise (Bundesministerium für Gesundheit (2022b)). The so-called vigilance system makes it mandatory for manufacturers to report serious and regularly occurring incidents or risks. The MDR also provides a unique device identification (UDI) for the traceability of medical devices (Schäfer, 2018)

*Table 2: Classification of medical devices (Bundesministerium für Gesundheit (2022b); Wabnitz, 2009; according to the MDR)*

| Class | Risk | Degree of invasiveness | Duration of application | Examples |
|---|---|---|---|---|
| I | Low | Low | Temporary (< 60 minutes) | reading glasses, wheelchairs, first-aid equipment, reusable surgical instruments |
| IIa | Moderate | Moderate | Short-term application (< 30 days), continuous/ repeated use of the same product | Single-use injections, ultrasonic equipment, X-ray film, MRT, dental fillings, contact lenses |
| IIb | Increased | Systemic impact | Long-term application (> 30 days) | Breathing apparatus, defibrillators, infusion pumps |
| III | High | Implantable and/ or highly invasive; direct application to the heart, central circulatory system or neurological system | Long-term application (> 30 days) | Heart catheters, stents, implants, artificial limbs |

However, the MDR has a few exceptions to the approval procedure described previously, which are discussed in detail below:

- Products manufactured and used internally by healthcare facilities located in the EU with appropriate quality management systems are exempt from the requirements of the MDR, except for the essential safety and performance requirements. However, it must be justified that there is no comparable product on the market that meets the target group-oriented requirements. Manufacturers of these customised devices shall prepare a continuously actualised document containing the following information:

- all essential data of the manufacturer;
- all essential data of the product (including characteristics from the doctor's prescription);
- a statement that the product is intended exclusively for a particular patient;
- the data of the person who prescribed the product;
- the statement that the essential safety and performance requirements are met.

*Figure 3: Development process of a medical device from the idea to the market launch (according to Risse, 2020)*

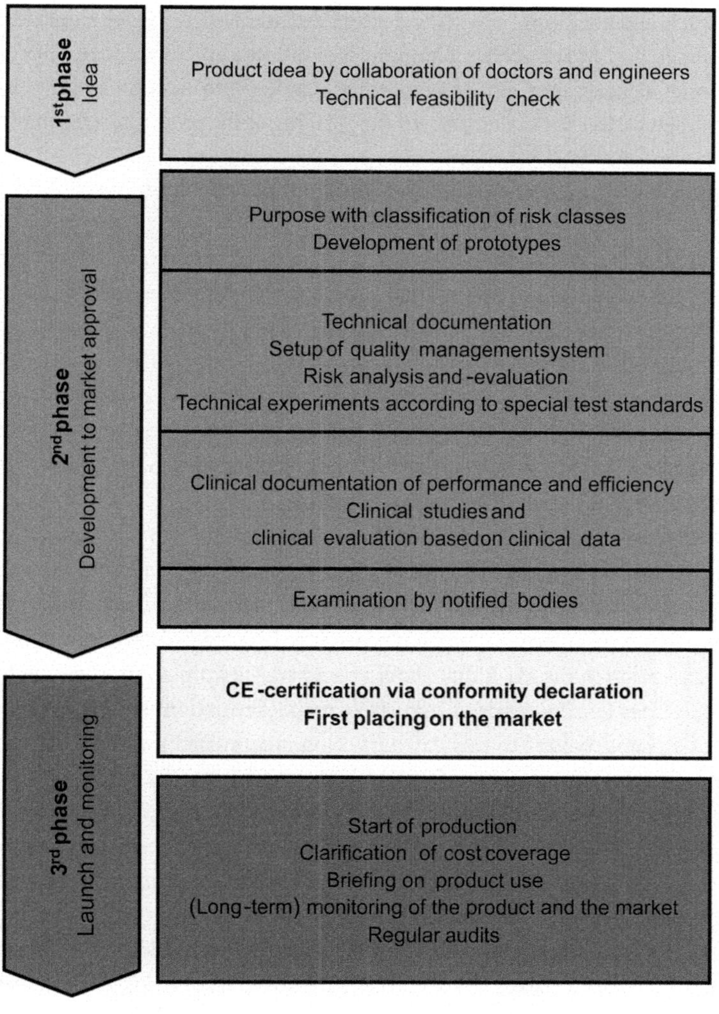

The document may also indicate that the safety and performance require ments have not been fully met.

- Customised products do not have to be CE certified but must have been prescribed by a doctor. An exception are individualised implants as Class 3 products. In this case, the manufacturer must involve a *notified body* for conformity assessment (according to the MDR).

Risse (2020) has summarised the entire development process of a medical product from the idea to the market launch (Figure 3). In Phase 1, doctors and engineers work together on an interdisciplinary basis to develop an idea for improving the healing progress or success of a given disease or injury. The doctor identifies a possible innovation potential so that the engineer subsequently develops and tests the technical implementation, which the doctor evaluates with regard to clinical criteria (Hermeneit et al., 2010). Phase 2 summarises the approval procedure described in the previous paragraphs. Phase 3 represents market introduction and monitoring, which follows CE certification and the first placing of the product on the market.

### 3.3 Approval of additively manufactured medical devices

Additive manufacturing can generate an enormous advantage in patient care through individualised products such as orthoses or dental prostheses, as already shown in Sections 2.3.1 and 2.3.3. In surgery, for example, additively manufactured, individualised templates have been used for years for drilling, cutting and sawing during operations on joints (Johner, 2019). Additive manufacturing also offers a clear advantage in the low-cost and, in particular, fast supply of medical aids, which can also be individualised. From a technological point of view, there is no reason why the supply should not be possible.

According to the MDR, individualised products are considered customised products, so that they may be used without CE marking in compliance with the safety and performance requirements (keyword: clinical testing). Thus, there is no need for a conformity assessment procedure by a *notified body*. However, there is one exception in the MDR that should be noted: Customised devices, which fall into Risk Class III. Customised, additively manufactured implants, such as osteosynthesis plates, belong to this category. Non-customised products or customisable products, where a basic variant is adapted to the specific patient, are treated according to the standard procedure of the MDR. This means that except in the case of Risk Class I, a *notified body* is involved in the conformity assessment and the product must be provided with a CE certification (Oppermann et al., 2020).

The establishment of a quality management system, in particular, requires great effort and expense for the manufacturer. The technology is still comparatively new so there are gaps in standards that still need to be closed and which also make it difficult for a manufacturer to be audited by a *notified body*. New fields also arise in risk analysis, such as handling powder material, biocompatibility of recycled powder or removal of support structures without leaving residues. Precise analyses are required for these risk areas, which may differ in the test methods compared to the analysis of traditional manufacturing. The standardisation of additive manufacturing must therefore be driven forward. In 2019, for example, the guideline DIN SPEC 17071 entitled *Additive manufacturing – Requirements for quality-assured processes at additive manufacturing centres* was published, which is industry-independent, i.e. not specifically tailored to the medical technology sector (Oppermann et al., 2020). DIN SPEC 17071 serves as the basis for the international standard DIN EN ISO/ ASTM 52920, published in 2021, entitled *Additive manufacturing – Qualification principles – Requirements for industrial additive manufacturing processes and production sites*, which defines and specifies both quality-relevant aspects in the process chain (Figure 4) and procedures in manufacturing. As the smallest changes in the process chain, such as the smallest differences in the starting material or the calibration of a system, it can affect the component properties and reproducibility. Production sites can be certified to this standard by *notified bodies* such as TÜV SÜD. Considering DIN EN ISO/ ASTM 52920 and DIN EN ISO 13485 certification, in principle every company is equipped for additive manufacturing of medical devices.

*Figure 4: Quality-assured process in an additive manufacturing facility (according to DIN SPEC 17071)*

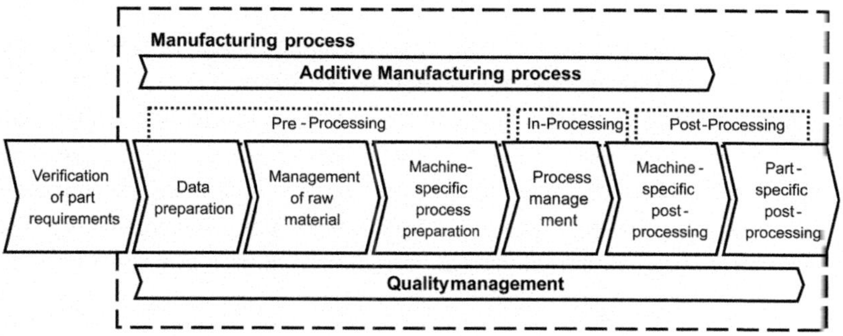


An important and noteworthy aspect of the process chain is the post-processing of additively manufactured medical devices. This is because post-processing steps, such as cleaning, sterilisation or packaging, can harm biological safety, surface quality or mechanical properties. The requirements for biological safety are specified in DIN EN ISO 10993, which includes tests for cytotoxicity or carcinogenicity. Sterilisation is regulated in DIN EN 556. Each product must be considered separately since there are four different sterilisation methods (gaseous or liquid chemicals, ionizing radiation and high temperature), which have different effects on the product and material (TÜV SÜD, 2021).

In addition to the approval of medical devices as defined, the question, arises as to which aspects involved in the process chain of additive manufacturing of medical devices can or must themselves be classified as medical devices. Software that, for example, optimises the geometry of an implant or tooth, or optimises the cutting pattern of templates, becomes a medical device because it serves a medical purpose. If this software was even integrated into the additive manufacturing system, the entire system would be declared to be a medical device. 3D scanners that have been specially developed for a medical application, such as scanners in the dental field with direct patient contact, are also considered medical devices (Johner, 2019).

When evaluating the initial materials for the respective additive manufacturing process and the corresponding medical device, there are different approaches taken by the manufacturers and *notified bodies*. On the one hand, the end product manufactured from the material can be classified as a medical device; on the other hand, there are material manufacturers who market their materials as medical devices. Furthermore, material manufacturers can market their materials as *medical grade* materials, which certifies that all basic safety and performance requirements at the material level, such as biocompatibility, are verifiably met (Johner, 2019).

One example of a certified company is 3D technology provider *Materialise*, which advertised its CE-marked, prescription-free, additively manufactured medical devices in the field of orthopaedics and oral and maxillofacial surgery on the *DeviceMed* medical device information platform in 2020. *Materialise* delivers thousands of individualised products annually, a comparatively large number in the industry, which would not be possible in this form without CE certification. This is because customised products can be sold without CE marking under the MDR, but in that case they must have been prescribed by a doctor, which stands in the way of larger-scale production. CE marking certifies that custom products meet the same quality requirements as commercially available products, helping to improve accessibility for surgery, among others, and ensuring patient safety and transparency in manufacturing. Ordering products without a prescription means less administrative work and more room for action for manufacturers offering individualised medical products (Lüttmann, 2020).

## 3.4 Accessibility for patients to individualised, additively manufactured products

The previous sections have dealt with medical devices and aids as well as the approval of additively manufactured medical devices in particular. Now, society's accessibility to individualised, additively manufactured medical devices, which are not subject to CE marking and conformity assessment according to the MDR as customised devices (with the exception of individualised implants), will be discussed. In addition, individualised, additively manufactured daily living aids, which are not medical devices, will be briefly discussed at this point. The question arises here as to how these products are or can be made available to patients or how they come into contact with the products and the technology, which, as described in the course of this article, certainly have advantages in terms of individualisation and rapid availability. In the following, various possibilities in surgery, orthopaedics, dentistry and dental technology and in connection with daily living aids will be examined as examples.

### Possibilities in surgery

In surgery, additive manufacturing can be used in conjunction with CAE (computer-aided engineering) methods based on CT (computed tomography) or MRI (magnetic resonance imaging) data in various areas, such as preoperative planning or patient information.

In surgical planning, the use of CAE methods creates a digital process chain, because both the patient's anatomy and the devices, prostheses or osteosynthesis plates, etc., adapted to the anatomy are available as a digital 3D model through feedback from the CT or MRI data. This makes the planning process more descriptive or visual, more precise and more efficient, making the work steps and the result more predictable and efficient (Risse, 2020). This can reduce the surgical time, which, for the patient, means a shorter time under general anaesthesia and a shorter wound exposure time with less blood loss (D'Urso et al., 1999; Guarino et al., 2007; Risse, 2020; Rozen et al., 2012), and, furthermore, costs can be saved. Additively manufactured models, e.g. in the form of reconstructed bones or joints, can play a role in planning, as the operation can be tested on the model in advance. During the surgical procedure, the surgeon can refer back to the models so that they provide visual and haptic support. During the operation, the surgeon can also make use of optimally matched, additively manufactured surgical templates, prostheses, osteosynthesis plates or other aids that do not have to be adapted to the patient's anatomy during the operation (Risse, 2020). In this way, in addition to increasing efficiency, risk can also be reduced, especially in complex interventions. Healing and rehabilitation can be improved. (Risse, 2020) The advantages in preoperative planning with additively manufactured models are shown, for example, in re-constructions in maxillofacial surgery (Azuma et al., 2014; Cohen et al., 2009; Lim et al., 2014; Liu et al., 2014) or also in reconstructions of the cervical spine (D'Urso et al., 1999).

Additively manufactured models are also used in the field of surgeon training or patient education. In this way, the patient can develop a better understanding through the tangible models and, if necessary, the acceptance for the intervention can be increased and the patient's fears or uncertainties can be reduced (Watson, 2014; Witschey et al., 2014).

## Possibilities in orthopaedics

In orthopaedic technology, individual prostheses, orthoses and other aids for the support of patients with disabilities or injuries can be manufactured using additive manufacturing. They serve to support and modify the structural and functional properties of the human neuromuscular and musculoskeletal system, thereby improving mobility and the patient's quality of life. In contrast to commercially available prostheses and orthoses, customised prostheses and orthoses have an improved fit. In addition, additive manufacturing offers rapid availability at lower cost, as fewer steps are necessary. The work steps for conventional and additive manufacturing are compared in Figure 5 using the example of an ankle joint orthosis. Traditionally, individually manufactured ankle orthoses are produced using a labour-intensive plaster casting technique. On the left side of the illustration, the various work steps of traditional production can be seen, from measurement, through moulding of the negative and subsequent casting of the positive plaster model, post-processing of the plaster model, and final moulding with thermoplastic film in a vacuum. The entire process usually takes one to two weeks. In contrast, a few days are usually sufficient for additive manufacturing, so that the patient is supplied more quickly. The 3D model to be manufactured is created within one day. For this, the affected part of the patient's body is 3D scanned or CT or MRI data is used and the geometry data obtained is further processed. Impressions, such as of the sole of the foot, can also be taken and then scanned. In the next step, the prosthesis or orthosis is digitally created for the model of the body part and additive manufacturing is digitally prepared. The prosthesis can then be manufactured. Only the last step – fitting to the patient – is similar to both procedures (Jin et al., 2015).

Another example from the field of orthopaedics is the online 3D printing marketplace *Protiq*[2], which offers shoe orthopaedic technicians a free online configurator for the production of shoe lasts. Shoe lasts are a 3D model adapted to a patient's foot and its needs, which is used as the basis for manufacturing a shoe that improves health. During online configuration, 3D scans of the foot or footprint are uploaded by the orthopaedic technician to determine the outline of the insole. Var-

2 https://www.protiq.com/3d-druck/anwendungsgebiete/3d-druck-orthopaedieschuhtechnik/

*Figure 5: Comparison of the manufacturing steps of classical and additive manufacturing using the example of an ankle joint orthosis (Jin et al., 2015)*

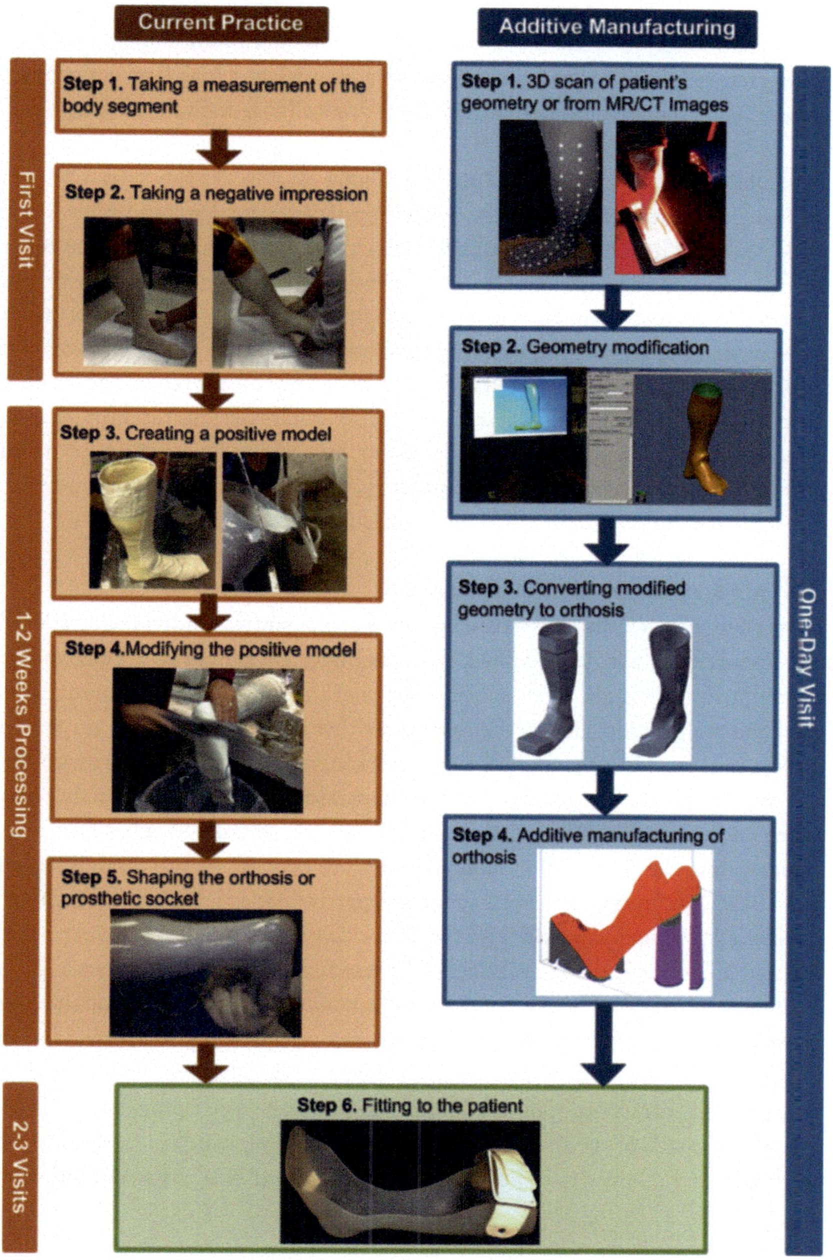

ious parameters can then be set, such as the leg axis, the twist or deformations at the shoe last. Once all the parameters have been defined, the orthopaedic technician can order the shoe lasts so that they can be additively manufactured and delivered within a few days, after which the actual manual production of the health-promoting shoe can begin. In this way, only a few days pass in comparison to several weeks in the traditional production of shoe lasts made of wood. In addition, the additively manufactured shoe lasts have further advantages, such as a high level of fitting accuracy, simple adaptability and reproducibility as well as individual markings.

### Possibilities in dentistry and dental technology

Additive manufacturing enables the production of dental implants and other dental tools. Complex dental crowns, bridges, orthodontic braces and also various other models, devices and instruments can be developed and manufactured with less time and lower cost. For this purpose, the patient's data is recorded with a 3D intraoral scanner and further processed using CAE methods (Javaid & Haleem, 2019). In addition to the 3D scanner, CT and MRI technologies are used to record patient data, as in surgery (Revilla-León & Özcan, 2019). It also enables the fabrication of removal dentures, aligners, surgical guides for implants, and models for treatment planning and preoperative jaw positioning (Azuma et al., 2014; Cohen et al., 2009; Engel et al., 2015; Javaid & Haleem, 2019; Lim et al., 2014; Liu et al., 2014; Tsai & Wu, 2014).

### Daily life aids for people with disabilities

People with physical disabilities can benefit enormously from individually tailored aids for everyday use. For example, eating utensils that cannot be gripped due to a hand malposition can be extended at the shaft by a geometry that counteracts the hand malposition. This counterpart can either be plugged onto the respective cutlery or it is additively manufactured as a coherent part (counterpart with, for example, a spoon). The geometry of the counterpart can be moulded using plasticine and scanned in (Richard et al., 2017). Individually tailored aids do not refer exclusively to the direct counteraction or improvement of physical disabilities but can also mean functional objects for the respective patient that are not commercially available, such as a holder for the wheelchair for a special object. Such items are available online on a wide variety of 3D printing model platforms such as *Libre 3D, Thingiverse, MyMiniFactory, YouMagine* or *RepRap* or can be modelled on the computer by the patients themselves, depending on the complexity. These models can be produced by the patients at home, if a 3D printer is available for home use, or in a 3D printing workshop, or ordered from a 3D printing service provider.

The approach of the *proDruck*[3] project (see Figure 6), which is funded by the German Federal Ministry of Education and Research (BMBF), is also interesting

3 https://www.prodruck-projekt.de/

at this point. Its overall objective is to develop a holistic employment model for people with disabilities using additively manufactured, individualised, daily living aids. This is because people with disabilities are often at a disadvantage when it comes to finding and keeping a job, which puts them at a social disadvantage. In this context, the project managers aim to develop a model for helping people to help themselves. In addition to training with the technology and 3D printers, a 3D printing lab tailored to people with disabilities is to be created. In addition, an online platform is to be set up for contact between experts and users and for exchanging 3D models or customising the models. These can be purchased or ordered there, undergo a quality check and are manufactured in the 3D printing lab that has been set up. The platform thus also serves to distribute developed aids or ideas and can also create an incentive for the industry to redesign production to meet the needs of the disabled and promote inclusion. In addition to the two areas of the laboratory and the online platform, an area dealing with ethics and security, such as data protection, is to be provided, which clearly sets the project apart from previously mentioned platforms such as Thingiverse. (Kruse & Mummert, 2019)

*Figure 6: Project objectives of "proDruck" for the supply of people with disabilities with individual assistive devices*

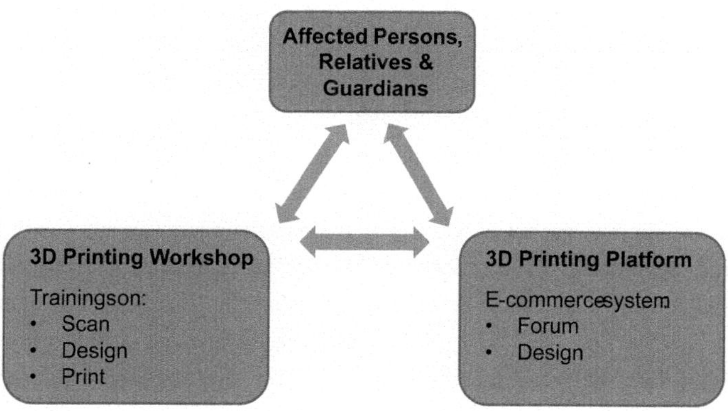


## 4 Additively manufactured finger prosthesis as an example in orthopaedic technology

In the following, an additively manufactured finger prosthesis developed within the framework of the NRW Research College will be presented as an example of individualised care through additive manufacturing in orthopaedic technology. This is a design and feasibility study. The product is not approved because the safety

*Figure 7: Stump of right index finger*

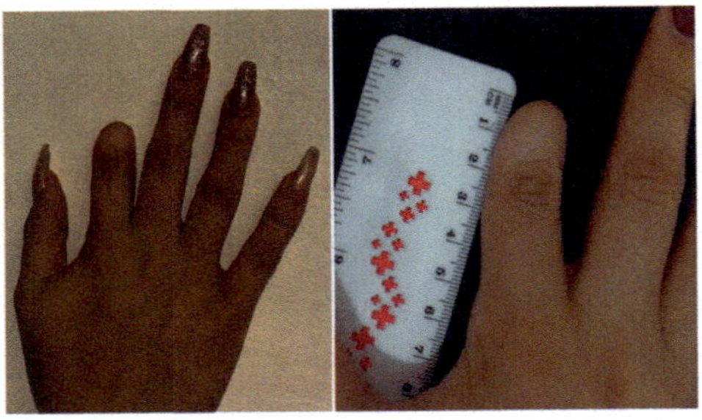

and performance requirements have not been fully verified, for example by a clinical evaluation. In the context of chapter 3, the individual prosthesis is a customised product according to the MDR, which is not subject to CE marking and the declaration of conformity of a *notified body.*

In the patient's childhood, the upper part of the index finger of the right hand just above its lower segment was amputated (see **Figure 7**). The stump has a length of approx. 5 cm. An individual digital model is to be created on the basis of the index finger of the left hand, which is to be manufactured additively with an overlap for attaching to the finger stump and for stabilization.

The patient's requirements for the prosthesis are essentially visual and functional. The dimensions should roughly correspond to those of the index finger of the left hand and fit into the overall appearance. The shape and colour should be based on the real limb for optical and psychological reasons. In addition, a high degree of comfort, a low or realistic weight, and a certain degree of flexibility are required. Resistance to various substances such as sweat, cleaning agents and disinfectants is also important.

## 4.1 Digital generation of the prosthesis

In order to be able to manufacture the prosthesis additively, a digital model must first be available. The model is essentially to be created by a 3D scan with following editing or modelling. However, since the patient was not physically available during the project, this method could not be applied directly to the "complete" index finger of the other hand. For this reason, it was decided to use wax casts of both hands that could be easily created (see Figure 8-left). The decisive factor was not the coarse outer geometry, but the more precise inner geometry, which was used to cast a model of the "complete" index finger from silicone latex or impression silicone. (see Figure 8 -right).

*Figure 8: Left: Wax pattern of hands (Orange colored model with amputation of index finger), Right: Silicone model of left index finger*

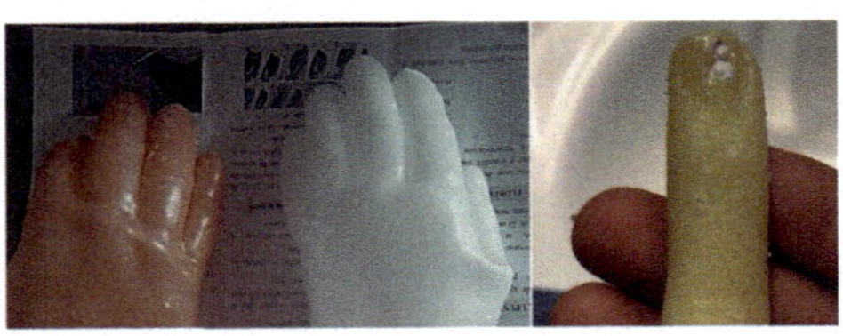

The silicone model of the "complete" index finger was digitised using 3D scanning. The data obtained was further processed in the scanning software (see Figure 9. -left), and the 3D model was exported in the STL data format commonly used for additive manufacturing (see Figure 9. -right).

*Figure 9: Scan file (left) and unprocessed STL file (right) of the finger prosthesis*

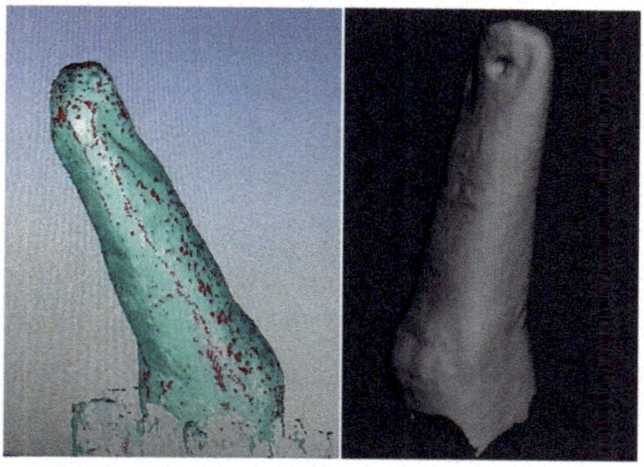

Subsequently, the data was further processed in modelling software. In this way, unevenness, as seen for example in the fingernail area, was removed and the correct length of the prosthesis of 5 cm could be set by removing the lower part. Furthermore, the rough surface resulting from the rough surface of the silicone model was smoothed. Details of the finger, such as the fingernail and the folds of the finger joints, were also created, and the tilt of the finger was adjusted. For placing the prosthesis on the finger stump, the lower part must be hollow for at least 2.5 cm so that the overall length of the finger fits and the hold on the stump is given. The modelling software was also used to create different variants of the finger prosthesis (see Figure 10). Both straight and curved versions, as well as completely hollow and shallow finger prostheses only in the lower region, have been produced. The hollowing and the variation of the wall thickness change the weight and the balance point as well as the stiffness. In addition, the wall thickness was varied between 0.6 mm, 1 mm and 1.3 mm. The different versions allow the patient to test the fit as well as the function.

*Figure 10: Final 3D model of the finger prosthesis in different variants (left: straight, right: curved)*

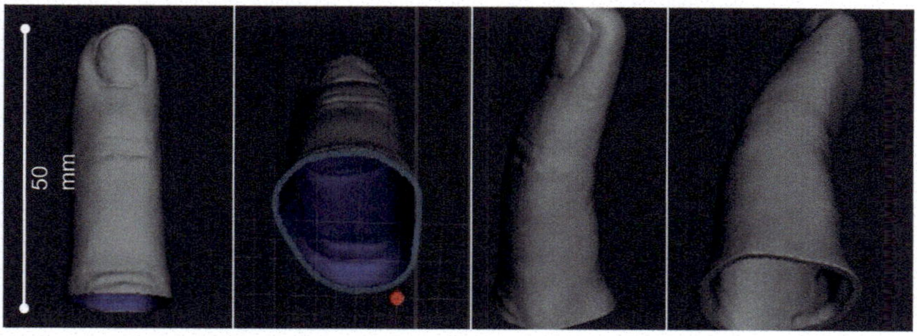

## 4.2 Manufacturing of the prosthesis

The finger prosthesis was manufactured using the additive manufacturing technology of laser sintering, a powder bed process that works with thermoplastics. A thin layer of powder is applied in a heated environment before a laser melts the required geometric information into this layer. In this way, the components are built up layer by layer.

For manufacturing the finger prosthesis, two materials were considered: polyamide 12 and thermoplastic polyurethane (TPU). Both materials are generally easy to process and can be subsequently smoothed and coloured.

Polyamide 12 has good chemical resistance, is biocompatible according to EN ISO 10993-1 and is certified for food contact (see database from EOS[4]). However, polyamide 12 is stiff and not very flexible. Both wearing comfort and function can be affected by this, which was subsequently verified by manufacturing and functional testing.

As a result, TPU with a shore hardness of 88A was used. The material is characterised by high flexibility, resistance to hydrolysis and various chemicals, and is UV stable. In addition, the TPU passes in skin contact the cytotoxicity test according to ISO 10993-5, the in-vitro skin irritation test according to OECD Guideline No. 439 and the in-vivo sensitization test according to ISO 10993-10 and OECD Guideline No. 429 (Material data sheet Ultrasint TPU 88A). The TPU finger prostheses manufactured and after-treated with glass bead blasting as standard are shown in two different variants in Figure 12 (condition: "as built"). In an initial assessment, the material exhibits a high level of wearer comfort due to its flexibility and good haptics ("soft" surface) and thus appears to be suitable for the intended use. In order to increase the surface quality of the rough surface resulting from the production process and thus further improve the wearing comfort and appearance, the prostheses were then chemically smoothed by solvent vaporising the surface (see Figure 12- 2nd from left). To make sure that the finger prosthesis fully meets the optical requirements, the prosthesis was then dyed in different skin colours (see Figure 12) In this way, the optimum colour can be selected directly by the patient.

*Figure 11: Finger prosthesis (curved and non-curved model) made of TPU*

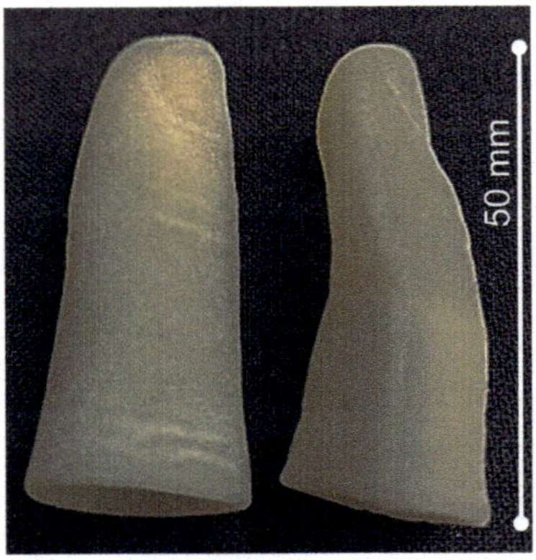


4 https://eos.materialdatacenter.com/eo/

*Figure 12: Finger prosthesis made of TPU (uncurved and hollow) in different stages of production: from left: 1. "as built", 2. chemically smoothed, 3.-6. chemically smoothed and dyed*

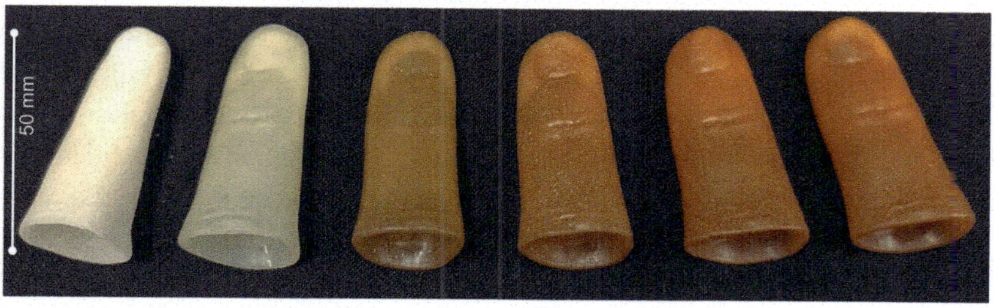


## 4.3 Conclusion regarding the additively manufactured finger prosthesis

From the manufacturing perspective, the laser sintering technology can be used to produce detailed, precise models which, with additional smoothing and colouring, can also meet the optical requirements and fit into the overall appearance of the hand. The flexibility of the TPU material also ensures the function. An initial haptic evaluation also confirms the requirements for wearing comfort.

Figure 13 shows the finger prosthesis being tested on the patient. It can be seen that the length and shape are appropriate for the patient. However, the shades provided do not match the overall appearance of the hand. The fit of the prosthesis is also not yet optimally adjusted. The opening at the contact area is slightly too small. All in all, the patient is nevertheless very satisfied with the first result. By making small adjustments, it is possible to create a very satisfactory finger prosthesis for the patient that fits into the overall appearance.

*Figure 13: One of the final versions of the finger prosthesis on the patient*

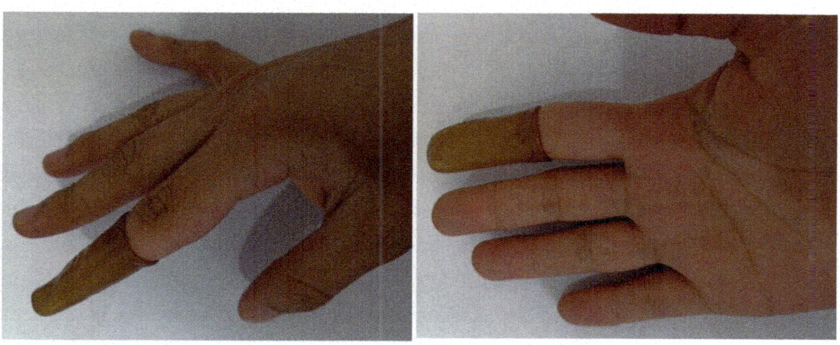

Looking ahead, the function of the prosthesis could be further developed so that it would be possible to bend the finger. The connection point between the prosthesis and the finger stump could also be adapted if necessary. To implement this, the interdisciplinary exchange with an orthopaedic surgeon or an orthopaedic technician could be advanced. The orthopaedic technician could support the engineer in the development of the design because generally there are not many limitations to the design from the perspective of the process and the software. In addition, in this case, the geographical closeness of the patient would have been useful for the final realisation, since no exact geometry data such as CT data was available. Even though it has been shown in principle that development is possible over a distance, the more intensive the transdisciplinary exchange between the interdisciplinary team and the patient, the faster the development can take place. In the best case, the patient is actively involved in the development. With the appropriate experience and training, the development process could be carried out in a few days, keeping the costs within acceptable limits.

## 5 Conclusion and challenges

This article highlights the possibilities of interdisciplinary collaboration in the additive manufacturing of medical devices and aids that are to be individualised, and has focused in particular on answering the following three central questions:

1. What does interdisciplinary collaboration mean for medical professionals and technicians or engineers?
2. Which challenges are currently still limiting the meaningful benefits of additive manufacturing for the use of medical devices in society?
3. What challenges are currently still limiting the benefits of additive manufacturing for the development of medical devices?

Medical technology generally means that there is interdisciplinary interaction between the disciplines of medicine and engineering and natural sciences. To achieve this, a common level of communication must first be created. For example, medical professionals such as doctors must familiarise themselves with the processes and properties of additive manufacturing, and engineers must familiarise themselves with the terminology and medical requirements as well as the approval of medical devices in order to work together efficiently and achieve a common goal in the best possible way. However, interdisciplinary cooperation also harbours dangers and potential for conflict in various aspects such as communication, object description, group dynamics, prejudices and methodology, so that team performance and project goals can lag behind expectations. However, such conflicts can be reduced through targeted intervention efforts (Brandstädter, 2019).

The accessibility of the technology to society, i.e. in this context to patients, has been demonstrated in this article by means of some examples from the medical fields of surgery, orthopaedics and dental technology as well as from the indirect medical field of daily living aids for people with disabilities. The geometric freedom of additive manufacturing, coupled with the unit-quantity-independent costs, makes it possible in the above-mentioned areas, but also beyond them, to manufacture individualised aids and medical products tailored to the disorders or disabilities of the respective individual in an advantageous and time-efficient manner (i.e. at short term and in some cases with shorter production times). For the optimisation and individualisation of the necessarily generated 3D data sets, it is also possible to draw on a large number of motion and stress studies, experience and literature. These enable the medical device and aid to be adapted to the individual in a way that is both precise and appropriate to the load. Thus, from a technological point of view, there is nothing to prevent the use of additive manufacturing. The use of additively manufactured individual medical devices must be initiated or prescribed by an authorized medical professional. In the case of everyday aids, the patient must initiate the process himself or herself or, for example, the care facilities must be sensitised to this. Especially in the case of the older section of society, stimulating and supportive intervention is required.

According to the MDR, individualised, additively manufactured medical devices are considered as customised products and, with the exception of individualised implants, are not subject to CE marking and conformity assessment as long as they comply with the safety and performance requirements. However, these products must have been ordered by an authorised medical professional in order to have a chance of being covered by the health insurance company.

For medical technology companies that manufacture not only individualised products but also mass-customised products and series products using additive manufacturing, in particular the certification situation, can be a challenge. To date, there is no guideline or standard for the additive manufacturing of medical products. A good orientation and basis for companies is provided by certification according to the standards DIN EN ISO/ ASTM 52920 (Additive manufacturing – Qualification principles – Requirements for industrial additive manufacturing processes and production sites) and DIN EN ISO 13485 (Medical devices – Quality management systems – Requirements for regulatory purposes). Challenges that could be collected in a standard for additive manufacturing of medical devices include materials, biocompatibility, reproducibility of properties and post-processing of additively manufactured components. In order to enter and implement additive manufacturing of medical devices, it makes sense for companies to join established networks in this field such as *Medical goes Additive*.

## References


Abke, J. (2003). *Verbesserung der Biokompatibilität metallischer Implantate durch kovalente Anbindung einer quervernetzten Kollagenschicht. Dissertation, Universität Regensburg.* https://doi.org/10.5283/epub.10102

Aboelela, S. W., Larson, E., Bakken, S., Carrasquillo, O., Formicola, A., Glied, S. A., Haas, J., & Gebbie, K. M. (2007). Defining interdisciplinary research: Conclusions from a critical review of the literature. *Health Services Research*, Vol. 42, Issue 1p1, 329–346. https://doi.org/10.1111/j.1475-6773.2006.00621.x

Azuma, M., Yanagawa, T., Ishibashi-Kanno, N., Uchida, F., Ito, T., Yamagata, K., Hasegawa, S., Sasaki, K., Adachi, K., Tabuchi, K., Sekido, M., & Bukawa, H. (2014). Mandibular reconstruction using plates prebent to fit rapid prototyping 3-dimensional printing models ameliorates contour deformity. *Head & Face Medicine*, Vol. 10, 45. https://doi.org/10.1186/1746-160X-10-45

Baldauf, M. (2016). *Biokeramische Werkstoffe.* https://docplayer.org/29426845-Biokeramische-werkstoffe.html

Beck, U. (1986). *Risikogesellschaft: Auf dem Weg in eine andere Moderne.* Suhrkamp. ISBN: 978-3-518-11365-3

Becker, J. (2021). Hilfsmittel. In *Gabler Wirtschaftslexikon.* https://wirtschaftslexikon.gabler.de/definition/hilfsmittel-35626/version-382709

Blecker, T., & Friedrich, G. (2006). *Mass Customization: Challenges and Solutions.* Springer New York. https://doi.org/10.1007/0-387-32224-8

BMWi (2015). *Industrie 4.0 und Digitale Wirtschaft. Impulse für Wachstum, Beschäftigung und Innovation.* Booklet.

Bogataj, M., Kosel, F., Norris, R., Krkovic, M., & Brojan, M. (2015). Biomechanical study of different plate configurations for distal humerus osteosynthesis. *Medical & Biological Engineering & Computing*, Vol. 53, Issue 5, 381–392. https://doi.org/10.1007/s11517-015-1247-1

Brandstädter, S. (2019). *Interdisziplinär erfolgreich – Modellierung, Validierung und Förderung interdisziplinärer Handlungskompetenz.* Dissertation, Universität Heidelberg. https://doi.org/10.11588/heidok.00029256

Gemeinsamer Bundesausschuss (2022). Richtlinie über die Verordnung von Hilfsmitteln in der vertragsärztlichen Versorgung (HilfsM-RL).

Bundesministerium für Gesundheit (2022a). *Hilfsmittel.* https://www.bundesgesundheitsministerium.de/hilfsmittel.html

Bundesministerium für Gesundheit (2022b). *Marktzugangsvoraussetzungen.* https://www.bundesgesundheitsministerium.de/themen/gesundheitswesen/medizinprodukte/marktzugangsvoraussetzungen.html

Butler, M. C. (1998). An integrating perspective on interdisciplinary, cross-cultural research. *Journal of Managerial Psychology*, Vol. 13, Issue 3-4, 199–205. https://doi.org/10.1108/02683949810215002

Choi, B. C. K., & Pak, A. W. P. (2007). Multidisciplinarity, interdisciplinarity, and transdisciplinarity in health research, services, education and policy: 2. Promotors, barriers, and strategies of enhancement. *Clinical and Investigative Medicine*, Vol. 30, Issue 6, E224-32. https://doi.org/10.25011/cim.v30i6.2950

Cohen, A., Laviv, A., Berman, P., Nashef, R., & Abu-Tair, J. (2009). Mandibular reconstruction using stereolithographic 3-dimensional printing modeling technology. *Oral Surgery, Oral Medi-cine, Oral Pathology, Oral Radiology, and Endodontics*, Vol. 108, Issue 5, 661–666. https://doi.org/10.1016/j.tripleo.2009.05.023

De Gruyter (1953). Allgemeine Anatomie. In A. Waldeyer & A. Mayet (Eds.), *Allgemeine Anatomie, Rücken, Bauch, Becken, Bein* (pp. 1–90). De Gruyter. https://doi.org/10.1515/9783111586687.1

Defila, R., DiGiulio, A., & Drilling, M. (2000). *Leitfaden allgemeine Wissenschaftspropädeutik für interdisziplinär-ökologische Studiengänge.* Allgemeine Ökologie zur Diskussion gestellt: Nr. 4. Interfakultäre Koordinationsstelle für Allgemeine Ökologie Univ. Bern.

Deutscher Dialogmarketing Verband (Ed.) (2019). *Dialogmarketing Perspektiven 2018/2019.* Tagungsband 13. wissenschaftlicher interdisziplinärer Kongress für Dialogmarketing. Springer Gabler Wiesbaden. https://doi.org/10.1007/978-3-658-25583-1

Frank, E., & Zitter, H. (1971). *Metallische Implantate in der Knochenchirurgie. Werkstoff · Verarbeitung, Operationseinsatz.* Springer Vienna. https://doi.org/10.1007/978-3-7091-8261-1

D'Urso, P. S., Barker, T. M., Earwaker, W. J., Bruce, L. J., Atkinson, R. L., Lanigan, M. W., Arvier, J. F., & Effeney, D. J. (1999). Stereolithographic biomodelling in cranio-maxillofacial surgery: a prospective trial. *Journal of Cranio-Maxillofacial Surgery*, Vol. 27, Issue 1, 30–37. https://doi.org/10.1016/S1010-5182(99)80007-9

Ehrenberg-Silies, S., Kind, S., Jetzke, T., & Bovenschulte, M. (2015). *Additive-Fertigungsverfahren / 3D-druck: Anwendungen und Potentiale.* Horizon Scanning. https://vdivde-it.de/sites/default/files/document/additive-fertigungsverfahren-3d-druck-2017.pdf

Engel, M., Hoffmann, J., Castrillon-Oberndorfer, G., & Freudlsperger, C. (2015). The value of three-dimensional printing modelling for surgical correction of orbital hypertelorism. *Oral and Maxillofacial Surgery*, Vol. 19, Issue 1, 91–95. https://doi.org/10.1007/s10006-014-0466-1

Epple, M. (2003). *Biomaterialien und Biomineralisation.* Vieweg+Teubner Publisher. https://doi.org/10.1007/978-3-322-80035-0

Ewinger, D., Ternès, A., Koerbel, J., & Towers, I. (2016). *Arbeitswelt im Zeitalter der Individualisierung.* Springer Fachmedien Wiesbaden. https://doi.org/10.1007/978-3-658-12753-4

Garland, D. R., O'Connor, M. K., Wolfer, T. A., & Netting, F. E. (2006). Team-based Research: Notes from the Field. *Qualitative Social Work*, Vol. 5, Issue 1, 93–109. https://doi.org/10.1177/1473325006061540

Gebhardt, A., & Schwarz, A. (2019). Additive Fertigung. In A. Gebhardt & A. Schwarz (Eds.), *Produktgestaltung für die Additive Fertigung (pp. 45–83)*. Carl Hanser Verlag. https://doi.org/10.3139/9783446461338.002

GKV Spitzenverband (2022). *Hilfsmittelverzeichnis*. https://www.gkv-spitzenverband.de/krankenversicherung/hilfsmittel/hilfsmittelverzeichnis/hilfsmittelverzeichnis.jsp

Grund, M. (2015). *Implementierung von schichtadditiven Fertigungsverfahren*. Springer Berlin Heidelberg. https://doi.org/10.1007/978-3-662-44266-1

Guarino, J., Tennyson, S., McCain, G., Bond, L., Shea, K., & King, H. (2007). Rapid prototyping technology for surgeries of the pediatric spine and pelvis: Benefits analysis. *Journal of Pediatric Orthopedics*, Vol. 27, Issue 8, 955–960. https://doi.org/10.1097/bpo.0b013e3181594ced

Haleem, A., & Javaid, M. (2020). 3D printed medical parts with different materials using additive manufacturing. *Clinical Epidemiology and Global Health*, Vol. 8, Issue 1, 215–223. https://doi.org/10.1016/j.cegh.2019.08.002

Hanawa, T. (2021). Metals and Medicine. *Materials Transactions*, Vol. 62, Issue 2, 139–148. https://doi.org/10.2320/matertrans.MT-M2020268

Heina, J. (1999). *Variantenmanagement: Kosten-Nutzen-Bewertung zur Optimierung der Variantenvielfalt*. Deutscher Universitätsverlag Wiesbaden. https://doi.org/10.1007/978-3-663-09093-9

Hermeneit, A., Steffen, A., & Stockhardt, J. (Eds.) (2010). *Medizinprodukte planen, entwickeln, realisieren – Der CE-Routenplaner*. TÜV Media GmbH. ISBN: 978-3-8249-1376-3

Huotilainen, E., Paloheimo, M., Salmi, M., Paloheimo, K.-S., Björkstrand, R., Tuomi, J., Markkola, A., & Mäkitie, A. (2014). Imaging requirements for medical applications of additive manufacturing. *Acta Radiologica*, Vol. 55, Issue 1, 78–85. https://doi.org/10.1177/0284185113494198

Ihle, J. (2007). *Ärztliche Leitlinien, Standards und Sozialrecht*. Dissertation, Universität Bremen. Nomos-Publisher. ISBN: 978-3-8329-2486-7

Javaid, M., & Haleem, A. (2019). Current status and applications of additive manufacturing in dentistry: A literature-based review. *Journal of Oral Biology and Craniofacial Research*, Vol. 9, Issue 3, 179–185. https://doi.org/10.1016/j.jobcr.2019.04.004

Jehn, K. A. (1995). A Multimethod Examination of the Benefits and Detriments of Intragroup Conflict. *Administrative Science Quarterly*, Vol. 40, Issue 2, 256-282. https://doi.org/10.2307/2393638

Jehn, K. A., Northcraft, G. B., & Neale, M. A. (1999). Why Differences Make a Difference: A Field Study of Diversity, Conflict and Performance in Workgroups. *Administrative Science Quarterly,* Vol. 44, Issue 4, 741–763. https://doi.org/10.2307/2667054

Thompson, J. (2022). *3D-Druck in der Medizintechnik: Neue Herausforderungen beim Datenschutz.* https://www.devicemed.de/3d-druck-in-der-medizintechnik-neue-herausforderungen-beim-datenschutz-a-999004/

Jin, Y., Plott, J., Chen, R., Wensman, J., & Shih, A. (2015). Additive Manufacturing of Custom Orthoses and Prostheses – A Review. *Procedia CIRP,* Vol. 36, 199–204. https://doi.org/10.1016/j.procir.2015.02.125

Johner, C. (2019). *3D-Druck in der Medizin: Anregungen bekommen, Fallen vermeiden.* Johner Institut. https://www.johner-institut.de/blog/regulatory-affairs/3d-druck-medizin/

Koren, Y. (2010). *The Global Manufacturing Revolution: Product-Process-Business Integration and Reconfigurable Systems.* John Wiley & Sons. https://doi.org/10.1002/9780470618813

Kruse, A., & Mummert, M. (2019). Mit 3D-Druck umfassende Teilhabe möglich machen. *Werkstatt:Dialog,* Vol. 4.2019. BAG WfbM (Bundesarbeitsgemeinschaft Werkstätten für behinderte Menschen e.v.). https://www.bagwfbm.de/wdg

Kumar, R., Kumar, M., & Chohan, J. S. (2021). The role of additive manufacturing for biomedical applications: A critical review. *Journal of Manufacturing Processes,* Vol. 64, 828–850. https://doi.org/10.1016/j.jmapro.2021.02.022

Kumke, M. (2018). *Methodisches Konstruieren von additiv gefertigten Bauteilen.* Springer Fachmedien Wiesbaden. https://doi.org/10.1007/978-3-658-22209-3

Lachmayer, R., & Lippert, R. B. (Eds.) (2017). *Additive Manufacturing Quantifiziert.* Springer Berlin Heidelberg. https://doi.org/10.1007/978-3-662-54113-5

Lim, C. G. T., Campbell, D. I., & Clucas, D. M. (2014). Rapid prototyping technology in orbital floor reconstruction: Application in three patients. *Craniomaxillofacial Trauma & Reconstruction,* Vol. 7, Issue 2, 143–146. https://doi.org/10.1055/s-0034-1371080

Liu, Y., Xu, L., Zhu, H., & Liu, S. S.-Y. (2014). Technical procedures for template-guided surgery for mandibular reconstruction based on digital design and manufacturing. *BioMedical Engineering OnLine,* Vol. 13, 63. https://doi.org/10.1186/1475-925X-13-63

Lüttmann, C. (2020). *Medizinischer 3D-Druck, sicher gemäß CE-Kennzeichnung.* https://www.devicemed.de/medizinischer-3d-druck-sicher-gemaess-ce-kennzeichnung-a-978791/

Mattmüller, R. (2012). *Integrativ-Prozessuales Marketing.* Springer Fachmedien Wiesbaden. https://doi.org/10.1007/978-3-8349-4470-2

Mello, A. L., & Rentsch, J. R. (2015). Cognitive Diversity in Teams: A Multidisciplinary Review. *Small Group Research,* Vol. 46, Issue 6, 623–658. https://doi.org/10.1177/1046496415602558

Oppermann, B., Hoyer, J., & Reischle, G. (2020). *Standards für das Regulatorische beim 3D-Druck in der Medizin sind schon in Arbeit.* Konradin-Verlag Robert Kohlhammer GmbH. https://medizin-und-technik.industrie.de/3d-druck/standards-fuer-3d-druck-in-der-medizin-sind-schon-in-arbeit/

Paul, J. (2007). *Einführung in die allgemeine Betriebswirtschaftslehre: Mit Beispielen und Fallstudien.* Gabler Verlag Wiesbaden. https://doi.org/10.1007/978-3-8349-9281-9

Pillar, F. T. (2006). *Mass Customization: Ein wettbewerbsstrategisches Konzept im Informationszeitalter.* Deutscher Universitätsverlag Wiesbaden. https://doi.org/10.1007/978-3-8350-9204-4

Revilla-León, M., & Özcan, M. (2019). Additive Manufacturing Technologies Used for Processing Polymers: Current Status and Potential Application in Prosthetic Dentistry. *Journal of Prosthodontics,* Vol. 28, Issue 2, 146–158. https://doi.org/10.1111/jopr.12801

Richard, H. A., Schramm, B., & Zipsner, T. (2017). *Additive Fertigung von Bauteilen und Strukturen.* Springer Fachmedien Wiesbaden. https://doi.org/10.1007/978-3-658-17780-5

Richard, H. A., Schramm, B., & Zipsner, T. (2019). *Additive Fertigung von Bauteilen und Strukturen: Neue Erkenntnisse und Praxisbeispiele.* Springer Fachmedien Wiesbaden. https://doi.org/10.1007/978-3-658-27412-2

Risse, L. (2020). *Präoperative Studien zur Gestaltung von patientenspezifischen, medizinischen Hilfsmitteln.* Dissertation, Paderborn University. ISBN: 978-3-8440-7745-2

Rozen, W. M., Ting, J. W. C., Baillieu, C., & Leong, J. (2012). Stereolithographic modeling of the deep circumflex iliac artery and its vascular branching: A further advance in computed tomography-guided flap planning. *Plastic and Reconstructive Surgery,* Vol. 130, Issue 2, 380e-382e. https://doi.org/10.1097/PRS.0b013e31825903d1

Schäfer, K. (2018). *Was sind Medizinprodukte? Definition, Medizinproduktegesetz, Zulassung.* https://www.devicemed.de/was-sind-medizinprodukte-definition-medizinproduktegesetz-zulassung-a-726920/

Schmidt, U., Penzkofer, R., Bachmaier, S., & Augat, P. (2013). Implant material and design alter construct stiffness in distal femur locking plate fixation: A pilot study. *Clinical Orthopaedics and Related Research,* Vol. 471, Issue 9, 2808–2814. https://doi.org/10.1007/s11999-013-2867-0

Schulin, B. (Ed.). (1994). Handbuch des Sozialversicherungsrechts. Bd. 1: krankenversicherungsrecht. Publisher C. H. Beck. *Zeitschrift für Arbeitsrecht und Sozialrecht,* Vol. 30, Issue 6. https://www.degruyter.com/database/IBR/entry/ibr.ID923996831/html

Schurawitzki, W. (1995). *Praxis des Internationalen Marketing: Grundlagen und Fallbeispiele.* Gabler Verlag Wiesbaden. https://doi.org/10.1007/978-3-663-05843-4

Stelzer, R. H., & Krzyzwinski, J. (Eds.). (2019). *Entwerfen, entwickeln, erleben in Produktentwicklung und Design 2019*. TUDpress. ISBN: 978-3-95908-170-2

Stember, J. (2020). *Innovative Wirtschaftsförderungen in Deutschland*. Springer Gabler Wiesbaden. https://doi.org/10.1007/978-3-658-28483-1

Ternès, A., Towers, I., & Jerusel, M. (2015). Konsumentenverhalten im Zeitalter der Mass Customization. Springer Gabler Wiesbaden. https://doi.org/10.1007/978-3-658-09846-9

Tsai, M.-J., & Wu, C.-T. (2014). Study of mandible reconstruction using a fibula flap with application of additive manufacturing technology. *Biomedical Engineering Online*, Vol. 13, 57. https://doi.org/10.1186/1475-925X-13-57

TÜV SÜD (2021). *Validating additive manufacturing processes to meet medical regulations: Ensure safe and reproducible manufacturing results*. TÜV SÜD. https://www.tuvsud.com/en/resource-centre/white-papers/additive-manufacturing-validating-processes-to-meet-medical-regulations

Ullrich, S. (2011). *Internetbasierte Internationalisierung: Entscheidungsfindung, Umsetzung und Erfolgsmessung*. Gabler Verlag Wiesbaden. https://doi.org/10.1007/978-3-8349-6177-8

Wabnitz, T. (2009). *Medizinprodukte als Hilfsmittel in der gesetzlichen Krankenversicherung*. Springer Berlin Heidelberg. ISBN: 978-3-540-88549-8

Wagner, R., & Knittel, S. (Eds.). (2022). *Soziale Krankenversicherung, Pflegeversicherung: Kommentar*. C.H. Beck. ISBN 978-3-406-45832-3

Watson, R. A. (2014). A low-cost surgical application of additive fabrication. *Journal of Surgical Education*, Vol. 71, Issue 1, 14–17. https://doi.org/10.1016/j.jsurg.2013.10.012

Weigel, B. & Nerlich, M. L. (Ed.). (2011). Praxisbuch Unfallchirurgie: Mit 161 Tabellen (2., vollst. überarb. und aktualisierte Aufl.). Springer.

Wettlaufer, L. (2021). *Medizinprodukte als Hilfsmittel: Eine zusätzliche Einnahmequelle?* Johner Institut. https://www.johner-institut.de/blog/gesundheitswesen/hilfsmittel/

Wintermantel, E., & Ha, S.-W. (2009). *Medizintechnik*. Springer Berlin Heidelberg. https://doi.org/10.1007/978-3-540-93936-8

Witschey, W. R. T., Pouch, A. M., McGarvey, J. R., Ikeuchi, K., Contijoch, F., Levack, M. M., Yushkevick, P. A., Sehgal, C. M., Jackson, B. M., Gorman, R. C., & Gorman, J. H. (2014). Three-dimensional ultrasound-derived physical mitral valve modeling. *The Annals of Thoracic Surgery*, Vol. 98, Issue 2, 691–694. https://doi.org/10.1016/j.athoracsur.2014.04.094

Zentralstelle der Länder für Gesundheitsschutz. (25.01.22). Zentralstelle der Länder für Gesundheitsschutz bei Arzneimitteln und Medizinprodukten. https://www.zlg.de/medizinprodukte/dokumente/stellenlaboratorien/benannte-stellen-eu-2017745-mdr

## Standards:

| | |
|---|---|
| DIN SPEC 17071 | Additive manufacturing – Requirements for quality-assured processes at additive manufacturing centers |
| DIN EN ISO/ASTM 52920 | Additive manufacturing – Qualification principles – Requirements for industrial additive manufacturing processes and production sites |
| DIN EN ISO 14971 | Medical devices – Application of risk management to medical devices |
| DIN EN ISO 13485 | Medical devices – Quality management systems – Requirements for regulatory purposes |
| DIN EN ISO 10993-17 | Biological evaluation of medical devices – Part 17: Establishment of allowable limits for leachable substances |
| DIN EN ISO 10993-1 | Biological evaluation of medical devices – Part 1: Evaluation and testing within a risk management process |
| DIN EN ISO 10993-5 | Biological evaluation of medical devices – Part 5: Tests for in vitro cytotoxicity |
| DIN EN ISO 10993-10 | Biological evaluation of medical devices – Part 10: Tests for irritation and skin sensitization |
| DIN EN 556-1 | Sterilization of medical devices – Requirements for medical devices to be designated "STERILE" – Part 1: Requirements for terminally sterilized medical devices |
| OECD Guideline No. 439 | In Vitro Skin Irritation: Reconstructed Human Epidermis Test Method, 2021 |
| OECD Guideline No. 429 | Skin Sensitisation: Local Lymph Node Assay, 2010 |

# Conclusion

*Ilona Horwath, Swetlana Schweizer, Thomas Tröster*

> "Our inventions change the world, and the reinvented world changes us"
> *(Jasanoff 2016:1).*

In this last chapter, we reflect on the impact of our work, i.e. our results, their societal value and effectiveness. Our reflection is guided by Lam et al.'s (2021) consideration of four aspects central to the knowledge generation processes in transdisciplinary research and hence to the question of its impact. These areas, context dependencies, scientific effects, societal effects, and innovative formats and methods, form the categories along which we have structured this conclusion.

As we have not conducted a full evaluation of FK LEM activities, what we provide here are the results of the evaluation of the Re-Use and Recycling cluster undertaken with our project partner Hebie GmbH & Co.KG, as well as FK LEM team reflection on framework conditions and the impact of our work. Thereby, we draw some general conclusions from our scientific practices and transdisciplinary experience.

Generally, the societal impact of transdisciplinary research includes short and long term effects, and is hard to measure. As Lux at al. (2019:185) point out, the major framework conditions are crucial for the chances to achieve meaningful societal impact, i.e. the historicity of the addressed problem, the heterogeneity of actors, the general environment, and the funding conditions. Hence, the framework conditions in which transdisciplinary research processes are embedded are of high relevance in fostering or hindering its societal effectiveness (ibid). The framework for transdisciplinary research at the FK LEM outlined in the Introduction illustrates our design to foster societal embeddedness, particularly in regional and organizational contexts, and with regard to building up capacities for further scientific cooperation.

We will first present the evaluation of the Re-Use & Recycling Cluster in the style of an interview with our project partner, followed by our reflection along the dimensions of context dependencies, scientific effects, societal effects, and innovative formats and methods.

## Evaluation of the transdisciplinary research collaboration with Hebie GmbH & Co. KG

1. **What was your motivation to participate in the cooperation?** With over 150 years of history, Hebie is a family-owned company with a long tradition. We set ourselves high sustainability goals and face the challenging task of reconciling these goals and the associated measures with the company's core competencies and economic aspirations. Hebie sees sustainable and socially responsible action as the prerequisite for long-term success. The reduction of resource consumption can be excellently combined with economic endeavours by using renewable or recycled materials. Therefore, the goal of manufacturing one of our products from a combination of sustainable and recycled material was obvious. In addition, we believe it is important to support research with the aim of preserving finite resources.
2. **What goals did you want to achieve with the project or cooperation?** The goals of the cooperation were to expand our knowledge of the specific application of materials, but also the "further education" with regard to the scientific examination of a question about the selection and application of new types of materials. As a medium-sized industrial company, we usually lack the personnel and time resources to discuss the requirements with regard to an alternative use of materials. The cooperation with the Paderborn University was an ideal solution for us, especially since the FK LEM researchers could certainly benefit from the company's experience and handling of the task.
3. **What are the most important results of the project from your point of view?** It is important for us to have gone through the process once, in order to be able to approach such a problem better and in a more planned way in the future and to become more confident in dealing with the cooperation partners. Another insight is that completely different materials can be an alternative to conventional materials.
4. **Were all goals achieved? If not, which objectives could not be achieved and what do you think was the reason for this?** The fact that not all goals could be achieved is not due to the cooperation, but rather results from a sales perspective. The alternative material as well as the specific restrictions regarding surface, colouring etc. have so far prevented the use of the tested material.
5. **How did the cooperation process work for you?** The cooperation with the FK LEM researcher was excellent and quite well organised. In future projects, it could certainly be possible to optimise the company-side contribution.

5.1 **How did the communication process work for you? Were there any particular challenges?** Special challenges arise from the novelty of the process, as usually the development or the design determines the material that fulfils the product-related requirements in the best possible way. The fact that the product must be adapted to a given material is a new approach for us and must first be established.

5.2 **What learning effects could you gain from the cooperation?** Good internal preparation as well as the early and intensive involvement of affected departments, especially development/design and production, are absolutely relevant for results.

6. **Did you already implement or use the results from the cooperation?** See question 4.

7. **In your view, to what extent is the result ecologically, economically and socially sustainable?** The bicycle is established as an essential part of daily mobility and has become an elementary component of the changing modal split. Especially in urban mobility and logistics, under the keyword "last mile", the bicycle is becoming increasingly important as an ecological, clean and modern means of transport. Since we manufacture products for this environmentally sustainable means of transport, which is accessible to everyone, it is both an obligation and a challenge for us, especially in this context, to combine ecology, social obligation and economy. In addition to the durability of the products, the conservation of resources is an essential sustainability criterion for us.

8. **Were the values and mission statement of your company sufficiently taken into account in the cooperation and in the result?** Hebie pursues a sustainability strategy that is fundamentally integrated into the corporate guidelines, but whose contents are also explicitly laid down in the form of a CSR (Corporate Social Responsibility) target catalogue. Our mission statement defines our standards in terms of reliability, down-to-earth-ness, and pronounced employee orientation. We live a cooperative approach among colleagues and with our business partners. We act responsibly and emphasise long-term, moderate management, high quality standards with regard to administration, as well as comprehensive transparency with regard to economic activity. These requirements were also implemented in the cooperation.

9. **Do they see the results as having added value for society?** From an ecological point of view, added value has certainly been achieved for society, but quite fundamentally, cooperation between companies and universities is also sensible from a social and economic point of view and beneficial for society as a whole.

10. **(What) added value do you think such research collaborations have for society?** The bundling of opportunities and resources and the combination of real economy and research lead to synergy effects that can enormously expand the range of services of all partners, often with only little additional effort.

## Framework conditions and reflection of the research team

**a) Context dependencies**

Context dependencies refer to factors which influence the research design as well as the interpretation of results. In transdisciplinary research, certain context dependencies can be expected (Lam et al. 2021:244). A common problem definition, for instance, entails that research objects are highly dependent on the particular context to which they relate. Thus, the transferability and generalizability of (some) results may be limited (Lam et al. 2021: 245), as in the case of studies II and III. On the other hand, both projects resulted in collaborations characterized by a continuous and substantial mutual learning process including the exchange of data, expertise, and perspectives. Both research partners—Weber Hydraulik GmbH and Hebie GmbH & Co. KG—also act as multipliers in their respective fields. It is likely that the results will be transferred into the design of new products, which was not possible within the time frame of FK LEM.

A second expectable challenge is the diversity of knowledge bases, experience and perspectives that need to be integrated during the research process (Bergmann et al. 2012, see also Introduction). Importantly, an integration of different perspectives provides the opportunity to not only foster mutual understanding for practical requirements, thought styles, functional logics and limitations in the participating societal and scientific fields. Often, such differences also point towards the gaps between theory and practice, or between competing theories that are not necessarily compatible in the first place. An iterative integration makes it possible to synchronize the goals, means, and values of participants, and to address gaps and apparent incompatibilities as focal points for linking theory and practice, science and society. Moreover, such focal points help us to discuss and advance disciplinary concepts of "objectivity" (Harding 2015), adding layers of situated knowledge and social context to the constitution of positions and perception. Importantly, all people participating in our projects are treated as "experts" for their particular domains. This conceptualization aims to oppose a reduction of the role of "lay people" in scientific processes, because the term is charged with associations of less valuable experience and a low capacity to judge on technological developments in the face of scientific knowledge (Nowotny 2005, Horwath et al. 2018).

Further dependencies were the structural, cultural and epistemic imbalance of the FK LEM (see Introduction).The mitigation of the imbalance in order to facilitate a fair collaboration posed a continuous challenge throughout the whole research period. However, through collaborative endeavours and the work accomplished in the research seminar, we managed to draw on appropriate sociological methods and perspectives across the participating disciplines and to integrate them in the research clusters. One key outcome of this approach is the fact that this generation of PhD researchers received a truly interdisciplinary education, including an acquaintance with different theories, methodologies, and epistemologies. In their future work, they can draw on this experience.

Unexpected dependencies included the rise of the climate protection movement. The urgency the societal movement bestowed to issues of sustainability and climate protection further legitimated and enhanced our aim to take sustainable and responsible engineering seriously and elaborate on corresponding strategies both empirically and practically, beyond marketing buzzwords. As our research also illustrates, sustainability is not a completely unambiguous state of things that simply can be "applied"; rather, it is a concept that has to be associated with specified goals. These need to be developed and co-constructed, within, and between particular societal contexts – including differentiated empirical analyses, informed and transparent trade-offs, and evidence-based practices. In this view, the climate protection movement motivated and reinforced our performance and the impact of our activities

*The* unexpected dependency, however, was the outbreak of the COVID-19 pandemic in early 2020 which profoundly changed the conditions of our work. To shift communication and research activities online required additional time; research designs had to be modified as events such as firefighter trainings did not take place and social distancing prohibited methods such as participant observations. The medicine cluster was able to respond directly to societal demands, i.e. protective gear, whereas the pandemic hampered the progress of their research within FK LEM. Lockdowns of the university, laboratories, and interrupted delivery chains further compromised time schedules and planning. At that point, the flexibility and support of the funding agency, theMinistry of Culture and Science of the State of North Rhine-Westphalia, ensured the possibility to continue with our work. With the establishment of new digital collaboration formats, however, positive effects include increased efficiency, reduced travelling times and thus less $CO_2$ emissions resulting from project meetings.

Furthermore, the research methods we designed and the multimethod approach to problem definition and solving respond to the challenge of integrating social context in transdisciplinary research: participant observation, survey studies in the field, and continued collaboration which help to foster societal effects.

**b) Societal Effects**

Societal effects describe changes within the close and wider spatial and temporal context of a transdisciplinary research project, e.g. network formation, learning, structural effects (Lam et al. 2021:246).

Although the pandemic interrupted the continued cooperation of FK LEM with climate activists, several workshops held previously had been productive in terms of developing and promoting concepts for a $CO_2$ free Paderborn University. The cooperation with Hebie GmbH & Co. KG on sustainable materials and the optimisation of the Turrix allowed the company to advance their professional expertise and to exhibit this progress in form of a demonstrator in their customer show room. The collaboration was enhanced by the network Lippe Zirkulär which facilitated the aim of transdisciplinary research to address real world problems, and the envisioned practical usability of the results.

More generally, societal effects in transdisciplinary research can be achieved via formats such as the Denkschule, participatory research methods and the building up of networks and structures for continued exchange and transfer. Such activities are time consuming and the resources of researchers and practitioners are limited. Hence, in line with the idea of "reverse communication" (Gibbons & Nowotny, 2001), we argue that stakeholders and organisations from the wider society should be encouraged to more proactively participate in university research, for instance, by suggesting relevant topics according to perceived challenges, and actively taking part in the definition of research problems. Researchers, on the other side, need to be accessible for societal concerns and accountable for the effects of their work (see also Introduction, results of the Thought School).

Over its course, transdisciplinary research repeatedly provides opportunities to bridge gaps between perceived problems and envisioned solutions, between overlapping but different knowledge systems, asymmetries in expertise, as well as a variety of professional and scientific values and assumptions. For instance, the approaches to optimize rescue tools draw on first responder experience, practical routines, and requirements articulated in technological norms for particular tools. Thus, through a triangulation of social scientific and engineering methods, the light weight optimisation of tools could be developed in line with training and rescue practices.

Participatory research on firefighting training sites turned out to be particularly rewarding, as researchers received positive feedback, and the practitioner's confirmation of the relevance of their work reinforced motivation and the ability to contextualize the functionalities of the tools in training and rescue scenarios. Although the prospect of demand-oriented lightweight tools is strongly welcomed by the members of rescue organizations, the benefits of such tools may not become rapidly available in the field. Technological development is often only possible with industrial partners due to the required resources such as expertise, patents, or data. Thus, the rules of market competition at the same time enable as well as limit the possibilities of transdisciplinary research, beneficial effects for society and the distribution of benefits in the field.

### c) Scientific effects

Scientific effects are changes in the structure of research problems, research practices, results, or scientific institutions (Lam et al. 2021:246). The interdisciplinary and transdisciplinary problem definition, the constitution of the research questions, helped to identify challenges and address them in ways that facilitated the integration of practical experience into the research context. Continued exchange with practitioners (including such diverse groups as economists, constructors, teachers, ...) fostered researcher understanding of the (immanent) logics of scientific systems and how they link to effects in the respective field of practice. Reflected exchange on practical requirements formed a substantial element in the iterative process of refining our research questions, and allowed for a more detailed description of research goals and possible outcomes. For instance, more nuanced criteria for additively manufactured products or additional desirable features as a result of patient's direct involvement in the design and manufacturing process. It also allowed to identify and utilize focal points to link individual research topics with transdisciplinary activities (see Introduction and Horwath et al. 2018).

Scientifically, the methods applied were not necessarily new; but they were applied and (re-) combined in systematic ways to tackle new research questions and perspectives. For instance, our experiments and the qualification of materials require certain methods and have to follow scientific protocols and disciplinary standards. Yet, disciplinary approaches could be fruitfully (re-) combined to serve new purposes such as an integration of the LCA approach as a means to explore re-use and recycling potentials and to consider the selection of materials as a societally consequential choice.

In addition, the climate protection movement increased public expectations regarding resource efficiency and sustainable technologies. To meet this heightened interest, we were able to also draw on a range of previously conducted studies and results on sustainable materials and light weight design in the construction of automotives or buildings. Generally, the heightened awareness on the sustainable and responsible design of technology and materials facilitated an extension of the areas of application for light weight design, e.g. the building of ships or halls. However, one limitation of public involvement in our particular context is the fact that lightweight design with hybrid materials is already established as a technology trajectory. Hence, participants did not have the opportunity to generally "opt out" of hybrid light weight design; instead, our activities focussed on the exploration of (more) sustainable applications.

Regarding theoretical frameworks, the research design of the Re-Use and Recycling Cluster builds on a standard model (Ulrich & Hill 2016) but modified it by staying accountable for practitioners insights throughout the collaborative process of product development. Part of the methods applied in the rescue cluster are conventional methods in social scientific research performed by engineers after interdisciplinary methodological training. Implemented as a sort of "emergency strategy" to cope with the structural imbalance of the contributing disciplines, the resulting ability of PhD researchers to reflect on scientific problems from different angles, thereby being able to draw on a broader epistemological knowledge base, was an effect we certainly welcomed.

As stated above, the effects of interdisciplinary and transdisciplinary education and practice can be seen in the strength of mutual learning processes (not only between researchers and practitioners but also and importantly between the different disciplines involved), which FK LEM members and research partners alike have highlighted as one of the strongest benefits of transdisciplinary collaboration. According to our experience, scientific cooperation is particularly appreciated by smaller companies as they do not have their own research and development units and usually only very limited access to scientific knowledge and approaches.

On the flipside, the networking effects of our work may be stronger at the regional societal level compared to scientific networks, as we chose regional networking as a strategy to foster transdisciplinary participation and the transfer of knowledge and results. While PhD researchers were driving this vivid exchange, it was difficult to gain acknowledgement for basic research, regional networking, and empirical results as valuable scientific contributions. This is a challenge resulting from interdisciplinarity as well as from transdisciplinarity, as the criteria for valuable results are not limited to the particular disciplinary forms of academic publishing and impact factors (see Introduction). Thus, a scientific effect is also the need to advocate for the acknowledgement of the specific quality criteria promoted in transdisciplinary research within our own disciplines and scientific environments.

**d) Innovative Formats and Methods**

Formats structure the whole transdisciplinary process. They include various methods such as interviews, visioning workshops, experiments,... (Lam et al. 2021:244). As explained in the introduction, we developed a serious of formats to facilitate a continuous and meaningful exchange with the public and within FK LEM, but also to mitigate for the high fluctuation among the FK LEM PhD research group. In mainstream discourse, a high fluctuation of researchers at universities is depicted as a driver of innovation (for a critical perspective see Bahr et al. 2022). In contrast, we experienced how fluctuation actually hampers innovative progress: knowledge, expertise and connections get lost, trainings have to be repeated, and commitment has to be (re-)established.

The structural imbalance between social science, 'hard' science, and engineering made it necessary to train engineers and natural scientists in social scientific research methods and paradigms, for instance to perform participatory observations, survey studies, and expert interviews. Although this training was met with enthusiasm and expanded the participating engineers' expertise and scientific horizon, the scope and depth of data analysis remains limited. This means that due to the structural imbalance we were not able to fully elaborate on particular sociological issues but that sociological concepts and methods were nonetheless driving our research activities. Through the intense collaboration in the research cluster, we gained significant interdisciplinary results. For instance, the joint endeavours of plastics technology, mechanical engineering, and product development generated interdisciplinary results which could be transferred to a local company to enhance sustainable strategies and product development in the future.

The selection and design of formats incited vital discussions among FK LEM researcher. The more heterogeneous the research group, the more time was needed to process the stream of inputs and knowledge in order to advance our research. Openness to unusual ideas, logics and unfamiliar approaches formed the precondition for a fruitful outcome. A general conclusion regarding formats and methods is that language and attitudes are always crucial elements for a successful interdisciplinary as well as transdisciplinary exchange. The prevailing expert culture in science can undermine a meaningful exchange, for instance, when participants *"tend to feel excluded or even patronized by a specialist disciplinary discourse that strikes them as unnecessarily opaque and distant from their lived experience"* (Jasanoff 1999: 63, see also Horwath et al. 2018).

Meaningful exchange outside the "disciplinary comfort zone" thus requires a certain degree of intellectual diplomacy (Jasanoff 1999: 65) and modesty: in inter-and transdisciplinary research, due to the complex nature and mutual constitution of the research objects, no single disciplinary repertoire or expertise can solve the problems – it is only possible through collaborative endeavours. Regarding language, deconstructivist approaches form the state of the art in many strands of technoscience as well as in cultural studies and sociological fields. Deconstructivist approaches are important, e.g. to critically advance scientific concepts, categories, and theoretical approaches. However, in a research environment characterized by strong interdisciplinarity, deconstructivist approaches turned out to be less suitable for the practical development of technologies and for an open exchange that involves different epistemologies, disciplines, and lived experience. This is not to say that the critical potential of deconstructivist thinking should not be used in transdisciplinary research collaborations but to suggest that it is necessary to get beyond the rhetorical and analytical devices of deconstruction in order to bridge traditional disciplinary and epistemological gaps with constructive language and approaches (Jasanoff 1999).

Transdisciplinary research does not per se deliver any additional value to scientific results (Nowotny 1999:106), just as the participation of stakeholders, actors, lay people, or practitioners does not automatically result in stronger objectivity and more robust solutions. Transdisciplinary research, taken seriously, requires a systematic integration of different knowledge bases and types of expertise. This is not only a scientific question but a political one as well: "Participation alone does not answer the problem of how to democratise technological societies" (…) "What has to change is the *culture* of governance, within nations as well as internationally; and for this we need to address not only the mechanics but also the substance of participatory politics. The issue, in other words, is no longer *whether* the public should have a say in technical decisions, but *how* to promote more meaningful interactions among policy makers, scientific experts, corporate producers, and the public"(Jasanoff 2005:383, original emphasis).

While we have contributed to the development of new formats and the modification of methods and attitudes to allow for a meaningful involvement of the public, and while we have opened up spaces for society to co-construct some areas of application of lightweight design together with scientists, an important limitation lies in the fact that lightweight design with hybrid materials is already established as a technological trajectory. Real democratic decision-making would also include an option for the public to reject certain technologies and materials altogether (Nowotny 1999, Jasanoff 2016). However, we hope that our work helps improve the role that science plays in society, and to bring society into the everyday relations and practices of science, in a shared commitment to solve the big challenges of our time together.

## References

Jasanoff, S. (1999). STS and Public Policy: Getting Beyond Deconstruction. *Science, Technology, and Society,* Vol. 4, Issue 1, 59-72. https://doi.org/10.1177/097172189900400104

Jasanoff, S. (2005). Technologies of Humility: Citizen Participation in Governing Science. In A. Bogner & H. Torgersen, (Eds.), *Wozu Experten? Ambivalenzen der Beziehung von Wissenschaft und Politik (pp. 370-389).* VS Verlag. https://doi.org/10.1007/978-3-322-80692-5_17

Jasanoff, S. (2016). *The Ethics of Invention. Technology and the Human Future.* W.W. Norton & Company. ISBN: 978-0-393-07899-2

Lam, D. P.M., Freund M. E., Kny, J., Marg, O., Mbah, M., Theiler, L., Bergmann, M., Brohmann, B., Lang, D. J., & Schäfer, M. (2021). Transdisciplinary research: towards an integrative perspective. *GAIA - Ecological Perspectives for Science and Society.* Vol. 30, Issue 4, 243-249. https://doi.org/10.14512/gaia.30.4.7

Lux, A., Schäfer, M., Bergmann, M., Jahn, T., Marg, O., Nagy, E., Ransiek, A.-C., & Theiler, L. (2019). Societal effects of transdisciplinary sustainability research—How can they be strengthened during the research process? *Environmental Science & Policy,* Vol. 101, 183-191. https://doi.org/10.1016/j.envsci.2019.08.012

Nowotny, H. (2005). Experten, Expertisen und imaginierte Laien. In A. Bogner & H. Torgersen (Eds.), *Wozu Experten? Ambivalenzen der Beziehung von Wissenschaft und Politik (pp. 33-43).* VS Verlag. https://doi.org/10.1007/978-3-322-80692-5_2

Nowotny, H. (1999). *Es ist so. Es könnte auch anders sein.* Suhrkamp Publisher. ISBN: 978-3-518-12104-7

# Authors

Researchers of the Forschungskolleg „Light-Efficient-Mobile" 2018 – 2023 and their Departments at Paderborn University

Emine Fulya Akbulut Irmak, Automotive Lightweight Design
Wolfgang Bremser, Prof. Dr. rer. nat., Technical Chemistry
Thomas Borgert, Forming and Machining Technology
Julius Bürger, Nanopatterning - Nanoanalysis - Photonic Materials
Najmeh Filvan Torkaman, Technical Chemistry
Iris Gräßler, Prof. Dr.-Ing., Product Creation, Heinz Nixdorf Institut
Anusha Lakshmi Innem, Technology and Diversity
Jörg Lindner, Prof. Dr. Nanopatterning - Nanoanalysis - Photonic Materials
Hendrik Hanses, Technology and Diversity
Alexander Henkes, Dr.-Ing., Engineering Mechanics
Philipp Hesse, Product Creation, Heinz Nixdorf Institut
Werner Homberg, Prof. Dr.-Ing., Forming and Machining Technology
Ilona Horwath, JProf. Dr. rer.soc.oec., Technology and Diversity
Kay-Peter Hoyer, Dr. – Ing., Materials Science
Alexander Klingebiel, Engineering Mechanics
Rolf Mahnken, Prof. Dr., M.Sc., Engineering Mechanics
Dennis Menge, Particle Technology Group
Dennis Milaege, Materials Science
Elmar Moritzer, Prof. Dr.-Ing., Plastics Technology
Maximilian Richters, Plastics Technology and Plastics Processing
Mirko Schaper Prof. Dr.-Ing. habil., Materials Science
Hans-Joachim Schmid, Prof. Dr.-Ing., Particle Technology Group
Swetlana Schweizer, Dr.-Ing., Automotive Lightweight Design
Thomas Tröster, Prof. Dr. rer. nat., Automotive Lightweight Design